Plate I

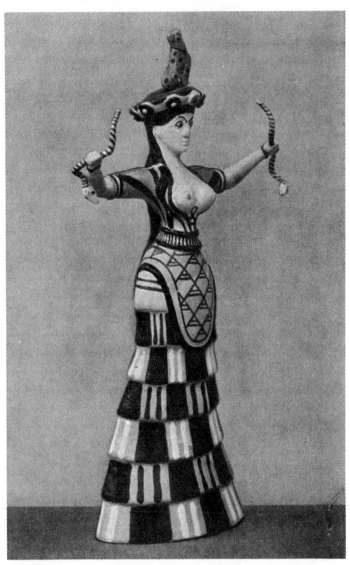

CRETAN SNAKE-GODDESS
Period 2000 - 1500 B.C.

A HISTORY OF COSTUME

BY

CARL KOHLER

EDITED AND AUGMENTED BY
EMMA VON SICHART

TRANSLATED BY
ALEXANDER K. DALLAS M.A.

with over 600 illustrations and patterns

DOVER PUBLICATIONS, INC.

NEW YORK

Published in Canada by General Publishing Company, Ltd., 30 Lesmill Road, Don Mills, Toronto, Ontario.

This Dover edition, first published in 1963, is an unabridged republication of the English translation first published by George G. Harrap and Company, Limited, in 1928. The sixteen full-page plates were reproduced in color in the 1928 edition.

This Dover edition is published by special arrangement with George G. Harrap and Company, Limited.

Standard Book Number: 486-21030-8
Library of Congress Catalog Card Number: 63-16328

Manufactured in the United States of America
Dover Publications, Inc.
180 Varick Street
New York, N. Y. 10014

PREFACE

WHEN we stand before the showcases in museums and look at the precious relics of bygone styles of dress which have been preserved by the skill and loving care of collectors our interest is aroused by more than shape and colour and material. What can have been the impression produced by this or that garment when worn by the actual person ? we ask ourselves, and How were these dresses cut and made so as to satisfy the ideal of form that prevailed at the time and found expression in them ? I hope that an answer to the first of these questions—as far as that is possible—will be supplied by the numerous photographs from life which are contained in this book. The second has already been answered by Carl Köhler, who as far back as sixty years ago worked with expert knowledge and great industry in the rich field of costumiery.[1] This book is meant to rescue his labours from unmerited oblivion, to supplement and adapt them to the needs of the present day. What distinguishes the works of Köhler above others of a similar kind is not only the detailed completeness with which they cover the entire development of costume, but also the author's extensive knowledge of the practical side of the subject and his thorough familiarity with technique and cut. His work contains complete answers to all the questions that deal with the practical side of the tailor's art in bygone periods.

In editing Köhler's writings for the present work I have omitted some passages and shortened others. In particular I have discarded his introductions, which deal with the history and the civilization of the various periods. Max von Boehn[2] has given in a superlatively excellent manner the historical background of dress, and as in his volumes a portion of my task has been incomparably carried out I have been able to devote my attention principally to the technical side of the subject. This has been neglected by all the books on costume with which I am acquainted. An attempt has been made to provide answers to questions which other writers have entirely ignored or dealt with only incidentally, but which all the same are important. In matters of costume theory does not carry us very far.

[1] Carl Köhler, painter, born in Darmstadt in 1825, died at Almoshof, near Nürnberg, in 1876. See the Bibliography, p. 457.
[2] *Die Mode : Menschen und Moden vom Beginn unsrer Zeitrechnung bis zum Ende des neunzehnten Jahrhunderts nach Bildern und Kupfern der Zeit.* 8 vols., with 1800 plates and illustrations, many of them in colour.

A HISTORY OF COSTUME

The cut of a garment cannot be described in words : we must actually see how its lines run before we can appreciate the effect.

The measurements which I have borrowed from Köhler and those which I have myself provided are in all cases given in centimetres. When the patterns are to be utilized the measurements must of course be altered to suit the figure of the person who is to wear the garment, but the proportions must be retained. The numerous new patterns which have been added to the already large number given by Köhler have been either taken directly from photographs of the costumes or borrowed from the fashion journals of the period in question. For technical descriptions of the original costumes shown in the illustrations I refer readers to the list of illustrations.

For the photographs of costumes worn by models only genuine ancient garments were used, and every detail was arranged as far as possible in keeping with the style of the period. The lace, the ornaments, the shawls, etc., are all genuine. On the other hand, for the footwear it was necessary to use for the most part faithful copies of the exhibits in the National Theatre in Munich. The same expedient had to be resorted to in the case of the trousers of some of the men's suits. These substitutions are indicated in the list of illustrations.

Facilities in regard to the use of ancient costumes were very generously accorded to me in a number of directions. The National Theatre lent its rich store of garments from the eighteenth and nineteenth centuries. Herr Kommerzienrat Max Bernheimer of Munich placed at my disposal not only several valuable ancient costumes, but also very convenient rooms, including the photographic studio of the firm L. Bernheimer, so that the men and women who assisted me could be dressed and photographed there. Genuine costumes and other requisites for taking photographs were also provided by the firms F. and A. Diringer and Rosa Klauber, of Munich, by Herr von Kramer at Ludwigshöhe, near Munich, Consul Löwy, of Venice, and not least by Professor Löwith, of Munich, who kindly gave me the benefit of his wide knowledge of costume.

In connexion with the fitting on of the women's dresses much help was received from Fräulein Hermine Moos, well known in connexion with her exhibition of costumes in the Bavarian National Museum. The men assistants were dressed by Meister Volpert, of the National Theatre. Accuracy in matters of *coiffure* was secured with the aid of Herr Schuster, of the same institution, and his staff. The photographs themselves were taken by Herr Hanns Holdt.

The excellent photographs of exhibits in the Bavarian National Museum were taken by Herr A. Beringer, of the Museum, with the courteous permission of the Chief Director, Herr Geheimrat Halm. Other photographs I owe to the kindness of the Curators of the Germanisches Museum in Nürnberg, of the Provinzial Museum in Hanover, and of the museums at Bern and Zürich. I have also received much help from Dr Friess, of Nürnberg.

PREFACE

For valuable hints regarding Greek costume I am indebted to Dr Weickert, of Munich. M. Jacques Heuzey, of Paris, lent the fine and instructive photographs from the work of Léon Heuzey, his father, which illustrate clearly how the ancient forms of dress were worn. Frau Professor Margarethe Bieber, of Marburg, supplied the photograph of the Greek tunic on p. 102.

Finally, my grateful thanks are due to the twenty-seven men and women who so kindly undertook to act as models in the costumes.

EMMA VON SICHART

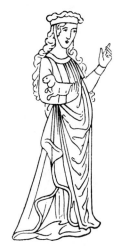

GERMAN FEMALE DRESS OF THE
TWELFTH CENTURY

CONTENTS

A HISTORY OF COSTUME

ILLUSTRATIONS

The names in italic indicate the source of the illustrations (fuller details of this are given in the Bibliography) or the owner of the originals. The illustrations for which no acknowledgment is made are taken from Carl Köhler's " Die Trachten der Völker in Bild und Schnitt."

PLATES

86 cm. ; length of back, 48 cm. ; length of front, 24 cm. ; length from shoulder, 47 cm. ; width of trimming round neck (80 cm.), 9 cm. The small coat-tail is cut on to the back gores of the skirt. The lining is coarse grey linen. The bib is about 25 cm. deep ; the width at the neck is 28 cm., at the waist 12 cm. ; it has a baroque embroidery design in yellow, blue, and rust-brown silks on blue silk ; it is edged with narrow gold braid. The material of the skirt is white cotton *piqué*. The embroidered flowers are worked in fine wool. The bodice is of blue taffeta. *Von Kramer, Ludwigshöhe, near Munich.*

About 1780. Waist (open), 96 cm. ; chest, 114 cm. ; width of back, 33 cm. ; length of sleeve, 61 and 53 cm. ; length of back, 114 cm. Material, yellowish-green cloth. All seams covered by rich braid, 6½ cm. wide, in blue, black, and bronze on cream ground. Double braid on sleeves, used as cuffs, is edged with dark blue cloth with two *passementerie* buttons. Height of collar, 11 cm. Eight buttons on the front. Front length, with cut-away, 122 cm. The lining is of green-yellow cotton. Breeches are of beige linen. The waistcoat is of white cloth. (Copies.) *Bernheimer, Munich.*

Dress Coat. About 1730–40. Pink with white pattern. Length of upper portion, 57 cm. ; total length, 108 cm. ; width of back, 33 cm. Cuffs, 12 cm. wide ; they are ornamented with three buttons, as are the pockets. Fastened with thirteen buttons, which are covered with the material ; only a few of the buttons, from waist upward, are meant to be done up. Material, white-pink damask ; lining, grey linen. Depth of collar, 2 cm. On the pocket-flap are sham buttonholes. Waistcoat (original) is of cream satin ; collar only 3½ cm. deep ; cut away at foot ; pockets pointed and stitched ; ten buttons covered with satin, which appear to form a double row, as the buttons on the one side are sewn on to the other end of the button-holes, which are closed by sewing. *Waistcoat : von Kramer, Ludwigshöhe, near Munich.*

Silk Gown. Lilac rococo dress. Waist, 66 cm. ; bust, 74 cm. ; length of skirt, 92 cm. Round the neck are frills of real lace. Below the skirt is a small hoop (panier). Material, soft lilac silk with reddish sheen, with white patterns of lacy sprays and small greenish-blue and rust-coloured bouquets of flowers. Width of skirt, 3 m. ; two pieces of trimming in the middle of skirt, at the knees 9 cm. wide, 75 cm. long ; below the knees, 25 cm. wide and 75 cm. long, are small ruches, about the width of a finger, which are finished off with narrow white silk braid. Over-dress worked upon lining of grey linen ; trimming of ruches as above, widening from 5 cm. at top to 15 cm. below. Total length of over-dress, 125 cm. ; frills at sleeves of white taffeta, 5 cm. in front, widening toward back of sleeve to 15 cm. The ruched bib at the back is fixed to paper ; inside is a (presumably new) trimming of rust-red colour. Lower width of over-dress, 395 cm. Watteau pleat. The over-dress has a coarse grey linen lining. Stockings (original) are cream coloured, of openwork with lace pattern. Pink silk slippers. *Munich, National Theatre.*

About 1740. Length of skirt, 92 cm. ; width, about 340 cm. ; depth of embroidery, 43 cm. ; width of waist, 86 cm. (enlarged) ; front of bodice, 34 cm. long ; from shoulder to waist, 47½ cm. ; bust, 96 cm. (enlarged) ; width of back, 30 cm. ; length of shoulder, 9 cm. ; length of sleeve, 58½–48½ cm. The short flap of the back piece is cut in a wide bell-shape with the back of the bodice. The lining is of grey linen ; the bodice of light blue taffeta ; the skirt of satin. Bodice and skirt are quilted in trellis form. The embroidery is 43 cm. deep, and represents large-leaved flowers richly worked. The bodice-lining

ILLUSTRATIONS

is slightly stiffened with whalebone ; it is closed by lacing. Round the neck was worn a fichu of dainty muslin, with a spray of flowers worked in colours (so-called *follette*). Grey shoes of deerskin. *Von Kramer, Ludwigshöhe, near Munich.*

X. LOUNGE COAT FOR INDOOR WEAR AND SLEEVED WAIST-
COAT 350

About 1750. Length of coat, 117 cm. ; width, 250 cm. ; back, 49 cm. ; each front piece, 37 cm. ; length of sleeves, with turned-back cuffs, 62 and 46 cm. ; depth of collar, 3½ cm. Material, white taffeta with pattern of stripes and flowers ; the lining is pale green silk. The gown fits closely round the body ; from the waist it is bell-shaped, with two gussets. With the coat was worn a sleeved waistcoat of the same material, with sleeves of pale green taffeta. Length, 70 cm. ; lower width of tails (which are wider from waist), 27 cm. each. From waist at back is a slit of 18 cm. The back is in two pieces. Waistcoat is cut away in front ; has two small pockets, 23 cm. long ; eleven buttons covered with silk ; wide buttonholes. With this coat and waistcoat were worn breeches of dark rose-coloured satin and a skull-cap of pink taffeta richly embroidered. *Professor Löwith, Munich.*

XI. LIGHT BLUE STRIPED ROCOCO COSTUME 354

About 1750. Length of skirt, 105 cm. ; width, 275 cm. ; width of front trimming, 23 cm.
Upper Garment. Length from shoulder, 146 cm. ; at back, 180 cm. ; width, 360 cm. ; shoulder, 10 cm. ; width at neck, which is cut square, 84 cm. ; length of bodice under the arm, 17 cm. ; length of sleeve, 15 cm. ; sleeve-frills, 13 cm. deep. Trimming of gown widens from 4 cm. to 16 cm. Round neck and on sleeves is white silk lace. The sleeve-frills are lined with pale yellow taffeta and trimmed with coloured silk braid. The bib is made of the same material as the gown, and is 22 cm. wide at the top, 8 cm. at bottom ; length is 25 cm. This bib is also trimmed with silk lace and with small silk flowers made of braid and chenille. The loops of ribbon are of pale blue taffeta 7 cm. wide. On the inside of the gown there is an arrangement for drawing the skirt up. The lining has been renovated and the upper garment widened.
Von Kramer, Ludwigshöhe, near Munich.

XII. COAT OF RED BROCADE 358

About 1760. Waist, 102 cm. ; chest, 110 cm. ; front length (measured along the curve), 117 cm. ; length of back, 106 cm. ; width of back, 43 cm. ; cuffs, 13½ cm. deep ; height of collar, 3 cm. On each back piece are two rows of pleats (in one of the rows the pleats are double) ; double pleat at slit. The buttons at the slit are 33 cm. apart. Length of sleeve, 63 cm. and 47 cm. Material, a ground of carmine satin, with flowers of velvet and rich gold and silver ornamentation inwoven. At front of coat, on both tails, on the sleeves, the pockets, the edges, and the waistcoat there are ribbon and floral patterns. At the right side there are twelve buttons, made of cardboard covered with gold cloth ; also buttons on sleeves and pockets. White satin lining throughout. Waistcoat length, 84 cm. ; cut away ; curved pockets, each with three points. Breeches of pink rep.
Grey deerskin shoes with straps and red hooks. Three-cornered hat. (Copies from the National Theatre.)
Bernheimer, Munich.

XIII. LIGHT BLUE GOWN WITH ROSE DESIGN, 1770 ... 364

(Cf. Figs. 445 and 446.) Width of back, 30 cm. ; waist, 68 cm. ; bust, 52 cm. ; length of upper garment, 125 cm. in front, 240 cm. at back. Material, pale blue taffeta with inwoven border of white, pink, and mauve flowers interspersed with white marguerites ; this floral border is trimmed with small blue points edged with silver. Width of this trimming, 19 cm. ; width of patterned material at

A HISTORY OF COSTUME

back, 82 cm. ; length of floral trimming at each side of back, 65 cm.
Similar trimming at front.   Pointed flounces in two rows round
sleeves, finished off with blue chiffon ribbon.   Below the front bib,
which is trimmed top and bottom with pointed taffeta, the bodice
is fastened with hooks.   Lining of white cotton.   Square neck.
The skirt, a faithful copy of original, is made of heavy white satin
and is trimmed with wide ruches.   Red leather shoes.   *Owner of
gown : Bernheimer, Munich.   Skirt and shoes : copy at National
Theatre, Munich.*

XIV. DRESS COAT OF LIGHT BLUE SILK.   DRESS COAT OF LILAC
VELVET   382

About 1790.
Dress Coat of Light Blue Silk.   Material, pale blue satin lined with
cream taffeta.   Waist, 96 cm. ; chest, 110 cm. ; length of sleeve,
42 cm. and 68 cm. ; width of back, 36 cm. ; total front length,
103 cm.   On right side seven buttons ; no buttonholes.   Two
buttons at back.   Height of collar, not counting turn-over, 9 cm.
Size of pockets, 27 × 12 cm. ; pockets slightly curved, with three
points ; three buttons below pockets.   Narrow cuffs without buttons.
Waistcoat.   Plainly cut, straight, of cream taffeta ; narrow, straight
pockets ;   no collar ;   turned-over corners are embroidered with a
narrow border of flowers ;   very small silk buttons, embroidered.
Length, 55 cm. ; lining of back of grey linen.
Black satin breeches (copy at National Theatre, Munich).   Hose
(original at National Theatre, Munich), beige-coloured, with red
stripes about 1 cm. wide.   Jabot and sleeves have frills of batiste.
Buckled shoes.
Bernheimer, Munich.
Dress Coat of Lilac Velvet.   Dress coat of the Duke of Leuchtenberg.
Front length, 105 cm. ; length from waist at back, 42 cm. ; back
length, 100 cm. ; width of back, 33 cm. ; shoulder, 12 cm. ; width
of coat (half) at front, 20 cm.   Lower edge of collar, 50 cm. ; upper
edge, 37 cm. ; height, 8 cm.   Length of sleeves, 50 cm. and 67 cm. ;
cuff, 11 cm.   Width of pockets, 20 cm. (upper) and 17½ cm. (lower) ;
depth of pocket, 9 cm. ; pocket has three buttons.   Lower edge of
tails, 27½ cm. ; under-flap at back, 12½ cm., making a doubled-over
tail.   Width of embroidery, 12–13 cm.
The coat is very slender, bulging at chest and then smartly cut back.
Above the left pocket a slit for the sword.   The whole is the type
of the elegant dress coat of the late eighteenth century, and still
fashionable at the beginning of the nineteenth century.   Material,
black-purple silk velvet ; lining, heavy white satin ; the embroidery,
12–13 cm. wide, is worked in white and in several shades of green,
representing geranium-leaves.   There is a narrow waistband, stitched
to the back, which was fastened below the waistcoat.   This coat
belonged to the Duke of Leuchtenberg, and became the property of
the National Theatre, along with several other beautiful rococo dress
coats from the same source.
Waistcoat belonging to this Leuchtenberg Coat.   Length from shoulder,
50 cm. ; length of front, 34 cm. (cut-away edges) ; height of collar,
7½ cm. ;   six silk buttons, 4 cm. apart, of which only two were
buttoned.   (The pockets, 19 cm. long, are sham pockets.)   Waist,
62 cm. ; below shoulder, 23 cm. ; length of back, 51 cm. ; width
of back, 37 cm.   With this costume went pale lilac breeches of
moiré (copy at the Court Theatre, Munich) ; also buckled shoes and
a black three-cornered hat trimmed with swan's down.
Munich, National Theatre.

XV. EVENING GOWN OF WHITE SATIN, 1865   430

Front length of skirt, 105 cm. ;   back length, 130 cm. ;   width,
460 cm. ;   waist, 68 cm. ;   bust, 96 cm. ;   length of back (bodice),
31 cm. ;   from shoulder, 38 cm. ;   front length (bodice), 45 cm. ;
shoulder length, 2 cm.   Epaulettes, 10 cm., finished with two frills
of silk lace, each 10 cm. wide.   Frill of tulle round neck ; this frill
is 6 cm. wide, has slot for a ribbon, and an edging of Valenciennes

lace, 2 cm. wide. Trimming consists of plaited braids of red satin, 1½ cm. wide, sewn on in loop form. The bodice has a divided front piece with a deep point; the back has two strongly curved seams. Neck, sleeves, and seams are stitched over. The lining, of fine white silk, is stiffened with whalebone; lining of skirt is of thin white satin; round the lower edge of this lining runs a trimming of lace (*ballayeuse*). The material of the skirt is laid in deep folds in front and at sides and drawn together at back.

To this dress belongs a shawl of red cloth, edged with a strip of white satin (4 cm. wide) trimmed with braiding of red velvet piping. Width of the rounded back, 59 cm.; near neck, 40 cm.; over shoulder, 45 cm.; lower width, 130 cm. The front pieces have a length of 97 cm.; they are laid into folds, 3 cm. deep, at shoulder; width of these front pieces, 48 cm.; lining, white jap silk.
Von Kramer, Ludwigshöhe, near Munich.

XVI. TOWN COSTUME WITH MANTILLA, 1860   438

Width of skirt, 415 cm.; bust, 102 cm.; waist, 88 cm.; back, 44 cm.; length of skirt, 105 cm. Material, green taffeta rep with black oak-leaves (reverse side shows black with green design). Lining, brownish sateen. From the side-seams forward the lining has a small corslet, made for lacing up; at sides, 9 cm. deep; in front, 17 cm. deep. At back three double inverted pleats; at each side of these three single pleats. Round waist is a narrow silk belt, 2½ cm. wide. Back of bodice seamless; narrowed toward waist by six small tucks. Front piece of bodice V-shaped; closed with hooks. Sleeves are bell-shaped and gathered on shoulder; their lower width is 75 cm. They are finished inside with black taffeta and a ruche of chiffon ribbon; outside they are trimmed with a braid of black-green silk and narrow silk fringe. This trimming widens out from 6 cm. to 15 cm. to look like a cuff. Inside the skirt is a trimming of sateen, edged with woollen braid. With this was worn a three-cornered collar, embroidered on white batiste. Sleeves are hand-embroidered. Headdress of lace worked on silk net, with yellow ribbons. Handkerchief of batiste. Black sunshade lined with satin; ivory handle. Mantilla (the property of *von Liel*) of black taffeta trimmed with narrow silk fringe; length at back, 90 cm.; at front, 85 cm.; lapel, 33 cm., widening to 41 cm.; a frill with curved silk fringe from 25 to 40 cm. deep. *Bernheimer, Munich.*

ILLUSTRATIONS IN THE TEXT

A HISTORY OF COSTUME

ILLUSTRATIONS

ILLUSTRATIONS

ILLUSTRATIONS

ILLUSTRATIONS

ILLUSTRATIONS

> Silk-embroidered velvet; dark brown. Full length of front, 48 cm.; length of basque, 11·5 cm.; back length, without basque, 37 cm.; basque, 11 cm.; width of back, 29 cm.; waist, 74 cm.; half width of basque, lower edge, 52 cm.; size of collar, top and bottom, 41 cm.; height of collar, 7 cm.; shoulder, 10·5 cm.; padding (in middle of front), 17 cm. wide and 57 cm. long. Three buttons at collar; eighteen down.
>
> The brownish-black velvet of which this doublet is made is much worn. The cut and workmanship are of unusual excellence. Originally the stiff linen lining was covered by a second lining of black silk. The doublet is covered with very rich embroidery. It is supposed to be of French origin. If that be so, several items of ress must have been worn with it—viz., an under-garment with sleeves, a Spanish ruffle, the wide, spherical breeches called *tonneaux*, reaching to the middle of the thighs, tight-fitting leggings (presumably stockings), and low shoes. *Nürnberg, Germanisches Museum.*

> Orange-coloured velvet with embroidery. *Consul Löwy, Venice.*

ILLUSTRATIONS

358. DOUBLET AND BREECHES OF DUKE PHILIP LUDWIG OF
PFALZ-NEUBURG (*d.* 1614) 290

From the mausoleum at Lauingen. Chest, 103 cm. ; waist, 96 cm. ;
front length, 36 cm. (the front has the neck well cut out) ; length of
back, 36 cm. ; width round the neck, 47 cm. ; shoulder, 13 cm. ; length
of doublet from armhole to waist, 12 cm. On each side there is a sort of
basque, or skirt, 15 cm. long, 12 cm. wide.at waist, and 25 cm. wide at
foot. Length of breeches, 70 cm. ; width, 150 cm. Each front part of
the doublet is cut in one piece. The seams are braided. The doublet
is fastened in front with loops and buttons. The double girdle, made of
narrow ribbons, ends in a tassel. The breeches are tied round the knees.
The material is of soft striped silk now brown in colour. *Munich,
National Museum.*

359. TWO PEA-JACKETS WORN BY PAGES, ABOUT 1607 291

Of black linen and red silk. Front length from shoulder, not counting
the flaps, 44 cm. ; back length, 43 cm. ; chest, 72 cm. ; shoulder,
4 cm. ; neck, 46 cm. There are eighteen flaps, each 4 cm. wide and 7 cm.
long ; they are ornamented with woven braid in red and gold.
Embroidered crests on the front. *Nürnberg, Germanisches Museum.*

360. FRENCH MEN'S DRESS, BEGINNING OF THE SEVENTEENTH
CENTURY 291

361. GREEN VELVET SUIT AND SHOES OF DUKE MAURICE OF
SAXE-LAUENBURG 292

End of the sixteenth or beginning of the seventeenth century. Length
of bodice, 40 cm. in front, 54 cm. at back ; chest, 129 cm. ; height of
collar, 6 cm. ; width of flaps, 7 cm. Braid is 2 cm. wide. Length of
sleeves, 77 cm. ; at their widest part they are 72 cm. wide. Length
of breeches, 85 cm. ; width, 133 cm. Material, green velvet. The
braid is of gold with silver herringbone work. Black shoes. *Hanover,
Museum.*

362. BAGGY BREECHES (PLUDERHOSE), 1620 293

Munich, National Museum.

363. RED VELVET SUIT AND SHOES OF DUKE MAURICE OF SAXE-
LAUENBURG 294

End of the sixteenth or beginning of the seventeenth century. Length
of bodice, front, 37 cm. ; back, 53 cm. Chest, 131 cm. ; height of
collar, 7 cm. ; width of flaps, 8 cm. The braid is 2 cm. wide. Length
of sleeves, 71 cm. ; width, 66 cm. Length of breeches, 84 cm. ; width
round waist, 129 cm. Material, patterned velvet, red, ornamented with
gold braid interwoven with silver threads. *Hanover, Museum.*

364. FRENCH-SPANISH DOUBLET, BEGINNING OF THE SEVEN-
TEENTH CENTURY 295

365. OLIVE GREEN DOUBLET OF QUILTED SILK, ABOUT 1630–40 296

Front length, including basque, 62 cm. ; basque in front, 27 cm. ; back
length with basque, 70 cm. ; basque alone, at back, 26 cm. ; width of
each basque, at foot 21–23 cm., at waist 18–23 cm. Neck-band,
upper width 49 cm., lower width 56 cm. ; shoulder, 18 cm. ; height of
collar (neck-band), 5 cm. in front, 6 cm. at back ; length of sleeve,
65 cm. ; width of half of under-sleeve, 16 cm. One button with loop
at collar ; sixteen buttons in front ; six buttons on sleeve. *Munich,
Germanisches Museum.*

366. CLOAK OF PALE YELLOW VELVET, ABOUT 1630 297

Front length from shoulder, 89 cm. ; back length, 84 cm. ; half neck
width, 32 cm. ; shoulder, 16 cm. ; half of lower width, 132 cm. ; length
of slit at back, 34 cm. ; straight-cut collar, 32 cm. wide and 22 cm.
deep ; width of armhole, 50 cm. ; slit of sleeves, 10 cm. All edges are
trimmed with braid (*Wetzlitze*) of the same colour as the material. The

ILLUSTRATIONS

(*b*) CORSLET (MIEDER) WORN WITH OVER-DRESS OF THE COUNTESS PALATINE DOROTHEA SABINE OF NEUBURG (*d.* 1598)

From the mausoleum at Lauingen. Waist, 57 cm.; back, 29 cm.; bust, 77 cm.; length from shoulder, 37 cm.; length from neck to point, 39 cm.; length from armpit to waist, 14 cm. From each side toward the back are six flaps. The back has five rows of stitching on each side of the arrangement for lacing. The front is very low, with short intakes, 4 cm. wide, under the armpits. Both at the front and back are two stitched eyes which allow a piece of braid to be run through. Stitchings in corslet shape ornamented the front piece. Material, rep-like silk of brownish colour.

(*c*) CHILD'S FROCK OF COUNTESS MARIA MAGDALENA OF HILPOLTSTEIN (*d.* 1629), DAUGHTER OF DUKE JOHN FREDERICK

From the mausoleum at Lauingen. Front length of bodice, 15 cm.; back length of bodice, 12 cm.; width of skirt, 100 cm.; length of skirt, 32 cm.; shoulder, 6 cm.; padding of sleeve, 2½ cm. Length of flaps over sleeves, 48 cm., reaching to hem of skirt, where they were 4 cm. wide. Width of sleeve at wrist, 12 cm. The sleeves were open in front, so that the under-sleeves were seen; they were sewn at the back of the wrist to a width of 3½ cm. The material was originally (presumably) soft green silk; the colour now appears brown. The trimming was narrow silver braid, continuing across the back. Laced at back.

All three at Munich, National Museum.

A HISTORY OF COSTUME

FIG.   PAGE

418. FARTHINGALE FRAME   341
Munich, National Museum.

419. DRESS OF A GIRL OF THE MIDDLE CLASSES, ABOUT 1720   342
Length of skirt, 95 cm.; width of skirt, 300 cm.; waist, 66 cm.; front length of bodice, 52 cm.; back length of bodice, 59 cm.; bust, 92 cm.; length of basque, 44 cm.; lower width of basque, 27 cm.; upper width of basque, 19 cm.; shoulder, 4 cm. Chemisette and apron are added. The skirt is of rust-red linen with white floral sprays, the bodice of glazed rust-coloured linen with white and blue floral pattern. Where the bodice is laced the edges are bound with blue *moiré* ribbon. The bodice is quilt-lined, and ornamented with stitched patterns. The skirt has a lining of stiff, yellowish, lattice-patterned muslin. The basques are cut into the bodice. *Von Kramer, Ludwigshöhe, near Munich.*

420. CORSET OF THE FIRST HALF OF THE EIGHTEENTH CENTURY 343

421. MEASUREMENTS AND CUT OF CORSET SHOWN IN FIG. 420 343

422. CORSET, FIRST HALF OF THE EIGHTEENTH CENTURY 344

423. LADY, FIRST HALF OF THE EIGHTEENTH CENTURY 344

424. DRESS OF YELLOW DAMASK, MIDDLE OF THE EIGHTEENTH CENTURY 345
Length of skirt, 103 cm.; skirt at its widest, 115 cm. in each part; entire width of skirt, about 350 cm.; length of bodice from shoulder, which is set well back, 58 cm. There are six basques, 21 cm. long and 44 cm. wide Length below shoulder, 14 cm.; bust, 97 cm.; length of back, 34 cm.; across back, 30 cm.; front length of sleeves, 24 cm.; back length of sleeves, 50 cm. The lower width of the sleeves is 45 cm. Diameter of skirt at hips, 150 cm. The material of this magnificent garment is, for the skirt, lemon-coloured damask, trimmed with a border of silver lace 6 cm. wide. The bodice is of yellow damask with linear patterns and floral designs in red and pale blue. The edges of the bodice and sleeves are trimmed with silver lace 2 cm. wide. Inside the lacing in front is a yellow bib stitched with red silk. The lining of the sleeves and basques is of pink glazed cotton. *Munich, National Museum. Lent by the wife of General von Taeter, Munich.*

425. LADY WEARING A CONTOUCHE (MORNING GOWN), FIRST HALF OF THE EIGHTEENTH CENTURY 346

426. WOMEN'S DRESS, FIRST HALF OF THE EIGHTEENTH CENTURY 346

427. HALF OF FRONT PIECE OF THE SCHLENDER 346

428. CONTOUCHE OF WHITE LINEN COVERED WITH DESIGNS IN QUILT STITCHING, MIDDLE OF THE EIGHTEENTH CENTURY 347
Front length from shoulder, 144 cm.; back length, 143 cm.; across back, 23 cm.; width round foot, 455 cm.; length of sleeves, exclusive of lace, 55 cm.; half the width of sleeve, 17 cm. There is a slit 21 cm. long below each sleeve where it is set in. The gown is for house wear. It is worked all over in quilt stitching. Two deep folds come down each side from shoulder to bust and open out below the breast. The back has a yoke, to which is attached a Watteau pleat. *Nürnberg, Germanisches Museum.*

429. STECKER (BIBS) AND SET OF TRIMMINGS WITH GOLD AND SILVER LACE. SHOES OF PINK VELVET 348
Middle of the eighteenth century. *Munich, National Museum.*

ILLUSTRATIONS

39

Roll collar, 126 cm. all round, 64 cm. measured from shoulder to waist (reaching far down at back); width of front piece of coat, 22 cm.; width of back piece of coat, 26 cm.; length of back, 103 cm.; length of sleeve at back, 81 cm. Each front has six metal buttons and six buttonholes. Depth of cuff, 5½ cm.; front length of waistcoat, 46 cm.; length of trousers, 75 cm. The material of the coat is dark blue cloth; the waistcoat is grey with a green pattern; the trousers are of white silk stockinette. The waistcoat does not belong to the suit.

Hat. Black top hat of straw in Florentine plaited work. Diameter of head, 18 cm.; height of crown, 14 cm.; width of brim, 6½ cm.
Munich, National Museum.

Front length of skirt, 125 cm.; length of train, 230 cm.; length of bodice, 12 cm.; shoulder, 2 cm. The bodice consists of one front piece and two strongly curved back pieces; it is closed at the back by two draw-strings, one at the top, one at the waist. The front and back parts of the skirt are straight pieces, joined by two gores on each side, the narrower of which ends almost at the top of the train. The material is very thin, very soft cotton stockinette, finely patterned, and of great elasticity. Round the head a turban of blue silk was worn. An underdress of a contrasting colour belongs to the gown. *Professor Löwith, Munich.*

Munich, National Museum.

Length of skirt (front), 120 cm.; back length of train, 240 cm.; lower width of skirt, 440 cm.; depth of embroidery on skirt, 15 cm.; belt, 2 cm.; shoulder, 2½ cm.; measurement round neck, 125 cm.; length of sleeves, 27 cm.; depth of embroidery round neck and sleeves, 2 cm. Eight small buttons on sleeve, about 3 cm. apart. The sleeve has long slashes half-way down, similar to the chiton sleeve. The skirt is made of three pieces, and is widened at the foot by two small gores. A drawstring runs through the top of the bodice and round the neck to regulate the width. The bodice is fastened by draw-strings at waist. The side-seams of the bodice are placed far toward the back. The material is finest lawn, soft and silky to the touch. The under-dress (slip) is of the same material; it has a sleeveless bodice; the width of its skirt is 380 cm. The embroidery both of the slip and the dress proper is worked in a flat design with loose, soft thread. *Von Kramer, Ludwigshöhe, near Munich.*

Width of lining at back, 15 cm.; sleeve-length, 27 cm. The sleeves of the lining are set in well toward the back, so that the back appears very narrow. Length of bodice in front, 10 cm.; from shoulder, 28 cm.; at back, 21 cm. The sleeves of the bodice are 30 cm. long, gathered on shoulder, and drawn in by a draw-string at the lower edge. The neck is fairly high at the back. The lining of the bodice is fastened by hooks. The skirt is made of two parts, each 126 cm. wide, and is trimmed round the foot with a frill 8 cm. wide. The front piece is 102 cm. long and 70 cm. wide at waist, arranged for pulling in. At the upper edge of the skirt a bib, 12 cm. wide and ending in two straps, is attached ; these two straps extend up to the shoulders, and are attached there with a small button. The gathers of the skirt at the back are 15 cm. wide. The bodice is 22 cm. long at the back. The bodice and the front of the skirt are buttoned together, and the skirt adjusted to the required width. Material, white muslin with narrow dark blue lines. The bodice-lining is of white linen. *Winterer, Munich.*

     Waist, 82 cm. ; bust, 106 cm. ; length, 107 cm. Material, greyish-white cotton with a wedge-shaped pattern in green, blue, yellow, and red worked on it. In the front of the lining are three intakes. The dress material is gathered on to the lining on both front pieces and at the back to a width of 15 cm. The puffs of the sleeves at the shoulders are 25 cm. wide ; below these are puffs 5 cm. wide. The belt, with ribbon ends, is 2½ cm. wide. There is a double puffed ruche at the neck ; a single puffed ruche at the turn-over ; another, 7 cm. wide, in front of the skirt ; and still another ruche, 5 cm. wide, round the foot of the skirt, which is 280 cm. wide. *Munich, National Theatre.* Cap of hand-made *filet* net by *Rosa Klauber, Munich.*

(b) WHITE DRESS WITH GREEN AND PINK PATTERN AND TRIMMING, 1815

Length of bodice, 27 cm. ; length below bust, 82 cm. ; length of skirt, 107 cm. ; width of same, 226 cm. ; length of the plain, long sleeves, 68 cm. (with a small addition), with a band 1½ cm. deep. Material, white nettle-cloth, with a conventional pattern of scattered flowers, green and pink. Round the hem runs a border, 20 cm. wide, of a rich pattern in the same colours. The bodice is fastened in front with hooks. The seams of the bodice are sewn over with a trimming made of a plait of the material of the frock. The skirt is plain at the back, and is gathered in front to a width of 13 cm. on each side of the opening. With this was worn a pale pink shawl of silk with an inwoven border of one colour. The reticule is covered with hand embroidery. The shoes are of white silk, without heels, and with crossed white silk ribbon. *Winterer, Munich.*

     Waist (measured below bust), 74 cm. ; bust, 86 cm. ; length, 101 cm. ; length of sleeves, 64 cm. Material, green striped taffeta with small

scattered flowers. Seams and narrow belt trimmed with dark green taffeta. Open in front. Much gathered at back. There is a drawstring round the neck. *Bernheimer, Munich.*
The necklace is of gold disks with the signs of the Zodiac. *Winterer, Munich.*

497. WHITE EMPIRE DRESS WITH GOLD EMBROIDERY, ABOUT 1806   401

Length of bodice, 13 cm. ; length from shoulder, 22 cm. ; length of skirt, 107 cm. ; length of sleeve, 22 cm.—7 cm. under arm ; width of sleeve, 45 cm. ; waist, 84 cm. ; width of skirt, 174 cm. A yoke, 1–1½ cm. wide, joins the front and back parts of bodice. The neck has a draw-string. This is tied in front, and also on each shoulder. The waist also is drawn in by a string or lace. The skirt is made of three pieces, and is gathered at the back to a width of 17 cm. to the right and left of the opening, which is in the middle of the back. The material is very fine lawn with hand-worked flat embroidery, with inset leaves of tulle outlined in gold. The embroidered border is 22 cm. wide. Below it is a narrower one of embroidered tulle. A small gold cord hides the seam where the wider border is attached to the dress. *Frau von Muchmeyer, Munich.*

498. GREY TAFFETA DRESS AND TAFFETA BONNET, ABOUT 1820 401
Professor Löwith, Munich.

499. GREY FROCK COAT, ABOUT 1830   403

Chest, 96 cm. ; waist, 82 cm. ; length, 91 cm. ; from shoulder to waist, 44 cm. ; length of frock, 47 cm. ; width of frock, 133 cm. Material, black and white woollen material, bound with black binding. Ten black patterned buttons, in a double row. There is a small slit at back with three buttons. On the right and on the left are three pockets bound with black binding. Also are shown black trousers of woollen stockinette, black silk neckcloth, and beige-coloured top hat. *Diringer, Munich.*

500. (*a*) BEIGE-COLOURED DRESS OF BARÈGE WITH TURQUOISE-BLUE TRIMMING   404

Waist, 76 cm. ; bust, 92 cm. ; length, 102 cm. Material, sand-coloured barège with ruching of turquoise taffeta. The skirt is made of four pieces. Lower width, 260 cm. ; length of bodice from shoulder, 34 cm. There is a seam in the middle of the front. The back is made of three pieces ; the fastening is by lacing. There are sleeve puffs laid in box-pleats 15 cm. deep ; the rest of the sleeve is plain. Round the neck is a taffeta ruche, 5 cm. wide, of turquoise blue ; also round the sleeves. The square buckle is of gold bronze. The yoke is of fine lawn, hand-embroidered, with narrow collar of same material. *Munich, National Theatre.*

(*b*) COAT OF KING LUDWIG I, ABOUT 1835

Length of bodice, 48 cm. ; entire length, 128 cm. ; width of bell-shaped skirt, 270 cm. (round cut out of the material). Double-breasted, with two rows of five black buttons. The edges are bound with black silk. Material, dark green cloth ; lining, black cotton. The tall hat is of sand-coloured silk (original). The neckcloth is black silk, tied in front. The grey trousers are strapped. *Munich, National Theatre.*

501. BROWN " BIEDERMEIER " TAIL COAT, ABOUT 1835 405

Entire length, 97 cm. ; tail to waist, 58 cm. ; length of bodice, 42 cm. ; across back, 30 cm. ; waist, 84 cm. ; width of the cut-away part, 19 cm. ; length of tail in front, 60 cm. ; width of tail, with under-flap, 24 cm. at waist, 17 cm. at foot ; length of front of bodice from the point, 30½ cm. ; width of each front piece, measured from armhole, 45 cm. ; width from side to front at points, 38 cm. The seam across the shoulders is 26 cm., cut well toward back. The seam over the shoulder, strongly curved, is 15 cm. The length of the sleeve, which is cut like a leg-of-mutton sleeve at top, is 48 and 63 cm. Depth of collar at back,

14 cm., turned over to a depth of 7 cm. ; depth of collar in front, 9 cm. ; upper length of roll collar, 38 cm. to point ; lower length of roll collar, 35 cm. This tail coat is of strong, light brown cloth, heavily padded, and stitched up to the collar. Six buttons are placed in a curved line ; there are four buttonholes. With this was worn a pair of trousers which were very full at waist, a waistcoat of grey and lilac striped velvet, a dark blue cravat, and a beige-coloured silk hat. *Munich, National Theatre.*

Waist (below bust), 82 cm. ; length of bodice from neck, 24 cm. ; width of sleeves, 33 cm. ; length of skirt, 97 cm. ; width of same, 225 cm. The skirt is made of four lengths. The bodice is fastened in front ; a narrow belt, 3 cm. wide, joins it to the skirt. The front seams of the bodice have a double piping. In the back there are four intakes. The sleeves have at the ball-shaped top two steps, set in with piping ; to these the sleeves proper, of leg-of-mutton shape, are attached, with gathers of 2 and 3 cm. A narrow drawing-in hem with cord runs round the neck. Material, rust-brown print with darker lines and black garlands. The lining of the bodice is white linen, laced. *Winterer, Munich.*

(*b*) Brown Print House Dress, about 1840

Waist, 88 cm.; bust, 114 cm.; length, 104 cm.; width of skirt, 350 cm. Material, brown print with white flowers. The lining of the bodice is grey sateen. The sleeve shows a slight leg-of-mutton shaping near the elbow; the lower part is plain, with a white cuff; the sleeves are gathered in at the shoulder to a depth of 15 cm. The bodice is fastened in front; it is plain at the back, and in front is drawn into a point, and has several rows of gathers. The neck is round. The neckerchief is of white lawn, hand-embroidered. *Munich, National Theatre.*

trimmed on all edges and round the neck and sleeves with strips of contrasting silk, and was fastened with buttons to match. The low-cut neck was filled in with a finely pleated chemisette of lawn. The hat worn with this was like that in Fig. 574.

Length of bodice-lining, 38 cm. in front, 27 cm. at back ; shoulder, 4 cm. ; neck, 100 cm. Each half has two back pieces, one side-piece, and one front piece. There are three intakes in the front piece, the whole whaleboned ; fastened to back by hooks. (The lining of white cotton has been restored.) Material of bodice : waist, 72 cm. ; bust, 96 cm. ; front length, 50 cm. ; back length, 39 cm. There are two pieces, one side-piece, and one front piece. The material is closely fitted to the lining. Being 19½ cm. wide at the shoulder, it is gathered in toward the front. At the back the gathers are 4 cm. deep, are in rows 1 cm. apart from each other, and are 6 cm. wide. In front they are 14 cm. wide, and here also 1 cm. apart and 4 cm. deep. All the seams have piping. Neck, 53 cm. ; length of sleeve, 59 cm. and 38 cm. ; length of sleeve-frill, 15 cm. ; length of skirt, 100 cm. ; width of skirt, 350 cm. ; depth of skirt-frills, 22 cm. These latter are ornamented with tucks 1 cm. wide, and cover each other for 2 cm. The lace round the neck is 1¼ cm. wide. The material is white muslin. *Diringer, Munich.*

From *Le Moniteur de la Mode*, 1868.

Waist, 82 cm. (enlarged) ; bust, 101 cm. ; length of skirt, 108 cm. ; width of skirt, 390 cm. Material, brownish-pink shot taffeta with darker stripes. The skirt has a white gauze lining ; it is bound with thin cord. A hem of white sateen runs round it. The bodice has a lining of white sateen. Trimmed with pale lilac gimp ; this borders the scalloped frill, which is 2 cm. wide. There is a bib-shaped fichu back and front. The front point is gathered in six rows to a depth of 11½ cm., the rows 1 cm. apart ; at the back are five rows of gathers, 5 cm. deep and 10 cm. in width. The rounded basque is 10 cm. wide in front, 19 cm. at back, where it is laid in three deep pleats. The bodice is fastened at the back by hooks. The sleeves are of an open bell-shape, finished at wrist with gimp, frills, and lace. The lawn collar is hand-embroidered. *Diringer, Munich.*

The blouse is trimmed with embroidered pieces, which form a yoke round the neck and finish the blouse in front downward. A similar yoke, *d*, trims the sleeve, *c*, which has besides a second puff, *e*.

To be worn over tight under-sleeves. The basque is cut out of a single piece of material ; only one half is given here. The seam joining basque and bodice is covered by a belt. Material, brown cloth.

ILLUSTRATIONS

A HISTORY OF COSTUME

INTRODUCTION

IN this book I have tried to show by practical examples the history of the development of dress. This attempt is based on the conviction that nothing but the original costume, if that be accessible, can be considered definitive for the conception we may legitimately entertain regarding the ideas about dress that prevailed in any period. We are far too ready to carry back to the costumes of bygone days our modern conceptions of what is becoming, and in our reproductions of historical costumes so to obliterate their peculiarities of style that the results have only a superficial resemblance to the original model. It was therefore my endeavour with the modern auxiliary of photography to rescue the various precious original garments from the perishableness that inheres in every material thing and faithfully to preserve their peculiar charm for the benefit of later ages. Of course, the further back we go the more difficult it becomes to secure original specimens. For the costume of the people of the Bronze Age, as well as for that of the early Teutonic peoples and of the inhabitants of North-west Europe from the thirteenth to the fifteenth century, we have, thanks to research, a number of perfect specimens, although even here there are also many large gaps.

With reference to the knowledge derived from works of art regarding the dress of ancient times there is this to be said. The artist frequently uses a *motif* of dress which belongs to an earlier style, either because he likes this better or because his own environment has not kept pace with the universal evolution of fashion. The period to which a work of art belongs has therefore sometimes very little connexion with the costume that work portrays. For this reason works of art are not always reliable sources of information. The artist's imagination is at work in them, supplementing and embellishing points of the dress that are unpleasing to it, with the result that it rarely produces a picture that is completely accurate. This is specially true in the case of great masters—even of the greatest. We are very apt to picture to ourselves the people of a period in the styles portrayed by these masters, but who would find fault with a Titian or with a Raphael for not keeping strictly to the fashion ? The case is different with those others to whom the history of art has awarded a lower place in the scale of excellence. These are in many cases of great importance for the history of dress. Their carefulness in reproducing the fashionable details and accidentals of dress more than makes up in the eyes of the student of costume for their slighter artistic value.

When handling ancient original costumes I was frequently struck with the great difference between the stature of the people of earlier centuries and that of those of our own day. Men and women have apparently grown stouter and taller. Very few men or women of to-day can don the ancient clothing. This is the case even with garments of the nineteenth century. Clothes of the Empire period and those of the *Biedermeier* style [1] are astonishingly small, and numerous alterations have to be made before they can be put on by a model to-day. Even more astonishing are the small measurements of the sixteenth-century clothes discovered in the Wittelsbach mausoleum at St Martin-in-Lauingen in Würtemberg.

It arouses a peculiar sensation to handle these heaps of garments belonging to days long past. One seems to see the river of time flowing past with all the happenings and experiences it brings to mankind. The clothing from the mausoleum at Lauingen belonged to a collateral branch of the royal house of Wittelsbach, the Dukes of Neuburg, Counts-Palatine of Sulzbach. For two hundred years these princes had lain at rest with their wives and children in their coffins of tin ; in 1781, in 1846, and again in 1877 they were disentombed, and their raiment was rescued from decay. The ladies were dainty ; their children, who had died young, were small and weakly. Along with the clothing were found the beautiful ornaments which are reproduced in these pages. The young unmarried Countess Maria Magdalena of Hilpoltstein had still round her neck the beautiful tiny pendant with the greyhound in white enamel, set with small pearls and rubies. All these Dukes of Neuburg seem to have been fond of fine jewels. One wore an armlet inscribed with the initials of his dearly beloved wife, the letters being separated by black links patterned with gold ; another had an armlet of thick gold chains set with polished spherical rubies. Beside the slim Duke Otto of Sulzbach was found a heart-shaped hatpin of gold, between the sprigs of forget-me-not and clover-leaves of white, blue, and green enamel was inset the monogram DM in rubies—a delicate token of homage to his dearly loved wife. The earrings, in comparison with present-day fashion, were very small, but the garments were liberally studded with the gold buttons which were a favourite form of ornament at the time. The wide sleeve, lined with green silk, of a leather jerkin in the Bavarian National Museum has on the right upper arm a sword-cut, testifying to a duel or a knightly adventure. And the owner of a waistcoat patterned in red of the eighteenth century must have been wearing this beautiful garment when he met his death, for the ragged, dark-stained rent low down on the left side speaks of the shot that cost him his life. Carefully treasured children's garments,

[1] *Biedermeier* is the term used nowadays to denote " a would-be man of honour."—TRANSLATOR.

coloured stockings and garters with gallant inscriptions, gloves of polished rose-coloured leather, shoes of red and green velvet with gold embroidery and high heels, fans ornamented with miniatures —all this dainty finery brought joy to the hearts of these men and women in their day.

I also give illustrations of costumes and suits from the well-filled wardrobe of Ludwig I of Bavaria, of which the National Museum possesses a complete collection. The King himself had carefully preserved all these garments, together with some attire belonging to his consort Theresa, and had with his own hand written full descriptions of them. He was tall and handsome, but slim, as his clothes prove, and the clothes themselves show an amazing precision in cut and perfect tailoring. We reproduce a " Polish " coat that belonged to him, a dress coat in dark blue with breeches of silk stockinette, a tall straw hat, and a double-breasted coat and tall silk hat. His travelling cloak and his leather travelling cap are also in the museum. To whom would these not recall those journeys to Italy which this art-loving prince undertook ? It was on his return that he presented to his subjects the treasures of the Pinakotheks[1] and of the Glyptothek[2] and those buildings to which Munich owes its renown as a centre of art. Not far from these garments is a suit of his unfortunate grandson, Ludwig II—a black walking-suit and an umbrella whose clumsy shape is hardly in keeping with one's conception of that artistic monarch. This suit belonged to his last years, when illness had robbed his figure of its Apollo-like beauty.

When one compares the clothing of these two men, grandfather and grandson, one cannot fail to be struck with the baneful effect produced by the sewing-machine as compared with skilled hand-sewing. By the year 1859 the sewing-machine had gradually replaced sewing by hand, and one grieves to have to say that men's clothes of this period made a somewhat sorry show when compared with the carefully made garments of earlier times. It was not only the splendid colour of the rococo period and its gradual evanescence in the Empire period that gave charm to the clothing of those eras. It was the technical perfection, the careful handwork that produced the smart appearance and that still distinguishes the *Biedermeier* dress coats in spite of their plainer materials.

Neither Carl Köhler nor Max von Boehn undertook to describe working-class dress or national costume. I too have omitted these from this work. The careful reader will quickly see how numerous are the points of contact between historical dress and that of the people : how rustic fashions retain styles and forms of cut that really belong to periods long past (these are technically called " fossils "), and how connecting threads from distant centuries persist into modern times. Ecclesiastical and clerical dress also betrays similar

[1] Two picture-galleries in Munich.—TRANSLATOR.
[2] The museum of ancient sculpture in Munich.—TRANSLATOR.

connexions with bygone styles. For example, the attire of monks, nuns, and clergymen retains many features of the costume of the Middle Ages. We come upon very close connexions between distant Eastern civilizations and Western types of dress, and even more deep-reaching associations between peoples are disclosed. Some of these peoples, though contemporaries, were separated by large distances ; others were separated in time by centuries ; but they hand on from age to age old-time ideas in dress that alter only slowly, either for convenience sake or from æsthetic motives.

The tailor's art is one of proportionate measurements. Every curtailment or change of a garment in one way is compensated by a lengthening or an emphasis in another way. To carry out these adjustments and adaptations and to bring about the universal use of the types thus produced—that is what we mean by a fashion. The transitions from one style to another take place gradually. They exhibit an organic growth, reaching at times to the extreme limit of possibility and again slowly retrogressing. And then in some other point of style the same process is repeated in obedience to an unwritten law.

The clothing of humanity is full of profound significance, for the human spirit not only builds its own body, but also fashions its own dress, even though for the most part it leaves the actual construction to other hands. Men and women dress themselves in accordance with the dictates of that great unknown, the Spirit of the Time.

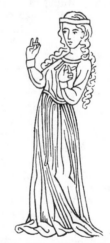

GERMAN FEMALE DRESS OF THE
TWELFTH CENTURY

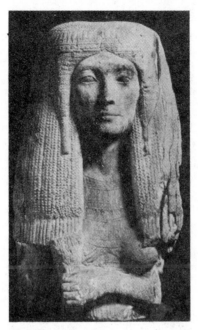

Fig. 1. STATUE OF A WOMAN—NEW KINGDOM

THE PEOPLES OF ANTIQUITY

THE EGYPTIANS

TO judge from the most ancient representation that we possess, the Egyptians of the Old Kingdom (*c.* 3000 B.C.) wore a loincloth (Fig. 8) made of woven material, which was wrapped several times round the body and kept in place by a girdle. In addition to this a wrap or a speckled skin was hung over the shoulders. This costume continued right up to the time when the so-called Old Kingdom reached its highest brilliance, and the beauty and costliness of material and draping were the only marks that distinguished monarch and nobles from the lower classes. By and by another item of dress was added—a somewhat close-fitting, one-piece skirt of expensive material, which was similarly fastened by means of a girdle. The so-called kalasiris (Figs. 3–5), a garment for both sexes, which was introduced shortly after the establishment of the New Kingdom (*c.* 1000 B.C.), was a long robe quite unlike those just mentioned, differing from them both in cut and in the materials of which it was made.

There was apparently more than one style of this garment. It was either a coat covering the body from the hips or the procardium to the abdomen, supported by a band passing over one shoulder, or it even reached as far up as the neck. Some forms of it were sleeveless

53

(Figs. 2 and 3), while others had short and narrow or long and fairly wide sleeves.

This garment also varied in width. Sometimes it was wide and

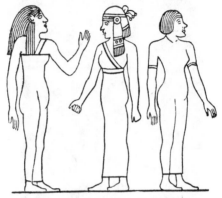

Fig. 2. EGYPTIAN FEMALE COSTUME

full, sometimes so close-fitting that it is difficult to understand how the wearer could walk.

Most probably, therefore, there were two ways of making the kala-siris. Either it was woven or knitted in one piece so as to impart to it some elasticity and cause it to cling closely to the lower limbs of the wearer even when he moved; or it was made of pieces cut separately and sewn together at the sides. In the former case it resembled a narrow bag of the same width throughout its whole length, sometimes with sleeves fitted to it or knitted in it. This elastic type of kalasiris seems to have been made of material which was in most cases of close texture, but occasionally very loose and transparent. It is of course possible that the transparency was due to the stretching of material that was originally close in texture and to the consequent tearing of the threads or stitches.

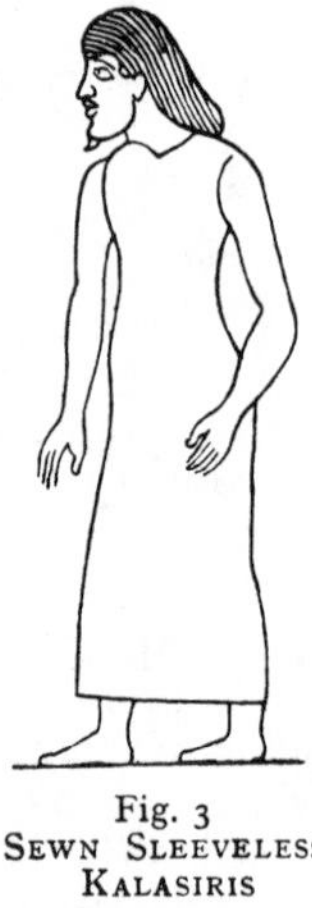

The sewn type of kalasiris was a short garment somewhat resembling a woman's petticoat. The width of the material determined the length of the garment, so that there was only one seam. The numerous folds were distributed at equal distances round the body. In some instances it was worn in apron fashion, and in that case it was not sewn at all.

Fig. 3
SEWN SLEEVELESS
KALASIRIS

The long type of kalasiris that covered the body up to the neck was made from a rectangular piece of material twice as long as the garment (see Fig. 4). It was folded in the middle, and a hole was cut out to allow the head to pass through. The sides were then

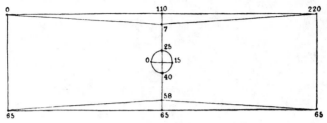

Fig. 4. Cut of the Sleeveless Kalasiris

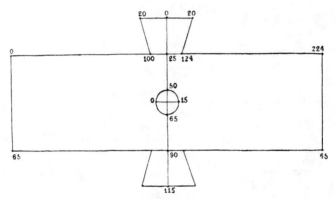

Fig. 5. Sleeved Kalasiris

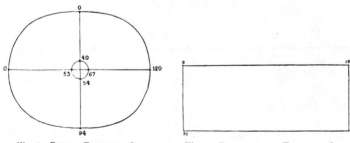

Fig. 6. Round Egyptian Cape   Fig. 7. Rectangular Egyptian Cape

sewn together, gaps being left unsewn at the top to serve as armholes.

When the garment was meant to be worn without a girdle the cut was

55

slightly altered so as to make the material over the shoulders narrower than that lower down. This is indicated by the interior lines in Fig. 4.

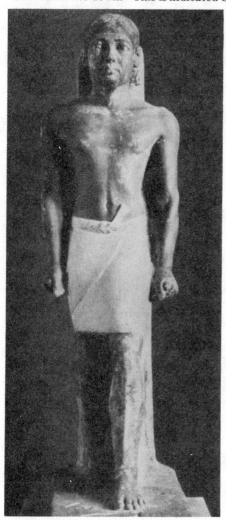

Fig. 8. Nofer the Brewer—Old Kingdom

For the sleeved kalasiris the sleeves were either cut separately and sewn on or a slight change was made in the garment itself (Fig. 5). The material on both sides of the opening for the head was left as wide as the intended length of the sleeves. The lower edges of the portions forming the sleeves were sewn together when the sides of the garment were sewn. The clothing of Egyptian women covered and concealed the person to a far greater extent than did the clothing of the men. The close-fitting, elastic type of kalasiris was the ancient national costume of the female population of the country. There were slight variations of style, but in all cases the garment was long enough to cover the ankles. In some it extended up to or beyond the breast (being held in place by shoulder straps), or even up to the neck. This last style was provided with sleeves.

The working class wore the same style of garment. In order to obtain greater freedom of movement they adopted various methods of tucking it up, and wore it much shorter than the upper classes did.

In addition to the garments described above, various kinds of capes were worn both by men and women of the upper classes. The earliest type, which was in regular use as far back as the time of the Old Kingdom, was an almost circular shoulder-cape (Fig. 6), either closed

56

or made to 'fasten behind. It varied in width, but never reached lower than the shoulder, and was made either of linen painted in diverse colours or of very costly network.

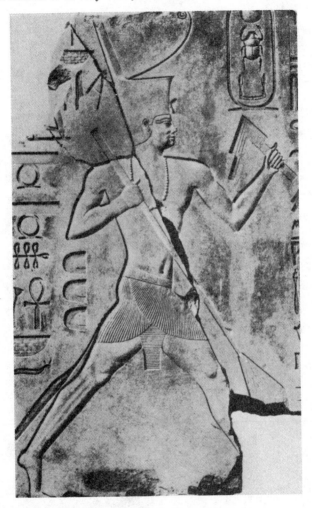

Fig. 9. KING SESOSTRIS I—MIDDLE KINGDOM

Another style of cape, made only of transparent materials, fell from the shoulders to a little below the elbows. This cape was either almost circular in shape, with a hole in the centre to allow it to be passed over the head (Fig. 6), or rectangular (Fig. 7). In the latter

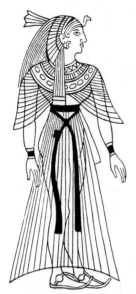

Fig. 10. EGYPTIAN QUEEN

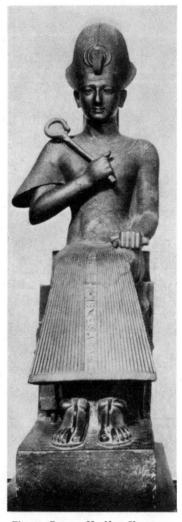

Fig. 12. RAMSES II—NEW KINGDOM

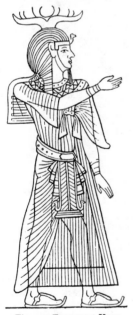

Fig. 11. EGYPTIAN KING

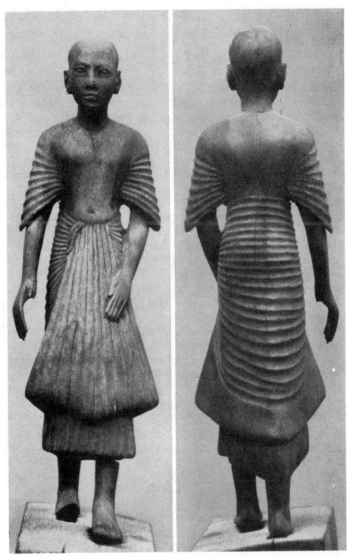

Fig. 13. STATUETTE OF THE LATE NEW KINGDOM

case the strips forming the cape were laid over the shoulders, gathered on the breast, and held in place by a clasp, so that the ends hung down loose.

In putting on the almost circular cape just mentioned the narrow

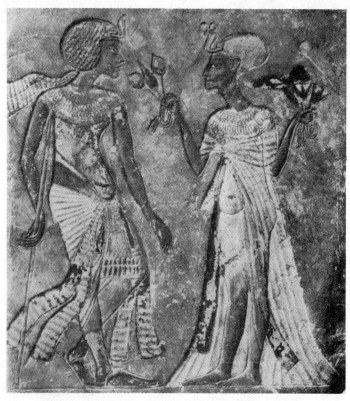

Fig. 14. AMENOPHIS IV AND HIS QUEEN—NEW KINGDOM

sides on breast and back were gathered, thus giving rise to diagonal folds.

As in the case of all ancient dress, the most important feature of the dress of the Egyptians was the draping. Each people had its own characteristic way of putting on garments that closely resembled each other in cut and style.

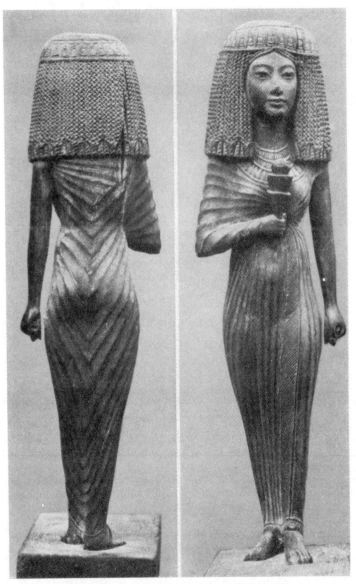

Fig. 15. STATUETTE OF THE LATE NEW KINGDOM

THE ETHIOPIANS

The dress of the Ethiopian peoples, whose territory lay to the south of Egypt, was on the whole identical with that of the Egyptians, although it had its own peculiarities largely due to racial separateness. Their original costume was a simple loincloth of wool or leather with a cloak-like garment worn over it. This costume gradually became

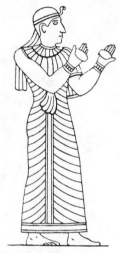
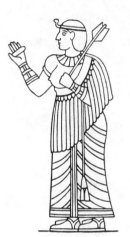

Fig. 16. LATER COSTUME OF ETHIOPIAN NOBLES

Fig. 17. ETHIOPIAN NOBLE LADY

more varied—girdles and jackets were added, the latter being of the elastic textile material already mentioned.

This was the usual wear of the people, but, as in Egypt, the dress of the upper classes was different, especially at a later period. As civilization advanced there was gradually evolved a style of dress entirely different from the Egyptian style. It had more of the character of the Asiatic or, more precisely, the Assyrian style. The loincloth came to be retained by the upper classes merely as a ceremonial dress; on ordinary occasions long garments were worn.

This clothing was made of opaque material, and at first did not extend higher than the breast. It was worn by both sexes, and consisted during the early period of a longish rectangular piece of cloth wide enough to cover the body from breast to feet. This was draped round the body and legs and was fastened over the shoulders and round the hips with straps or belts.

By and by the garment consisted of two pieces, the front being longer than the back.[1] The extra length of the front piece was gathered in deep folds, and these were fixed in such a way as to produce a graceful outline.

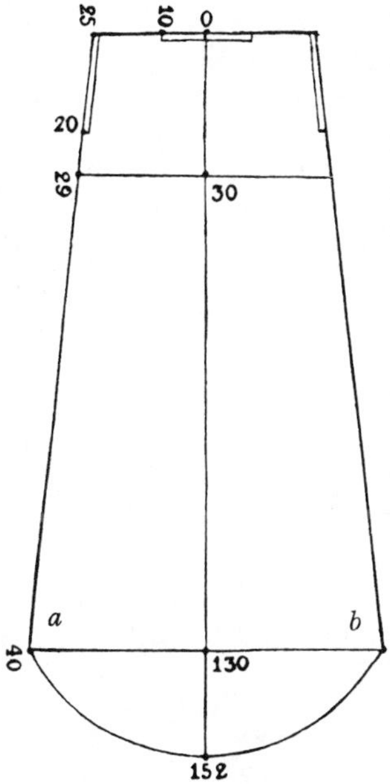

Fig. 18. ETHIOPIAN GARMENT

The gathering of the garment not only made it fit closer to the body, but also produced numerous oblique folds, which Ethiopian artists indicated by parallel strokes, which suggest patterned material rather than folds of drapery. In addition to those garments which were only hip-high the men wore on the upper body elastic jackets with short sleeves. Many, however, wore a garment reaching to the neck, with tight sleeves that came down to the wrists (Fig. 16). This had already come to be the chief garment of noble ladies. It was made of patterned materials and worn without a girdle. It was longer in front than at the back, and was gathered in folds and fixed in the manner already described.

The only difference between this garment and the one previously described was its greater length. When the two parts were sewn together they were also sewn at the top, except the opening for the head (see Fig. 18). At the sides were the armholes, and into them were fitted sleeves made separately. They were cut quite straight, and were sewn so as to narrow toward the wrists (Fig. 19).

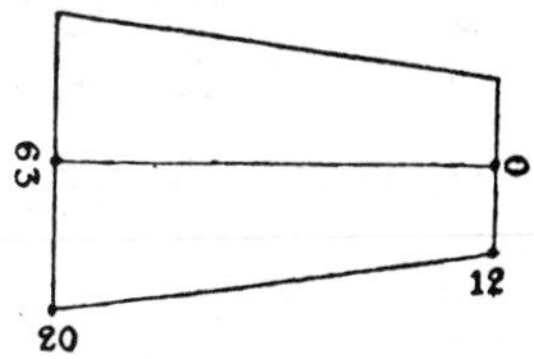

The lower edge of the long Ethiopian garments was trimmed with strong braid, which was patterned and decorated with small tassels. The braid was also brought up the front of the garment, and served to cover up the pins and stitches used to keep in place the gathered folds.

Fig. 19. SLEEVE OF ETHIOPIAN GARMENT

This long costume with its gathered folds was very unlike the Egyptian style, and this unlikeness was greatly accentuated by a broad tasselled scarf or sash (Fig. 17), which was hung over one shoulder and passed under the opposite

[1] The sleeveless garment is cut as in Fig. 18, but the length only comes down to the line ab. Fig. 18 shows the cut of the front piece. The back piece is cut straight at the foot (along the line ab), but is in other respects the same as the front piece. The double lines at the top of the pattern indicate the openings for the head and arms.

arm.   This gave to the dress of the Ethiopian nobles a character not unlike that of the Court dress of the Assyrians.

THE SYRIANS AND PHŒNICIANS

The most ancient known delineation of the peoples of Western Asia dates from about 2300 B.C., about the end of the Old Egyptian Kingdom.   It depicts people of the tribe or clan Aamu, whose territory lay

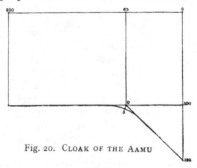

Fig. 20. CLOAK OF THE AAMU

presumably in Southern Syria.   Their clothing was the same for both sexes, and consisted of a fairly large rectangular piece of material

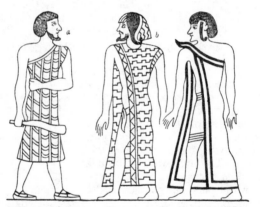

Fig. 21. (a) AAMU IN ANCIENT   Fig. 22. AAMU IN LATER
COSTUME. (b) RIBU   TYPE OF DRESS

(Fig. 20) which was wound twice round the body, covering it from the armpits to the knees.   One corner of this material, longer than the others, was thrown backward over the left shoulder and tied at the back to the other top corner (Fig. 21, a).

A garment similar to this, but more nearly square, was worn by men.   It was hung like a cloak over the back, and one of the upper corners was brought forward over the shoulder. When worn in this fashion it was probably fastened round the body by tapes attached to it for the purpose. Though the cut of these garments was simple, the material of which they were made was very beautiful, being

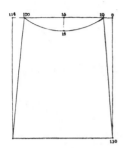

Fig. 23. CLOAK OF THE AAMU

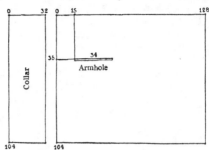

Fig. 24. CLOAK OF THE CHELI

patterned in various designs, usually stripes of green, blue, and red on a white ground.

On a picture five hundred years later, belonging to the New Egyptian Kingdom, we are again shown members of the Aamu tribe. Evidently the dress of the tribe had changed but little in that long interval. The women wear practically the same dress, but the men have exchanged the garment just described—covering the whole person except the arms—for a simple loincloth, and have added to it a cloak reaching nearly to the feet, one corner being pulled through under one arm and tied on the opposite shoulder (Fig. 22). This cloak differed from the more ancient Aamu garment only in the fact that the material was cut narrower at the top than at the bottom and was perhaps shaped at the upper edge (Fig. 23). The knotting of the ends was facilitated by broad tapes fastened to the upper corners.

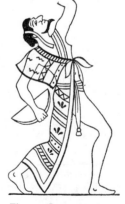

Fig. 25. COSTUME OF THE CHELI

Very similar to this style of dress was that of the Cheli, or Chari, who occupied the interior of Syria. Their sole dress was a cloak brought forward under one arm and tied at the breast and kept in place round the body by tapes. A slit was made to allow the arm to pass through (Figs. 24, 25), and a collar was sewn on to the cloak, adding greatly to its appearance. The cut of this cloak was a rectangle very nearly square, the shorter side being equal to the longer side of the rectangle out of which the collar was made. The collar was sewn on to the cloak, and was frequently of

65

a different pattern and colour ; the seam was hidden by a broad strip of patterned braid, the long ends of which served as tapes. The materials used by the Cheli were not inferior in beauty of colour to those of the peoples we have already discussed, and even excelled them in fineness.

To the north of the Cheli, probably on the Upper Euphrates between Taurus and Antitaurus, lived the Retennu-Tehennu, divided into various clans.

The dress of this people was different in the different clans. It covered the person to a far greater degree than did that of the inhabitants of Syria, and this seems to indicate that the Retennu

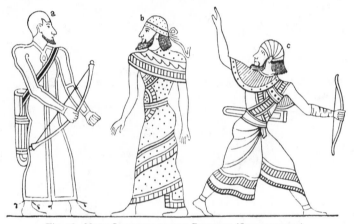

Fig. 26. MALE COSTUMES OF THE RETENNU (CAPPADOCIANS)

occupied a colder district. From the type of their dress it is possible to distinguish three clans or ranks. One wore the apron-like garment ; the second wrapped material round the body ; the third wore tailored garments. These differences, however, so far as our knowledge goes, are applicable only to men's dress. Women's dress consisted almost entirely of several coats put on one over another and kept in place by a girdle round the hips. In addition to these women also wore a large, circular shoulder-cape, which was fastened all down the front by means of clasps. Underneath this cape they wore dark-coloured ribbons crossed over the breast, with the long ends hanging over the back.

The apron-like garment of the Retennu was made as follows : an almost rectangular piece of material of suitable size (Fig. 27) was thrown round the loins and kept in place by a girdle and perhaps also by broad tapes crossed at the breast and back. With this was worn a fairly large shoulder-cape (Fig. 28), which covered one arm down to the elbow and left the other arm bare. This cape came right up to the neck, and seems to have been fastened down the short side by means of clasps.

If we judge from the richly patterned materials used, the wrap style of costume was a privilege of the wealthier classes. These garments had the shape of a very much elongated triangle, whose tapering

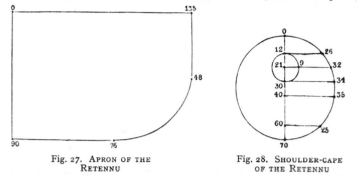

Fig. 27. Apron of the
Retennu

Fig. 28. Shoulder-cape
of the Retennu

end was kept in place by a girdle (Fig. 26, b). With this the Retennu wore what looks like a tight but elastic collar, which for the sake of freedom of movement was pushed high up at one shoulder. They seem also to have used shoulder-capes similar to those already mentioned. The third style of dress was so entirely different from the

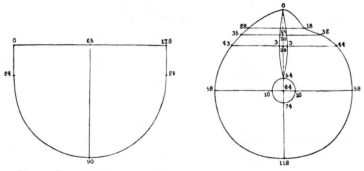

Fig. 29. Upper Garment of the
Phœnicians

Fig. 30. Cape of the
Phœnicians

other two that it must have been peculiar to one special clan—unless, indeed, it was the exclusive war-dress of this people (Fig. 26, a). This dress, made of very strong material (probably leather), consisted of a coat with long, tight sleeves, covering the body from the neck to below the calves. In cut it resembled the Egyptian kalasiris, with this difference—that along all seams and down the front it was covered with broad strips of coloured material and the bottom edge was trimmed with tassels attached by cords.

THE HEBREWS

We possess very few representations of Hebrew costume apart from some found in the ruins of Nineveh. Taken with the descriptions furnished by the Old Testament, these, however, enable us to make

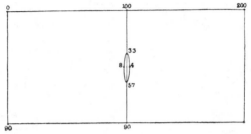

Fig. 31. HEBREW UPPER GARMENT MADE IN TWO PARTS

out quite clearly a distinct type. A sort of shirt and a cloak constituted the earliest dress. In the reign of David, under Assyrian and Phœnician influence, the material gradually became richer and finer,

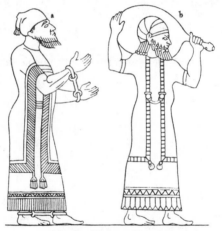

Fig. 32. HEBREW NOBLES

but, speaking generally, the original cut was closely adhered to (c. 1000 B.C.)

Men's dress consisted of a shirt-like under-garment of full length, with sleeves of varying length, and a rectangular piece of material which could be wrapped round the body as desired. One shirt was not always considered enough, and some men wore two, the one next the skin being of linen and longer than the upper one, which was of wool.

68

THE ASSYRIANS AND BABYLONIANS

A very ornamental item of Hebrew dress was the girdle, used to keep the under-garment in place over the loins. It was originally made of leather, but by and by it was made of expensive material inter-threaded with gold, or even of metal adorned with precious stones. Over these was worn the traditional cloak-like plaid. In later days, shortly before and during the Assyrian captivity, other upper garments came into use. One form was shaped like a caftan ; another was made in two parts and sewn together on the shoulders so as to form a front and back part. This last-mentioned garment, although certainly of Assyrian or Babylonian origin, was an important item in the wardrobe of the high priest, and, like the rectangular

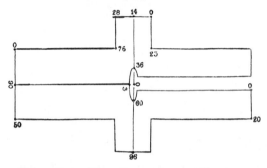

Fig. 33. GOWN (UPPER GARMENT) OF THE HEBREWS

cloak, was adorned at the four corners with purple tassels in remembrance of the statutes of Jehovah. At a later time, by an ostentatious enlargement of these tassels, the scribes and Pharisees sought to distinguish themselves from ordinary people as specially religious. [1]

This upper garment was very simple. It was merely two pieces of material identically alike, either rectangular (Fig. 31) or having the lower corners rounded. These were sewn at the shoulders so that the garment remained open at the sides (Fig. 32, *a*). The caftan-like costume, on the other hand, was also in two pieces, a front and a back, but it had sleeves, and was closed at the sides (see Fig. 33). It was, however, open all down the front, and was kept in place by a cord.

THE ASSYRIANS AND BABYLONIANS

Babylonian and Assyrian dress, although simple in cut, like that with which we have hitherto dealt, had reached a high degree of excellence in respect of material and trimming. The Babylonian Empire (about 2000 B.C.) had given place to the Assyrian Empire, which by the year 1300 B.C. had become the most powerful Asiatic state, and had absorbed the entire civilization of Western Asia.

[1] Matthew xxiii, 5.—TRANSLATOR.

The national dress both in Assyria and in Babylonia was a shirt with short, tight sleeves, cut very like the Egyptian kalasiris. The length varied. This was the sole garment of the lower orders for both

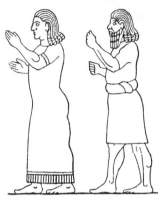

sexes. Some wore it with and some without a girdle (Fig. 34). Even during the time when the national prosperity was at its height the slaves of the nobles had no other dress than this, and, in their case, it was only long enough to reach to the knee.

Men of the higher orders also wore this short-sleeved shirt, but with them it reached to the feet. Most of them wore girdles trimmed with tassels, and, in keeping with the dignity of the wearers, the garments themselves were trimmed and embroidered more or less elaborately.

Fig. 34. NATIONAL COSTUME OF ASSYRIA AND BABYLONIA

Even the monarch wore this costume, and, in addition to it, on ceremonial occasions he put on a cloak-like over-garment, whose shape and trimming underwent many changes as time went on.

In its earliest form this garment resembled the shoulder-cape that was from primitive times worn by the nobles of the various peoples (including the Aamu and Ribu) inhabiting Western Asia. It consisted of a large, oblong piece of material of varying colour and pattern. This was either drawn forward under one arm and fastened on the other shoulder with an agraffe or clasp, or openings were made in it for the head and one arm, and it hung over both shoulders, being open of course on one side.

As time went on these cloaks became richer and more elaborate. The edges were trimmed with fringes and tassels. But the only change of cut was that the shoulder parts were lengthened so as to reach the middle of the upper arm. To allow this to be done the garment was made in

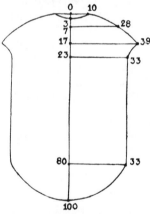

Fig. 35. ASSYRO-BABYLONIAN ROYAL ROBE

two pieces and sewn together at the top, a hole being left for the head (see Fig. 35). Both sides were now left open, instead of being open only at the armhole, and the front and back pieces were held together with tapes sewn for this purpose to the inside of the garment. (See Fig. 36.)

The usual badge of rank worn by all higher Court and State officials was a long fringed stole or shoulder-scarf, the ends of which were wound round the person. While rank was sometimes indicated by the amount of trimming on the full-length skirt, it was still more clearly shown by the scarf. The richness of the material and the

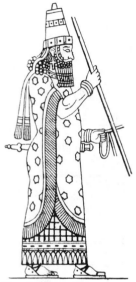

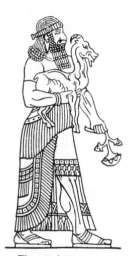

Fig. 36. Assyro-Babylonian Royal Costume

Fig. 37. Assyrian or Babylonian Priest

length (as well, perhaps, as the colour of the fringes and the manner in which the scarf was worn—plain or crossed) indicated the station of the wearer. For example, a scarf with long fringes worn crossed over the breast was the distinctive mark of the prime minister, or vizier. A double scarf with equally long fringes worn crossed indicated the master of ceremonies. The king's own personal attendants—armour-bearer, cupbearer, etc.—wore scarves with short fringes. Officials of still lower grade, like the parasol-bearer, wore no scarf at all. The monarch himself in early times donned the scarf over all his other attire, but in after days, from 750 B.C. onward, this ceased to be part of his state dress.

The official dress of the priests was quite unlike that of the high Court functionaries, and even the costume worn by the king as head of the priesthood was altogether distinct from that which indicated his royal rank. It is difficult to make out how far the priests' dress differed from that of ordinary laymen in respect of material and colour, but there is no doubt that there was a difference. In any case, the official costume of the priest was not less magnificent or imposing than that of the courtier. It seems probable that a special material —bleached linen—was used by the priests, and by them exclusively.

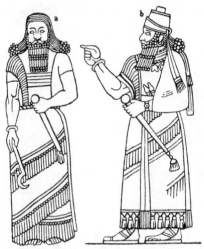

Fig. 38. (a) Assyro-Babylonian Priestly Costume. (b) Royal Dress

There were two styles of priestly costume, used in different ceremonies. In the one case the priest wore the long, short-sleeved shirt, and over it a garment that swathed the body from the feet

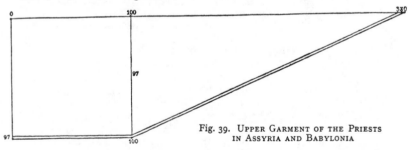

Fig. 39. Upper Garment of the Priests in Assyria and Babylonia

up to the loins or even to the shoulders. The shorter style (Fig. 38, a) was made of a piece of material in the shape of a right-angled triangle, one of the sides containing the right angle (Fig. 39) being of a length equal to the distance from the waist to the feet. The other side was considerably longer, and the third and longest side of the triangle was fringed. The garment was put on in this way. It was spread round the person so that the longer of the two sides containing the right angle encircled the waist at an equal height all round. It was kept in place by a cord passing round the body. The fringed side thus encircled the body in an ascending spiral.[1]

The piece of material, embellished by an embroidered inscription and with a fringe down one side, worn on the high priest's breast seems to have been made of thick cloth, and was hung over the shoulders, an opening permitting the head to pass through. The lower edge lay on the wearer's back, and the whole was kept in position by a girdle.

The dress worn by the king at the same religious ceremony, though apparently similar to this high priest's dress, was really very different. Whereas the high priest's robe was triangular in shape, that of the king (Fig. 38, *b*) was rectangular, the two short sides being of a length

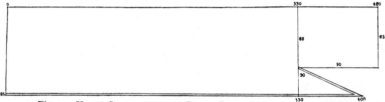

Fig. 40. Upper Garment of the Royal Priestly Costume in Assyria and Babylonia

equal to the distance from the loins to the feet. A piece was cut out of one of the two short sides, making two peaks, one rectangular and one triangular, the latter forming part of the lower portion of the garment and fringed all round like the bottom edge (Fig. 40).

This garment was swathed round the body as before, but in order that the bottom edge with the fringe should encircle the body in an ascending spiral the material was kept moving upward and disposed at the top in folds running obliquely round the body. These folds were concealed by a girdle. This swathing process was so carried out that the garment was pulled up across the back, and the back of the excision reached well up to the nape of the neck. The two peaks, held in position by the girdle, were then brought forward over the shoulders so that the triangular peak could be drawn over the right shoulder, covering the upper right arm, while the rectangular peak passed over the left shoulder, hiding almost entirely the upper left arm. The other type of ceremonial priestly dress also included the short-sleeved shirt as under-garment. This did not, however, reach to the feet, but only to the knee. As in all other forms of ceremonial dress, the bottom edge was trimmed with rich braid and with tassels (see Fig. 37).

The high priests, the head of whom was the king himself, wore over this a cloak-like garment cut all in one piece (Figs. 41 and 42).

[1] The double lines in Fig. 39 indicate the sides that were fringed.

It was drawn through under one arm and fastened on the opposite shoulder in such a manner that the front fell back over the upper arm.

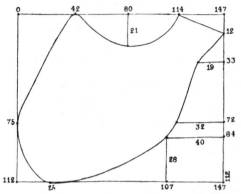

Fig. 41. CLOAK OF THE ASSYRIAN OR BABYLONIAN PRIEST

On the open side the back of the cloak was tied to the front with cords sewn to the inside, their tasselled ends hanging low down. This arrangement caused the garment to fit fairly close over breast and back.

There are also representations which show members of the priesthood wearing not this cloak-like upper garment, but a long apron of equally costly material. Reaching from the hips to the ankles, it covered only the back parts, leaving in view

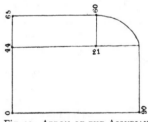

Fig. 43. APRON OF THE ASSYRIAN OR BABYLONIAN PRIEST

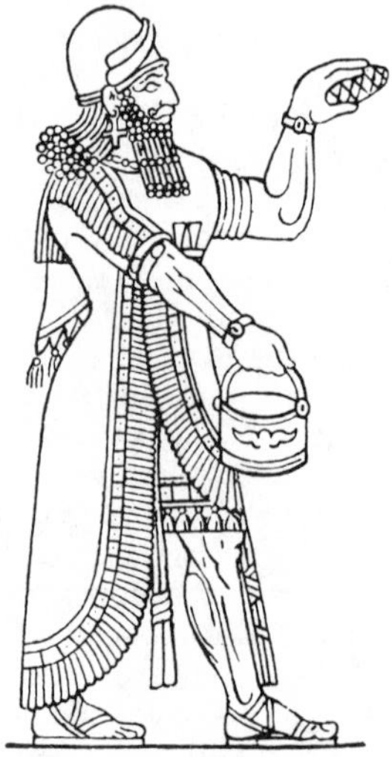

Fig. 42. PRIESTLY ROBES WORN BY THE KING IN ASSYRIA AND BABYLONIA

the front portion of the short, richly embroidered shirt (Fig. 37). All the edges of this apron, except that at the top, had a double row of tassels and fringes. These were attached in such a way that the tassels hung down behind the fringes, and were therefore visible only on the inside of the garment, while only the fringes could be seen on the outside.

74

THE MEDES AND PERSIANS

This apron was kept in position round the body by long cords, whose tasselled ends were long enough to reach the feet. Over the shoulders a long scarf or stole with long fringes was worn.

The priests occasionally wore a garment slightly different from this one. This was merely an apron reaching from the waist to the knee, adorned with braid and tassels. It was flung round the lower trunk and thighs and kept in place by cords with tasselled ends.

THE MEDES AND PERSIANS

An entirely different type of dress is met with when we turn to the Medes and Persians. In contrast to the costumes swathing the body

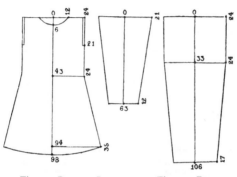

Fig. 44. PERSIAN LEATHER   Fig. 45. PERSIAN
COAT WITH SLEEVES   BREECHES

worn by the peoples already mentioned, we now find hose or breeches and a blouse-like shirt with sleeves.

The original Persian costume was made of tanned hides, covering not only the upper part of the body, but also the legs. At a later time (about 700 B.C.) the Persians used strong but soft materials to provide suitable protection in view of the climate of the country.

The tailoring of men's clothes in ancient Persia was somewhat complicated by the fact that it had to be adapted to the size of the hides available. Therefore not only had the body of the coat to be made in two or three pieces (Fig. 44), but the sleeves also had to be cut separately and then attached to the coat. This coat reached from the neck to the knees. It was open down the front, and fastened by a girdle. The sleeves were somewhat tight, and covered the whole arm down to the wrist.

The hose or breeches of the Persians (Fig. 45) were fairly wide. They reached sometimes to the knees and sometimes to the ankles, and were fastened round the waist. They were thus both simple and convenient, and their great width at the top made up for the lack of stylish cut.

The footwear of the Medes and Persians consisted either of pieces of leather or other material folded tightly round the feet and tied over the instep or of actual boots, which were just as primitively simple as the other type of foot-covering just mentioned.

The Persian headdress was a fairly deep cap, coming down in front to the eyebrows and at the back to the nape of the neck. It was

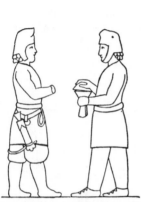

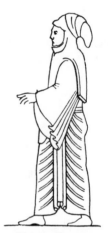

Fig. 46. National Costume of
THE PERSIANS

Fig. 47. Median
National Costume

made of stiff material, such as felt or leather, and had side-flaps which were often long enough to be tied under the chin.

The dress of Persian women differed little from that worn by the men. The primitive form of it was hides wrapped round the body. At a later time the cut was the same, but the garments were now made of fine leather or felt. The only real differences between the dress of the two sexes were that the women's coats were wider and longer than those of the men and were closed down the front except for a slit at the breast. When the Median type of dress became increasingly common among the Persians the ancient Persian female garments gradually disappeared, or were greatly modified. They were considerably lengthened and became more voluminous, and the sleeves were wider. Median styles of dress were in strong contrast to the Persian styles. In the latter the garments were close-fitting, short, and made of strong material; in the former they were wide, long, and voluminous, and were therefore made of finer materials.

The usual men's dress, called kandys, was much wider at the foot than higher up, and was so long that it had to be gathered in front and at the sides and held by a girdle (Fig. 47). The sleeves came to the wrists ; they were cut very wide near the wrist, but were tighter toward the armhole.

The Median coat consisted of two pieces, front and back, cut practically alike, except that the cut for the neck was in the front

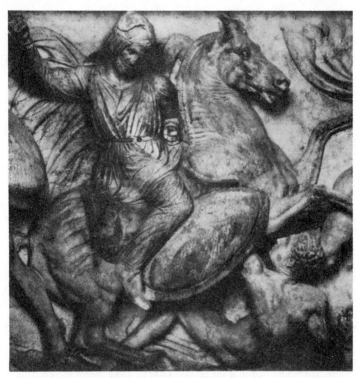

Fig. 48. PERSIAN ON HORSEBACK

piece. These pieces were much narrower at the top than at the foot (Fig. 49), and were sewn together at the shoulders and down the two sides. The sleeves were quaintly shaped, and were put in at the holes left for the purpose in the side-seams. As was almost universally the case in ancient times, the sleeve-seams were in line under the arm with the side-seam of the garment.[1]

This type of costume was worn by Medes of all classes, and was also the ceremonial garb of the monarch and his officials. It was Cyrus who introduced this Median dress into Persia. The ancient Persian national dress was retained only by subordinate Court officials.

The priests in Media and Persia, the " magicians," when performing

[1] The crosses in Fig. 49 indicate how the sleeve itself was sewn.

their official duties were clothed in white. The cut of their garments varied with their rank. The only item of dress which was worn by all priests was the sacred girdle. Priests were forbidden to wear any

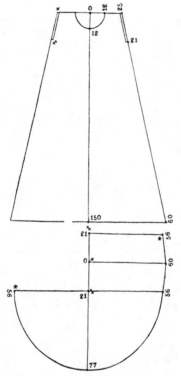

Fig. 49. MEDIAN GARMENT

kind of ornament during their celebrations, but they had to carry a cane rod in their hands. (See Fig. 51.)

In the ceremonies performed in honour of the sacred fire the retinue of the priests was dressed in purple. A purple robe—or at least a purple cape—seems to have been the distinctive dress of the chief priest (Fig. 51, a). When officially employed he wore the Median national costume and a headdress very similar to that worn by the king. The material and cut of the clothing of the rest of the priests bore greater resemblance to the Persian costume, or consisted of an under-garment and a wrap or plaid.

Like the cape of the high priest, the priest's upper robe was made in two pieces, a front and a back. In contradistinction to the former, however, it was not sewn from top to foot, but was open

78

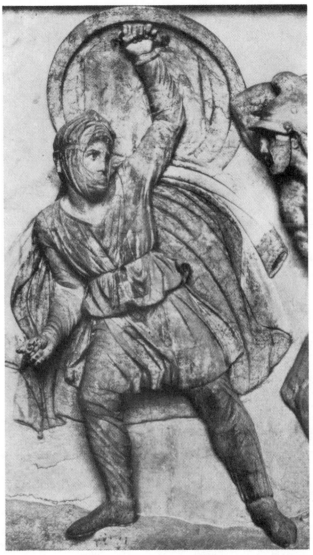

Fig. 50. PERSIAN WITH SHIELD
Fourth century B.C.

at the sides. Moreover, the front and back pieces of this robe differed from those of the other both in shape and size, and the garment itself had a hood-like collar, separately sewn on (Fig. 52, *c*). The front and back pieces were first sewn together at the shoulders ; then the

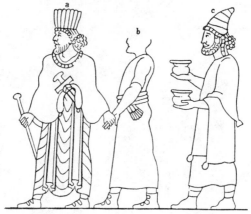

Fig. 51. MEDIAN AND PERSIAN PRIESTS

rest of the width of the back piece was turned over forward. The rest of its upper edges was sewn to the sides of the front piece. The collar was also sewn to the front piece so that the seams of this sewing met the seams connecting the front piece with the back.

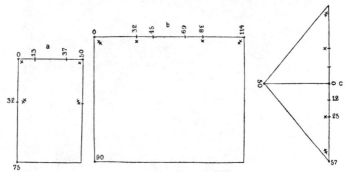

Fig. 52. UPPER GARMENT OF MEDIAN AND PERSIAN PRIESTS
(*a*) Sleeve ; (*b*) back piece ; (*c*) hood.

When the garment was being put on, the loose flaps of the front piece were fastened together underneath the back piece.

Median footwear, like the Persian, consisted of laced shoes made of leather or other strong material. Those worn by wealthy people were richly embroidered, trimmed with gold, and frequently light in colour.

The Median type of hose or breeches, when worn at all, was probably in all respects like that of the Persians.

On the other hand, the Median headdress was quite unlike that worn in Persia.   It was a hood that not only covered the head, but entirely surrounded the face, concealing even the chin.   From it hung down two broad strips, one falling over the breast and one over the back.   A different form of headdress was used by the upper classes. These wore round caps varying in height and increasing slightly in diameter upward, the crown being either flat or raised.   The crowns and edges of these caps, which were sometimes bestowed by the monarch as signs of distinction or of royal favour, were frequently covered with rich embroidery.   The wearing of a blue and white cord round the cap was a privilege strictly confined to relatives of the royal family.

THE SCYTHIANS

The dress of the Scythians, Sarmatians, and Dacians is specially interesting, because the cut and style of it show many points of

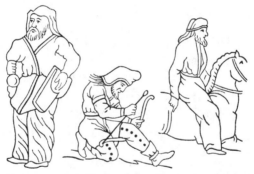

Fig. 53. Scythians

resemblance to the Teutonic fashions of prehistoric and early times. The Scythians (of about 700 B.C.) wore long trousers, smock-like shirts, and cloaks very like those worn by the Teutonic peoples.

All the Scythian tribes dressed in very nearly the same way.   The men wore fairly wide trousers and a coat open in front and held in place by a girdle.   Sometimes the coat hung down over the trousers, and sometimes it was tucked into them.   The feet were shod with short top-boots fastened round the ankles (Fig. 53).   The headdress was either a cap-shaped piece of material kept on by a string that passed round the head or a pointed cap like that worn by the Phrygians.

The material used by the Scythians varied with the degree of civilization attained by the different tribes. The majority of them, being nomads wandering about on the Steppes, had nothing but the material that their flocks supplied. They were exposed throughout a large part of the year to inclement weather, and therefore their clothes were made of tanned leather, the separate pieces being sewn together with narrow strips of leather. Some tribes wore clothing fashioned in the same way, but made of fur, while still others dressed themselves in material made from sheep's wool and felted.

The cut of the garments was as primitive as the material of which

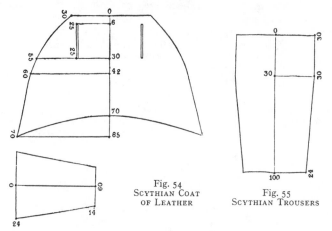

Fig. 54
SCYTHIAN COAT
OF LEATHER

Fig. 55
SCYTHIAN TROUSERS

they were made. The coat consisted of two pieces (Fig. 54) joined by a seam running down the back. In each piece a slit was cut for the arms, and the sleeves were sewn in separately.

The trousers were made of two oblong pieces of material (see Fig. 55). Each of these was folded lengthwise and sewn up the greater part of the length. These two bag-like pieces were then sewn together where the seam in each had stopped, this junction seam running up in front and at the back and between the legs. The extra width at the top was distributed round the waist during the process of dressing and kept in place by the girdle.

The headdress was a piece of leather or other material, which was given the necessary shape in the process of fulling.

As with most other Asiatic peoples, women's wear among the Scythians was almost identical with that of the men. The only differences were that women's clothes were longer and wider, made of finer material, and more daintily worked.

Widespread and numerous as the Scythians were, only one tribe among them attained any historical importance. These were the Parthians.

THE PARTHIANS

The Parthians were a savage race of horsemen. Speaking generally, their clothing was the same as that worn by the other Scythian tribes, especially by the monarchical Scythians who were settled round the

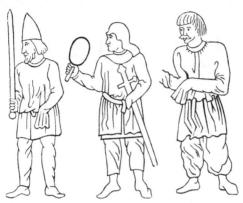

Fig. 56. PARTHIAN COSTUME

shore of the Black Sea. Like these last mentioned, the Parthians usually wore several coats one over another. When putting on these coats they pulled the upper one, which was cut wide and was long enough to reach to the knees, up under their girdle, so that the bottom edge of the coat underneath (which was much shorter and closer-fitting) could be seen (Fig. 56). They also wore long, fairly wide trousers. Their headdress was sometimes pointed and sometimes round, or shaped like the Phrygian cap. The shoes were of leather, frequently dyed a reddish purple.

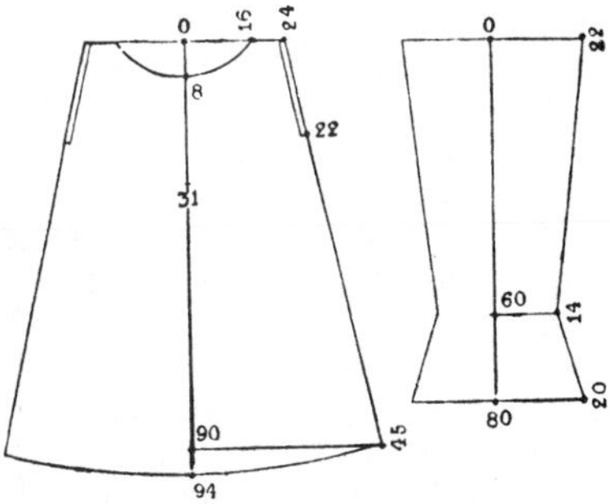

The trousers were made in the same manner as those of the other Scythian tribes, but in some cases the Persian style was followed (Figs. 45, 48, 50). The Parthian coat, on the other hand, which was made of coloured, soft materials, often

Fig. 57. PARTHIAN COAT WITH SLEEVE

of fine quality, resembled the Median garment. It consisted of two pieces, front and back, shaped alike. (See Fig. 57.) These were sewn together on the shoulders and at the sides as far as the sleeve-hole. The sleeves were conspicuously long. The hole for

83

the head was very wide ; round it was a broad hem for the tie-string, so that the garment could be drawn tight up to the neck or allowed to lie lower on the shoulders. In this way the top of the under-garment, which was similar, but, as said above, shorter and closer-fitting, could be seen to a greater or less extent, as the wearer pleased. The upper coat either had a slit at the breast or was divided in front from the foot up to the fork ; it might even be left completely open in front.

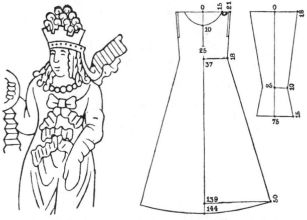

Fig. 58. Noble
Parthian Lady

Fig. 59. Parthian Woman's Coat
with Sleeve

This was the ordinary Parthian dress. That of the upper classes was made of splendid material, mostly coloured and richly adorned. Over it was also occasionally worn an oblong cape, fastened at the breast with an agraffe, or clasp.

The only differences between women's dress and that of the men were in the greater length of the former and the finer material of which it was made. The clothing of women of the upper classes was much more gaily coloured and more richly adorned (Fig. 58). A frequent addition to the costume was a cloak-like wrap, and some women wore a veil fastened to the head and falling down the back. For the rest, this long-sleeved garment was close-fitting at the top. (See Fig. 59.) No girdle was worn with it. The slit at the breast began at the neck, but was covered with bows of broad ribbon. In order to render the upper part of the garment close-fitting it was shaped at the waist, the lower part being cut considerably wider than the upper.

SARMATIANS, DACIANS, AND ILLYRIANS

THE SARMATIANS, DACIANS, AND ILLYRIANS

The dress of the Sarmatians closely resembled that of the Parthians, but there was this difference. When the Sarmatian wore two coats he put on the shorter one above the longer one, and only the longer one (which often reached to the feet) was fitted with long sleeves. The sleeves of the shorter one never came below the elbows, and often came no lower than the middle of the upper arm. Occasionally no upper coat was worn at all, and the Sarmatian costume then consisted of the trousers, the long coat tucked high up, and a cloak, which might be long or short, rectangular or semicircular. This cloak was fastened at the right shoulder with a pin, or brooch, or

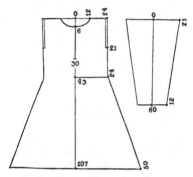

Fig. 60. DACIAN COAT WITH SLEEVE

even a thorn. The long coat was kilted sometimes high, at other times low. Sometimes it was slit at the sides, or it might be closed all round. The headdress was a cap almost identical with that worn by the Phrygians. In battle a helmet was worn. The trousers and footwear were similar to those in use among the Parthians and monarchical Scythians. The dress of Sarmatian women, who, well armed and mounted, followed their husbands into battle—among the Yaxamatians women formed the sole cavalry of their tribe, the men fighting on foot as archers—was almost the same as that of the men —viz., a long under-garment, with a shorter one over it. Both of these were sleeveless, and were girt high or low as the wearer pleased. The short upper garment sometimes had a long slit at the breast trimmed with ribbons, with which it could be tied. The female headdress was a tall cap like that worn by the Phrygians.

Dacian and Illyrian costume closely resembled that worn by the Sarmatians, and consisted of shoes, trousers, long coats, and oblong or semicircular cloaks. The main difference was in headdress. Whereas the Sarmatians wore Phrygian caps, the Dacians and Illyrians wore a fairly tall, stiff conical cap made of some kind of felt (see

85

Fig. 61). Another point of difference was that the Dacians, unlike the Sarmatians, did not wear several coats one over another, and,

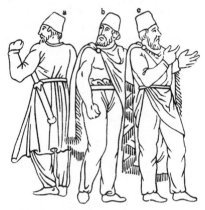

Fig. 61. (*a*) and (*c*) Dacians. (*b*) Illyrian

speaking generally, Dacian dress was not so long or so loose as the other.

In cut Dacian costume, made of fine or coarse woollen material, resembled that of the Parthians, but the coat, especially the upper

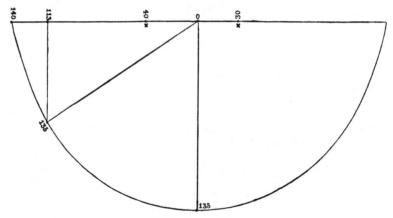

Fig. 62. Dacian Cloak

part of it, was considerably tighter than in the Parthian type. It had a slit at the breast, and at one side or even at both was open to half-way up the thigh.

Dacian trousers were shaped like those worn by the Scythians, but

THE CRETANS

were not nearly so wide, and were tied round the ankles after the Sarmatian style.

The Dacian cloak was almost semicircular (Fig. 62) ; the curved edge had long fringes. It was held together by a clasp on the right shoulder.

The chief difference between female dress in Dacia and Sarmatia was that the Dacian style had sleeves, while the Sarmatian coats had none. Dacian women followed the practice of wearing several coats ; the sleeves of the over-garments were shorter than those of the under ones, and were gathered and tied just above the elbow or half-way up the upper arm. The garments were very long and very full, the over one being usually shorter than the one beneath. Both had one or two tucks, and were in this way shortened. Quite frequently the girdle was replaced by a cloak, oblong or with a rounded lower edge, worn so that the upper edge passed round the body, the corners being knotted together in front. The Dacian women had a very peculiar fashion of disposing of the great width of the upper part of their clothing. They gathered a large part of the material at the back and arranged it in a knot, pinning it to keep it in place. Round the head they tied a kerchief, which fell to the nape of the neck like a hair-net.

The clothing of the Dacian women must have been made of fine material. In cut the garments consisted of two broad oblong pieces, a front and a back. These were sewn together at the shoulders and down the sides—except, of course, the openings for the arms. The opening for the head was finished with a wide hem, through which a string was passed for fastening. The sleeves had, as usual, only one seam, and were tighter at the wrist than at the shoulder.

THE CRETANS

An era of great development, contemporaneous with the civilization of ancient Egypt and Phœnicia, and which may be dated about 2000–1500 B.C., had preceded the civilization that came from Asia Minor into Crete and Greece. Such fragments of Cretan culture as have come down to us reveal a beauty of technique and a delicate sense of form to which no contemporaneous civilization provides any parallel. Owing to the lack of written records, the processes and methods of manufacture are still wrapped in obscurity, but although we are thus reduced to surmise regarding the materials used, the dress of that time is of the highest interest in view of its connexion with the costumes of other peoples. Our attention is especially attracted by the dress worn by the women. The slim, wiry figures of the men are clothed almost universally with a loincloth, richly patterned and splendidly decorated. Here and there we see wide cloaks that clothe the whole body, giving it a large appearance. Women also, it would

87

seem, wore the short loincloth, but we find them wearing in addition skirts put together in an almost fantastic manner that betrays a highly developed knowledge of the technique of dressmaking. These

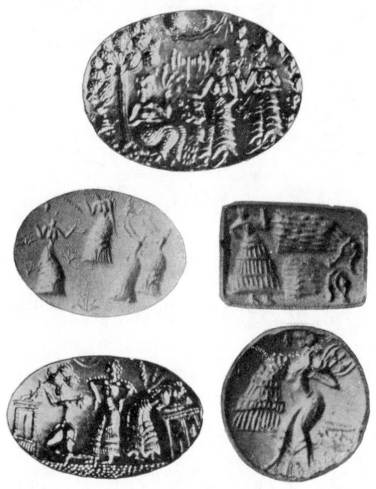

Figs. 63–67. CRETAN SEALS

skirts are constructed in tiers, separated by strips of rich ornamentation. There are even examples of what are called *volants*, or flounces —*i.e.*, narrow strips of patterned material, the upper projecting over the lower, and, if we are to judge from the perpendicular lines, disposed in fine accordion pleats. Over these falls a rounded kind of apron. The waist is slender, and surrounded by a rolled girdle. The upper part of the person is clothed in a sleeved jacket sewn at the

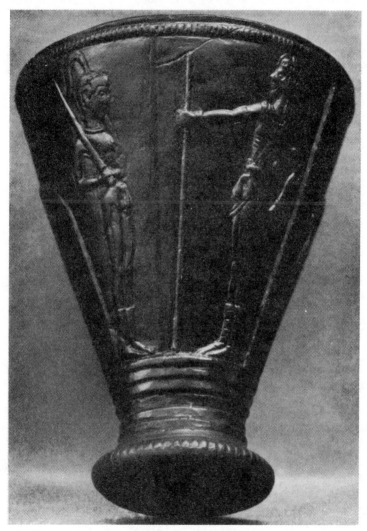

Fig. 68. CRETAN GOBLET

shoulder, but the breast is bare. (See Plate I.) Considering the shape and the rich trimming of gold disks, it has been recently suggested that the material of these jackets was leather.

The headdress of these splendidly attired women is a turban-like roll of patterned material or a tall cap. The figures of women of the lower classes are clothed only up to the waist—*i.e.*, they are without jackets.

It has been surmised that the skirts consisted of several skirts, somewhat like aprons, which were worn one above the other, and which the wearer wrapped round her. More probably, however, they were bell-shaped garments of elastic material, woven or cut in a

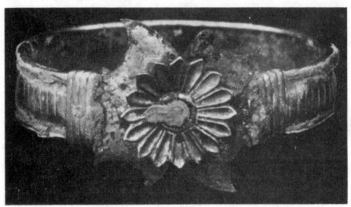

Fig. 69. MYCENÆAN BRACELET

circular shape, such as are still worn by Thessalian peasant women. The bell-shape is always pronounced—wide at the foot, tapering quickly upward, and fitting tightly at the loins. The jacket also was apparently close-fitting, giving no occasion for draping.

These women, in their charming, elegant costume, are delineated for us on a number of mural paintings and seal impressions (Figs. 63–67). These are full of interest. Even although we are still ignorant regarding the material of which the garments were made, we have good grounds for believing that the costumier's art was highly developed in the Ægean zone of civilization around the Mediterranean Sea, including the Etruscan territories. Many of the mural tablets look like prehistoric fashion-plates. One of these dainty works of art shows a slender woman (Fig. 67), dressed in a simple skirt, holding in front of her another highly ornamented skirt with diagonal stripes at the hips. Below these is a portion showing longitudinal folds, separated from the upper part by cross trimming. Round the part at the foot is a sort of *volant*, or flounce.

Another plaque (Fig. 66) shows a woman with two garments, the jacket being clearly recognizable. It is very evident that women's dress played a great part in this civilization. Jewellery was just as highly developed. Gold buttons beautifully chased and showing leaves and animal figures, daintily wrought golden necklaces, etc., give us a hint of the luxury that prevailed. Technical skill is shown at its best in the necklets of granulated gold.

Just as perfect in their way as the jewellery of the women were the weapons of the men—of the lithe bull-fighter, the wrestler, the javelin-thrower, and the men who hunted the lion and the stag and guided their teams of galloping steeds.

THE PEOPLES OF ASIA MINOR

The western peoples of Asia Minor, as depicted on ancient vases, wore clothing of extraordinary magnificence, and were distinguished by a great fondness for jewellery and splendid weapons. The beauty and variety of the ornaments referred to must not be credited wholly to the imaginative gifts of their craftsmen. They must be regarded

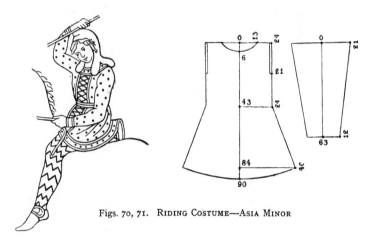

Figs. 70, 71. RIDING COSTUME—ASIA MINOR

as having been copied from actual specimens, and Homer's descriptions of the splendour of ancient Troy support this view.

The dress in which we may picture to ourselves the Trojan heroes was the same as that worn almost universally by the ancients—viz., a front piece and a back piece, both oblong, sewn together on the shoulders and down the sides, openings being left for the arms. The single seam in the sleeves was on the under-side. This costume underwent practically no change, except in the length and width of the coat. The sleeves were always close-fitting at the wrists, but the size of the neck-opening might vary a little.

Along with these coats men wore tight-fitting hose of richly patterned material, very like those worn by the Parthians. The material was presumably knitted, not woven, so that the garment fitted closely to the legs (Figs. 70, 73, 74). The material must also have been very costly, for it was delicately patterned and ornamented with gold.

The footwear was equally magnificent. The shoes were richly trimmed or embroidered, and enclosed the entire foot.

Very striking was the headdress worn by the Phrygians and Lydians and adopted apparently from them by the adjacent peoples. It was a tall, nearly conical cap knitted in one piece. It enclosed the entire head, and had a broad flap which hung down over the nape of the neck. Two other, narrower flaps came to the shoulders, and could be tied if necessary under the chin. The round top peak of the cap was stuffed with some material and made to lean forward.

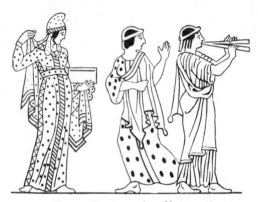

Fig. 72. WOMEN OF ASIA MINOR

Women's dress (Fig. 72) among the peoples in the west of Asia Minor had altered far less in the course of the centuries than that of the men. At the time of the Roman dominion it was almost what it had been at the time of the Trojan War. It consisted of a long, loose under-garment and a cloak-like plaid. Gay colours, rich patterns, and dainty trimmings constituted women's finery. As time went on the women of Asia Minor wore not merely the usual garments of wool or linen. Some wore the delicate, transparent dress of fine flax from the islands of Cos and Amorgos, through which the outlines of the body could be seen even when more than one garment was worn.

The cut of these female garments was the same as that of the men's. Occasionally, however, the coat was almost as wide at the shoulders as at the foot. Women's coats were at times very wide, but short ; frequently the sleeves were not tight at the wrist, but were left as wide there as at the sleeve-holes where they were attached to the coat. The Coan garments were very full, equally wide at top and foot. They were usually sleeveless, so that the arms were bare up to the shoulders.

THE GREEKS

The material of the cloak, which was worn by women only out of doors, was as richly decorated as that of which the coat was made. This cloak was roughly rectangular, and was slung round the person according to individual taste. Most women liked to have one arm free.

Women went barefoot far more frequently than the men. Their shoes when they did wear them were similar to those worn by the men, but were more dainty and more richly ornamented. The headdress too was the same for both sexes, except for the more lavish adornment and superior daintiness of the caps of the women and the more delicate fabric of which they were made. The flap at the back of the cap covering the nape was sometimes so large that it could serve as a mantle (Fig. 72). Of course, there were some women who were not content to follow the ordinary fashion. Some abandoned the back- and side-flaps, turned the edge of the cap outward, and instead of stuffing the top peak crushed it so that it did not rise so high. Some even went about without any headdress, and merely used a clasp to keep their hair tidy.

THE GREEKS

The chief items of Greek costume were three in number : a linen shirt (the chiton), worn mostly by the Ionians, an upper garment of

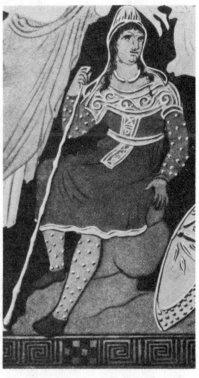

Fig. 73. FIGURE ON A VASE
Fourth century B.C.

wool (the peplos), worn only by women, and originally only by Dorian women, and a woollen cloak (the chlamys). From these three garments were gradually evolved by various methods of girding and gathering a considerable number of impressive styles of dress, each tribe having its own characteristic way of wearing and draping them.

Greek dress in the earliest period (about 600 B.C.) still bore the impress of Asiatic influence. Most men wore a cloak, with the right-hand corner flung over the left shoulder and covering the left arm. Under this they wore a long pleated shirt (chiton), braided at the neck

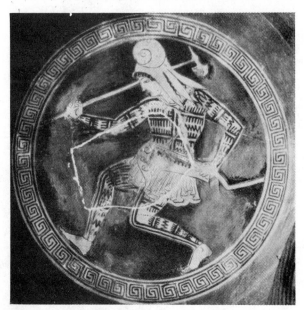

Fig. 74. PICTURE ON A GREEK VASE
Sixth century B.C.

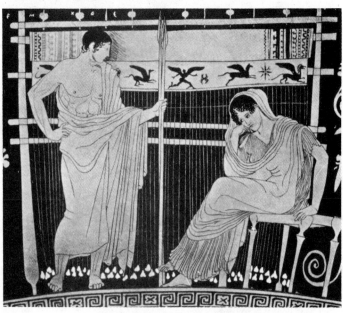

Fig. 75. DESIGN ON A GREEK VASE
The return of Odysseus: About 440 B.C.

and down the seam. In contrast to the fashion of later days, the material was gaily patterned. Sometimes the cloak was drawn

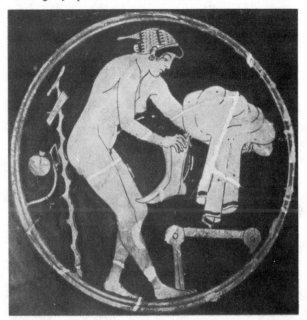

Fig. 76. VASE DESIGN
End of the sixth century B.C.

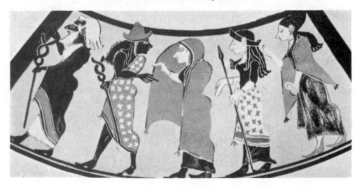

Fig. 77. DESIGN ON VASE
Sixth century B.C.

through under the right arm, so that this arm and the right shoulder were bare. The hair was curled and disposed round the face. At the back it lay smooth, or was arranged according to the wearer's taste.

95

Older men wore a full beard running to a point at the chin (see Fig. 77), while young men were beardless.

The peplos of Dorian women was in most cases made of richly patterned material. This garment seems to have been tubular in shape, the upper edge being turned down to the waist. It was put on over the head and made to fit closely at the shoulder with fasteners, the arms being left bare. It seems to have been fairly close-fitting. It was held at the waist by a girdle. The lower edge was finished

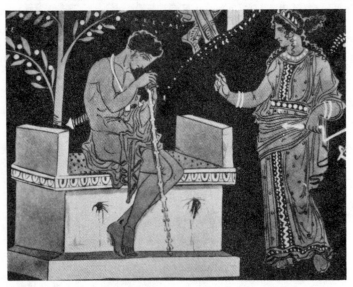

Fig. 78. Embroidered Chiton with Cloak
Design on vase from the end of the fifth century b.c.

with braid—it was sometimes left as a selvage ; the lower end of the turned-down part was similarly treated. The patterns were checks, wavy lines, stripes, or flowered designs. The wraps were also of dainty patterns, and were braided at the edges. These could also be used to screen the face. The hair was in curls tied at the nape and hanging down in waves to the shoulders (Fig. 77).

Before the date of the wars with Persia (sixth and beginning of the fifth century) the Ionian women wore a long girdled chiton with sleeves, which were taken from the main body of the garment and sewn up or tied at intervals. Over this was worn a narrow plaid (Fig. 80), which was either brought through under the left arm and fastened on the right shoulder, or had its edges tied together with tapes at intervals down as far as the elbows. From there it fell in front and at the back in two long peaks.

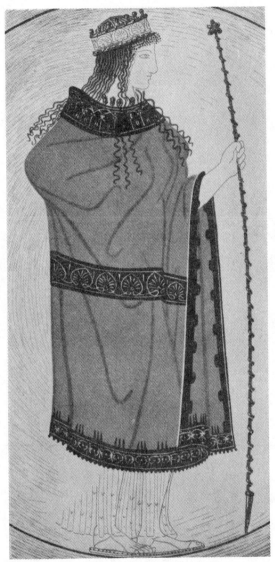

Fig. 79. CHITON WITH CLOAK
Design on vase of first half of the fifth century B.C.

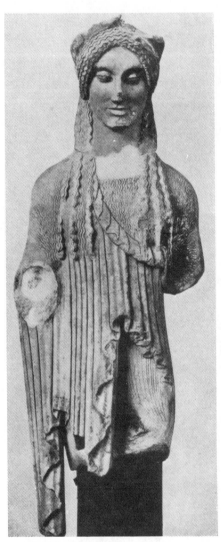

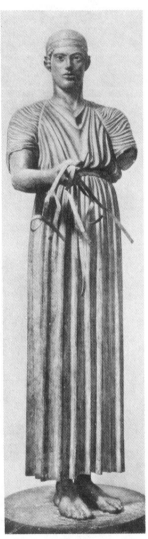

Fig. 80. CHITON WITH SHORT CLOAK
Statue of the end of the sixth century B.C.

Fig. 81. LONG MALE CHITON,
WITH GIRDLE
Charioteer of Delphi. First half of the
fifth century B.C.

The men of Ionia wore the same long chiton without a girdle, and over it the large plaid with braided edges. Leaving the right arm free, this lay on the left shoulder, the right-hand corner being flung over the left shoulder. The chiton of both sexes had a narrow coloured stripe half-way up the calf. Patterned materials ceased to be used

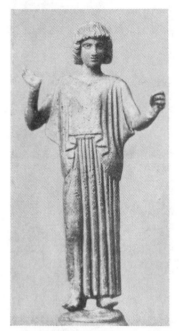 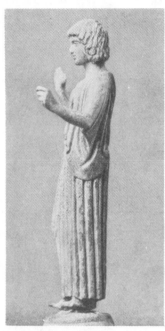

Figs. 82, 83. UNGIRDLED DORIAN PEPLOS, WITH OVER-FOLD
Statuette of about 470 B.C.

after the time of the archons, and did not reappear till toward the end of the fifth century. The peplos then began to have coloured stripes round the edges.

The chiton of the fifth century consisted of two rectangular pieces equal in length to the height of the wearer and in breadth to the distance from elbow to elbow (the narrow chiton) or from finger-tip to finger-tip when the arms were at full stretch. The long male chiton was also girdled below the breast, as in the figure of the Delphian charioteer (Fig. 81). The girdle was crossed at the back, brought over the shoulders, and fastened again at the back. This produced the sleeves, which consisted of the material at the top sewn together or fastened with tapes. The chiton was always closed at the sides, and made of very fine pleated linen. This style of girdling subsequently went out of use again.

The peplos, the garment of the Dorian women, was worn at first without a girdle. A piece of woollen material, about 3 metres wide and of a length equal to the height of the wearer, was folded at the upper extremity to form first a narrow and then a wider shawl or plaid. The material was brought through beneath the left arm and fastened with tapes on the right shoulder so as to

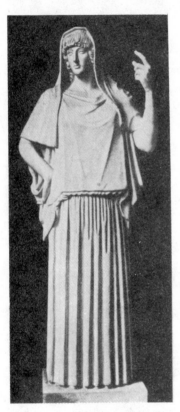

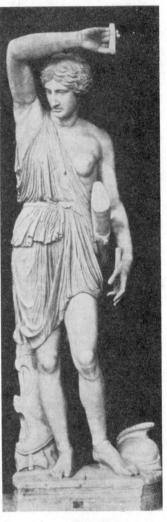

Fig. 84. Peplos, with Girdle under the Over-fold, and Headdress
About 480 B.C.

Fig. 85. Short Chiton with Double Girdle
Fifth century B.C.

leave a broad peak in front and behind. The peplos was open at the right side, and hung in broad folds from the shoulder. In course of time the shawl, or plaid, was so wide that it reached to the

Plate II

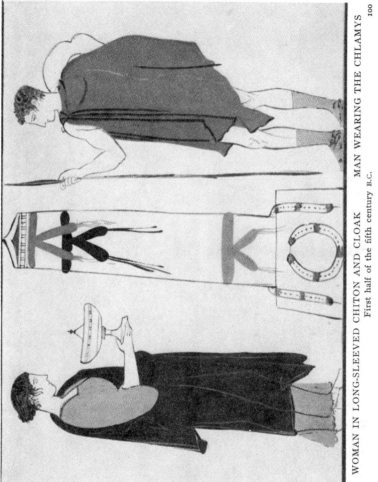

WOMAN IN LONG-SLEEVED CHITON AND CLOAK   MAN WEARING THE CHLAMYS

First half of the fifth century B.C.

100

hip; it was tied with tapes on both shoulders. The peplos was girdled beneath this shawl and pulled up over the girdle in a loose bunch. Under the arms the material was so wide that it formed a sleeve that often fell to the hips. (See the figure of the so-called *Hestia Giustiniani*, Fig. 84.) The headdress was a large kerchief. The men wore a short sleeveless chiton with a single girdle, and the same kind of garment was worn by the Dorian maidens. It was also the gymnastic

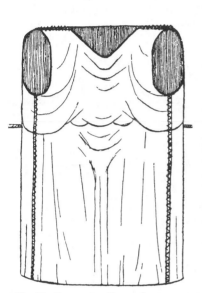

Fig. 86. CUT OF THE EARLY SLEEVELESS
CHITON

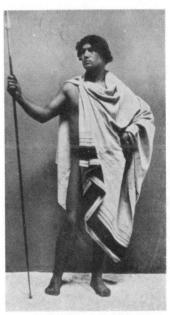

Fig. 87. CHLAMYS
Photograph from life by Heuzey.

dress. (See Fig. 91.) For this purpose it was usually fastened with tapes on the right shoulder, leaving the left breast bare (Fig. 85). The short male chiton was also the common dress of the country people, and this same garment, without a girdle, was worn by the soldier beneath his armour. The more ancient type of chiton consisted of two similar rectangular pieces, sewn together like a sack, but with openings left for the head and arms (Fig. 86). Over this short chiton the men wore the chlamys (in war it was put on above the armour), a woollen cloak (Fig. 87) about 1 metre in width and 2 in length, with broad coloured braid at the bottom edge. (See Plate II.) This chlamys was thrown over the left shoulder; the free ends were fastened with tapes on the right shoulder, so as to leave the right arm clear.

After the Persian wars (c. 480 B.C.) the Dorian style of dress was introduced among the Ionians, and this intermingling gave rise to a large number of most beautiful styles of dress.

The chiton of the fifth and fourth centuries was made of two rectangular pieces of linen equal in length to the height of the wearer, and of a width equal to the distance from elbow to elbow (the narrow chiton) or from finger-tip to finger-tip when the arms were extended (the wide chiton). One piece was laid over the other, and the two were sewn together down two-thirds of the long sides. At the point where the unsewn thirds ended, a third at each end of the narrow side was either sewn or tied. (See Fig. 88.) The centre

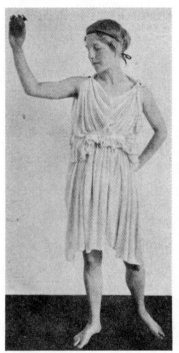

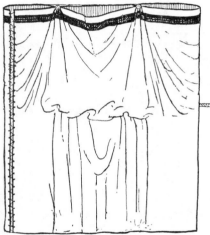

Fig. 88. Chiton with Double Girdle
Photograph from life by Margarethe Bieber.

Fig. 89. Cut of the Later Chiton

third was left unsewn, as the opening for the head. The arms were thrust through the slits in the sides, these slits thus serving as wide sleeves. Two girdles were put round the waist, quite close together, the lower one being concealed by the hanging folds. This is the type of chiton that is seen in the statues of the Amazons and on the frieze of the Parthenon. Examples are also found in the Parthenon frieze of a short chiton with long, narrow, pleated sleeves, which seem to have been sewn on to the main part of the garment.

The peplos also was modified by the Ionian peoples. They too wore it above the chiton. (See Fig. 98.) The turned-down part of the

Ionian peplos was very wide—nearly a third of the total length of the garment—and came down to below the hips, covering the upper

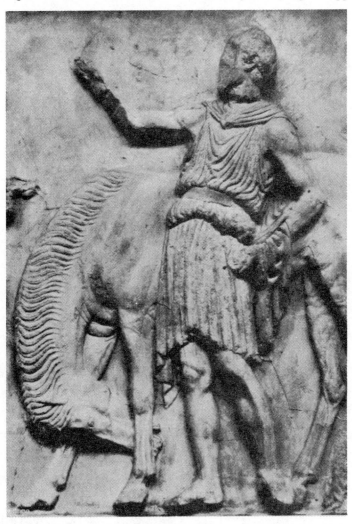

Fig. 90. MALE CHITON WITH DOUBLE GIRDLE
Fifth century B.C.

half of the thigh.   The girdle was worn by the Ionians not beneath the turned-down part, but over it (Fig. 92).

Thus arose a large number of variations of the same fundamental styles—viz., the peplos closed at the side and arranged with an over-fold, the open peplos (Fig. 98), the long, open chiton with over-fold,

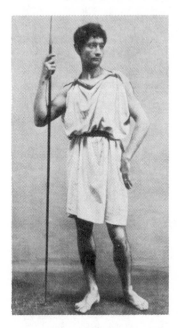

Fig. 91. SHORT MALE CHITON WITH
ONE GIRDLE
Photograph from life by Heuzey.

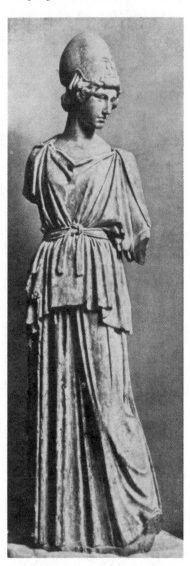

Fig. 92. PEPLOS WITH GIRDLE ABOVE
THE OVER-FOLD
About 450 B.C.

sleeveless and worn with one girdle, the same with double girdle (Fig. 100), the chiton girt high at the breast (Fig. 101), with and without sleeves, the chiton with double girdle. The cloak was either fastened on the left shoulder, leaving the right arm free (Figs. 93, 95) or was worn like a shawl over the head and held in position with the right hand (Fig. 96).

The vase designs of the fifth century show several female figures still wearing the kerchief and hair-bandeau (Fig. 78). In the later period these were

104

practically unknown. The only fashion was to curl the hair and put it up in various ways. For example, a circlet or comb held the hair (Fig. 99), the hair at the back of the head being bunched together into a kind of knot, or arranged in curls over the brow like a coronet.

From the time of the legislation of Lycurgus Dorian men had

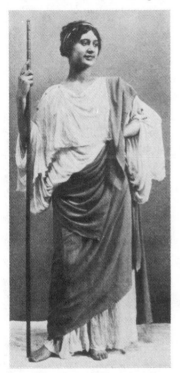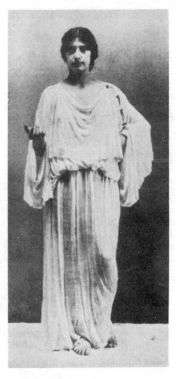

Figs. 93, 94. LONG-SLEEVED CHITON WITH OVER-FOLD, WORN WITH A SINGLE GIRDLE

With and without cloak. Photograph from life by Heuzey.

ceased to wear the chiton. They retained only the cloak (Figs. 102–105), and it was regarded as a sign of manly spirit to follow this fashion. At the same time, this custom was far from being universal, although the representations of that period might suggest that it was usual. These show us orators and poets like Demosthenes and Sophocles wearing only the cloak, but there is every reason to believe that the ordinary Greek of the best period wore the chiton under his cloak, and that the absence of it was due to affectation.

Both men and women wore sandals, but leather boots were also worn (Fig. 76). The most perfect representation of the sandal is that found on the foot of Hermes as sculptured by Praxiteles (Fig. 106).

Most of the works of art that have come down to us show the men

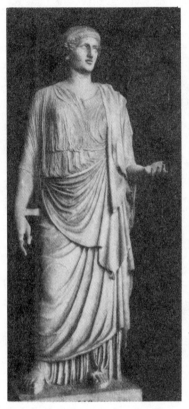
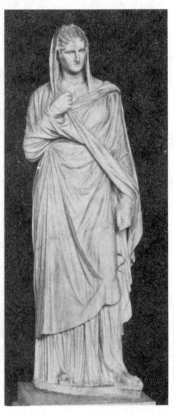

Fig. 95. CHITON WITH CLOAK
Greek ; second half of the fifth century B.C.

Fig. 96. CHITON WITH MANTLE
Fifth century B.C.

with short, curly hair. This and the absence of a beard were considered the best style, but there are also examples of a short beard on cheek and chin (Figs. 104, 105).

The materials of which Greek costume was made kept pace with the advancing civilization, and showed more and more improvement. Well-to-do people wore a chiton made from the finest textiles of Asia Minor —viz., the so-called " Coan " materials. All the woollen garments —peplos and himation and all the various cloaks or plaids—were richly coloured. A favourite colour (and one that indicated some distinction) was an intense dark red or purple. The trimming usually took the form of coloured stripes and braids with patterns either inwoven or embroidered.

Only scanty remnants of these ancient costumes have been

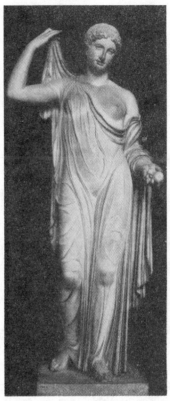 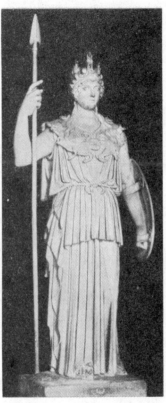

Fig. 97. CHITON WITHOUT GIRDLE
400 B.C.

Fig. 98. PEPLOS, OPEN AT THE SIDE, WITH SINGLE GIRDLE
Fifth century B.C.

preserved for us. Most of them are from graves of the fourth century B.C. But the excavations at Achmim in Upper Egypt and at Antinoe in Central Egypt have brought to light splendidly preserved garments from the second to the seventh centuries B.C. which greatly enrich our knowledge of ancient costume. For it is legitimate to transfer—with some limitations—to the costume of the ancient Greeks and Romans the conceptions we gain from these regarding the technique of weaving and ornamentation.

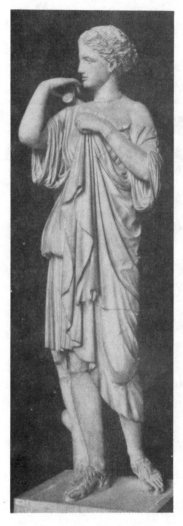

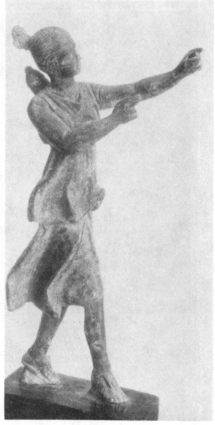

Fig. 99. SHORT CHITON WITH DOUBLE GIRDLE AND SLEEVES, WORN WITH CLOAK

Fourth century B.C.

Fig. 100. DOUBLE-GIRDLED CHITON WITHOUT SLEEVES

Statuette of the fourth century B.C.

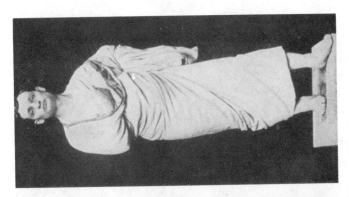

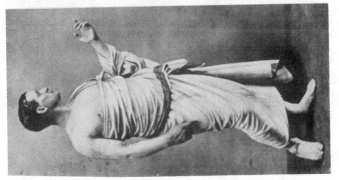

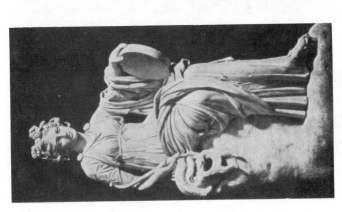

Figs. 102, 103. Greek Cloaks
Photographs from life by Heuzey

Fig. 101. Chiton with Sleeves,
girdled under the Breast
Third century b.c.

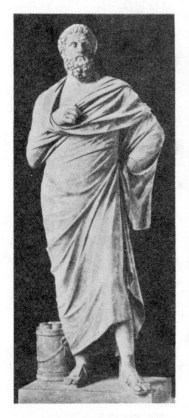

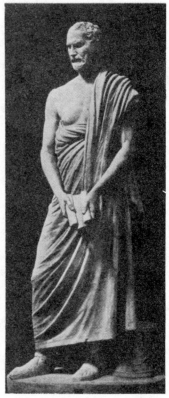

Fig. 104. GREEK CLOAK
Fourth century B.C.

Fig. 105. GREEK CLOAK
Third century B.C.

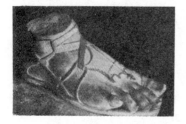

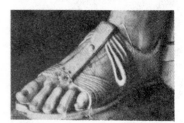

Figs. 106, 107. STYLES OF GREEK SANDALS

The dryness of the desert sand has preserved these garments from decay. Very few of them are of silk. The majority are of white or

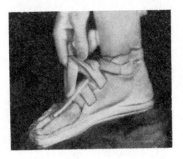

Fig. 108. Greek Sandal

dyed linen of finest thread, and the colourings of the embroidery are extremely beautiful. The abundant traces of colour on statues and reliefs prove that ancient costume was not in monotone and certainly not white.

THE ETRUSCANS

The oldest Etruscan type of dress had points of resemblance to that of the Greeks, both European and Asiatic. Like the Greeks, the Etruscans wore a cloak, the tebenna, a kind of plaid, sometimes rectangular and sometimes shaped like a segment of a circle. One end was brought forward over the left shoulder, and the plaid itself was carried round the back and drawn through under the right arm, the other end being flung back over the left shoulder. The segment-shaped cloak was all along the characteristic Etruscan type—it was the real tebenna. Even before they came into touch with the Romans at all the Etruscans wore a shirt-like under-garment similar to the Greek chiton.

The dress of Etruscan women was somewhat Oriental in character. It was a long, shirt-like robe, as tight-fitting as possible over the shoulders, and increasing in width down to the foot. It had half-length sleeves, and was worn without a girdle. (See Fig. 109.) Made of the finest materials, and trimmed with beautiful braid, this robe reached to the feet, and sometimes even trailed on the ground. (See Fig. 110.) As it was almost always tight at the neck, sometimes covering it right up to the chin, it had a slit at the back, about 20 centimetres long, fastened with ribbons or other fasteners.

Over this robe Etruscan women wore a cloak, which was usually in shape a long rectangle. These cloaks, which were also made of fine material, were either simply hung over the back or passed over the head so as to cover almost the whole person. Sometimes they were worn like a shawl over the shoulders, the ends being variously arranged in front, or crossed and fastened at the back.

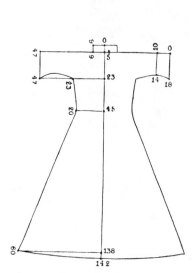

Fig. 109. ETRUSCAN WOMAN'S ROBE

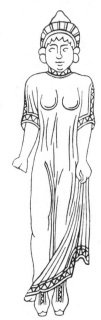

Fig. 110. ETRUSCAN LADY

THE ROMANS

Little as we know of the primitive Roman dress, there is no reason to suppose that it differed much from the representations we have of it on the most ancient Roman statues. If that be the case, men's dress consisted of a kind of shirt, the tunica, and a cloak worn over it, the toga. Sometimes this latter was the sole garment worn.

The toga, a distinctively Roman garment, resembled a double tebenna. It was in shape probably like two large segments of a circle, equal in size, placed with the straight edges together (Fig. 113), though other methods of cut have been suggested. The distinguishing feature of this garment was its amazing size. In length it was nearly three times and in width about twice the height of the wearer. These proportions were not, of course, invariable, and it is probable that in early times, when the garment was made of coarse stuff, and not, as in later days, of very fine woollen material, it was considerably smaller.

The toga was put on by folding it longitudinally about the middle, bunching it into thick folds, and hanging it over the left shoulder so that a third of the total length was suspended in front (Figs. 111, 114). The remainder was passed diagonally across the back, brought through under the right arm, and again thrown back over the left shoulder. Owing to its width it also covered nearly the whole of the left arm. Finally, the portion crossing the back was spread out so as to cover the right shoulder-blade, and the corner that hung forward over the left shoulder was shortened by drawing the toga up at the breast and letting it fall over

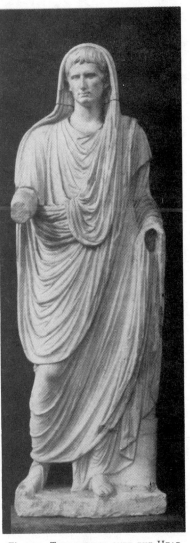

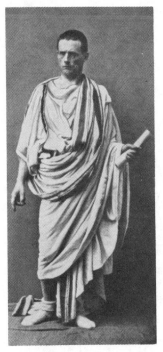

Fig. 111. Toga
Photograph from life by Heuzey.

Fig. 112. Toga draped over the Head
About the middle of the first century B.C.

the mass of folds. This mass of folds at the breast served as a pocket, and bore the name of *sinus*.

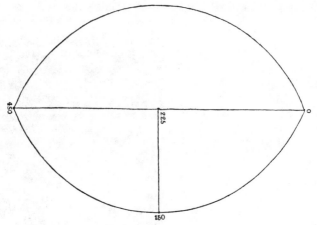

Fig. 113. CUT OF FIG. 114

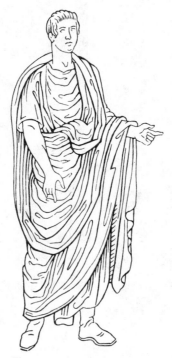

Fig. 114. ROMAN WEARING TOGA

The pænula (Fig. 115) was a bell-shaped garment, worn in inclement weather. In most cases it was closed all round, but occasionally it

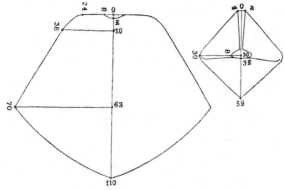

Fig. 115. ROMAN PÆNULA
(a) The cowl or hood.

was left open down the front. When it was closed all round it had to be lifted at the sides in order to allow free movement of the arms.

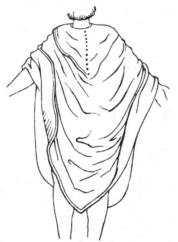

Fig. 116. HOW THE PÆNULA WAS WORN

As a rule it had a hood attached to it.[1] (See Fig. 116.) It had an opening at the breast which was fastened at the top with a pin. The

[1] There were numerous small variations in the cut of the pænula. Occasionally it had no hood. Sometimes it was the same length all round, sometimes it was shortened at the sides. The back sometimes ran down to a point, and sometimes this point was rounded off, and so on.

hood was joined to the garment round the neck, and the flaps were probably sewn down to the edges of the breast opening. The pænula was usually made of tightly woven, rough woollen stuff, but sometimes of soft leather.

The under-garment—and the actual indoor dress—of the Romans was the tunica (Fig. 117). This was a kind of shirt, cut fairly wide, closed all round, and reaching to below the knee. The sleeves (when the garment had these) covered the arms to the elbows. As a rule a girdle was worn with it. The tunica was sometimes so wide that when spread out it reached on both sides to the middle of the forearms. The sleeves were comparatively short, and were wide at the top, decreasing in width toward the wrists. The extra width of the garment—which bore a close resemblance to the ancient Ionian female coat—was caught up by the girdle and disposed in graceful folds. In course of time the tunica often became long enough to reach the feet, and was made not only of wool, but also of cotton or other materials. Such a garment was called *tunica talaris*. This was the usual marriage-dress for men, but was always looked down upon as common garb by more Spartan Romans, and it was not till much later days that it displaced the shorter tunica.

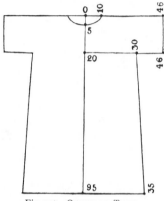

Fig. 117. ORDINARY TUNICA

As time went on several tunics were worn at the same time, the inner one always being closer-fitting than the one over it. The ancient Roman dress was always one single tunic, worn next the skin.

The long-sleeved tunic—*tunica manicata*—was always looked upon as *outré*, and did not become general till the time of the later Empire. Previous to that time, however, priests wore it, especially foreign priests, and it was a part of the usual actor's wardrobe.

To walk abroad dressed only in the tunica was considered bad form, and only working people did so. For them, of course, either the toga or any other over-garment would have been very inconvenient.

Both on the toga and on the tunica various badges were worn indicating the rank and calling of the wearer. Chief of these were two purple stripes, varying in width, called *clavi*. They were attached to the front and back of the garment, passed over the shoulders, and fell perpendicularly to the foot. According to the width of these stripes the garment was called *tunica laticlavia* or *tunica angusticlavia*. The former, with broad stripes, was worn by members of the Senate ; the latter, with narrow stripes, was worn by the *equites*. These tunics were usually worn without a girdle, as was also the *tunica palmata*, so called because it was embroidered in gold with palm-branches.   It was worn by victorious generals when celebrating their triumph.

Up till about the end of the Republic the Roman wardrobe did not include anything that could be called hose or breeches.   Only after they had seen these garments worn by their Gallic and Parthian foes did the Romans adopt them.   At first they were fairly close-fitting, and did not quite reach the knees, but by the time of the later Empire they were wider, and reached to the ankles.   The early type somewhat resembled those worn by the Gauls, but they were closer-fitting and considerably shorter.   The later type approximated more to those of the Persians and Parthians.   Both kinds, short and long, were more a part of military wear than of fashionable dress.   As the wearing of hose in the city of Rome was forbidden by law,[1] men of weak constitution wrapped bandages or something similar round their shins to keep themselves warm in rough weather, and gradually added to their dress various kinds of scarves and body-bandages.

In early days the Roman women dressed in exactly the same manner as the men, but the influence of the neighbouring Etruscans and the Greeks was not long in making itself felt.   As civilization advanced and brought to Rome the products of the whole known world, the material and adornment of women's dress underwent great changes at the dictates of the constantly varying caprices of fashion.

The chief items of female dress comprised a shirt or chemise worn next the person, a dress over it, a cloak-like over-garment, and a veil.

The first of these, the *tunica interior* or *intima*, or, as it was also called, *interala* or *indusium*, was worn next the skin.   It was closed all round except for the armholes.   It was of the same width throughout, and reached to the feet.   Usually it had short sleeves.   It was the woman's house dress, and was at first made of wool ; as time went on, however, it was usually of cotton or silk, or even, especially in the late days of the Empire, of transparent " Coan " material.   In the case last mentioned it was long and full, and had a long train, and was worn sometimes with a girdle and sometimes without.   In most cases it was adorned at the shoulders with clasps or buttons.

Over this was worn the stola, which was cut exactly like the garment underneath it.   The only difference was that the stola had sleeves, either wide or tight, covering the upper arm, especially if the under-garment was sleeveless.[2]   Although many devices were used to alter the shape and draping of the stola, such as varying its length, wearing one girdle or two, or even giving it the set of the Greek chiton, these variations were of little account in comparison with the manifold varieties of the materials of which Roman ladies made this garment and in comparison with the numerous means used for its adornment.

[1] Of course this prohibition did not apply to foreigners resident in Rome, but only to Roman citizens.

[2] Before putting on the stola the Roman lady usually put on a broad belt of soft leather to elevate the breasts.

One of the most popular ways of adding to the attractiveness of this wide, trailing dress, which for freer movement had to be tucked up to a greater or less extent, was to edge it with purple and trim it with pearls or gold spangles and to sew rich braid round the low neck-opening and the ends of the sleeves. If the stola was not sufficiently long for it to be tucked up at the waist to hide the girdle, the girdle itself supplied a further opportunity for the display of luxury. Instead of the ordinary plain ribbon, an expensive hoop was used, or a piece of valuable braid studded with precious stones or pearls. The greatest pains were taken to secure the most graceful possible draping. Young girls wore, instead of the stola, a garment somewhat similar, but not long enough to reach farther than half-way down the thigh. They wore no girdle.

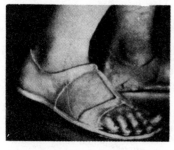

Fig. 118. ROMAN SANDAL

When the Roman lady went out of doors she put on a third garment, the palla. In early times this resembled the male toga, but at a later time both the shape and the material of it were altered. It was very voluminous, and might be either square or oblong. It had sometimes the shape of a very wide pænula, and sometimes it looked like two large plaids joined on the shoulders with clasps and fastened round the waist by a girdle.

The full dress of a Roman lady was incomplete without a veil. In early days it was called the *flammeum* ; the later name of it was *ricinium*. It was attached in various ways at the back of the head, and hung down over the back and shoulders.

As a rule a man wore no headdress. When the weather was rough he simply pulled his toga or the hood of some other over-garment —*e.g.*, the pænula—over his head. When he did wear a headdress of any kind, it was a felt hat, with a broad or narrow brim, like that worn by the Greeks. Hunters, sailors, and especially people who spent most of their time in the open wore caps of leather or plaited straw.

Women sometimes enclosed their hair in nets of gold or silver thread, but nearly all tied a kerchief round the head at night in order to keep their careful *coiffure* in order while they slept.

Footwear was an important—in fact, an indispensable—part of Roman attire. There were numerous styles, exhibiting all the gradations from the simple sandal to the complete boot reaching up to the calf. Equally numerous were the colours and the materials employed. For certain ranks and classes the kind of footwear was definitely laid down, and not only soldiers, but members of the Senate, consuls, and others had to wear, and were limited to wearing, the footgear prescribed for them.

DRESS OF THE BYZANTINE EMPERORS

On the whole the footwear of the women was like that of the men, but showed less variety. They preferred sandals and shoes that did not come above the ankles to boots reaching higher up the calf. They naturally paid even more attention than the men to daintiness of appearance, and their shoes were not only trimmed with gold, but embroidered with pearls and similar ornamentation.

THE DRESS OF THE BYZANTINE EMPERORS

The dress of the Byzantine or Greek emperors is not much older than the Eastern Roman Empire itself, for the Imperial raiment adopted by Diocletian and made still more magnificent by Constantine was soon disdained as " vain show " by the Emperor Julian, who ascended the throne only ten years after Constantine's death. Julian's immediate successors attached just as little importance to it as he had done. Theodosius (379–395) was the first who thought it necessary to manifest his dignity in his attire as well as in other directions, and it was he who introduced the splendour which was continued by all the Greek emperors who came after him.

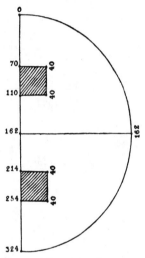

Fig. 119. BYZANTINE IMPERIAL MANTLE

This Imperial attire differed little in respect of cut and material from that of Diocletian. Like the latter, it consisted of a stola[1] of white silk heavily ornamented with gold at the breast and shoulders. It was, that is to say, a kind of shirt, long-sleeved and reaching to the feet (sometimes called *talaris dalmatica*), with a purple cloak, fastened at the shoulder with a precious clasp, adorned with a broad strip of gold embroidery (*clavus*), and with ornaments pointed or round, embroidered or attached. The royal attire also included shoes[2] of purple silk embroidered with pearls, a diadem with a rich setting of pearls, and the royal staff or rod of gold. This magnificent attire, it is to be kept in mind, was worn by the emperors not only on certain State occasions, but almost always, for the Byzantine Court was the most luxurious and dissolute of all Courts throughout the Middle Ages.

[1] From the beginning of the Roman Eastern Empire onward dress for the two sexes among the higher classes seems to have been the same. For both sexes it is sometimes called stola and sometimes tunica.

[2] The emperor alone was allowed to wear shoes of this kind, and therefore the phrase " This prince has assumed the shoes of purple " was equivalent to saying that he had ascended the throne.

In a large piece of mosaic work in the church of S. Vitale at Ravenna, representing the Emperor Justinian and his retinue about the year 547, the monarch is clad (see Fig. 120) exactly as we have described, except that he is wearing instead of the stola a white tunica, reaching only to the knee, trimmed at the side with gold, and held in position by a red girdle, and also has on very tight purple hose. The *clavus* of his purple cloak is of gold decorated with red

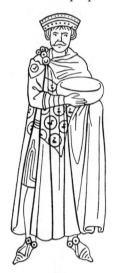 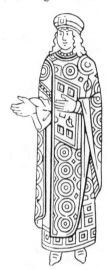

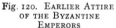

Fig. 120. EARLIER ATTIRE OF THE BYZANTINE EMPERORS   Fig. 121. LATER ROYAL ATTIRE OF THE BYZANTINE EMPERORS

rings, in each of which is set a green animal resembling a duck. Three gold bracelets are on his forearm.

The Imperial mantle, like those of other Byzantines of high rank, was in shape a semicircle or other large segment of a circle (Fig. 119). It was put on with the centre of the straight edge on the left shoulder. Then it was carried fairly tightly round the neck and pinned on the right shoulder so that it fell down on both sides of the right arm. This shape for the mantle and this way of putting it on were retained by all the Byzantine emperors. The ornamentation, however, underwent repeated change, and by and by the mantle became stiff and unpliant, owing to the gold embroidery, the jewels, and not least to the heavy border studded with pearls and precious stones with which the whole garment was hemmed. The *clavus* also was always put on this garment, and it too was lavishly adorned. Soon after Justinian's death the method of wearing it was changed. The left side was raised and allowed to hang over the arm (Fig. 121).

TEUTONIC PREHISTORIC PERIOD

TEUTONIC BRONZE AGE—THIRD TO FIRST CENTURIES B.C.

THE earliest remains of costume from which we gain a faithful picture of the dress of the Teutonic peoples are those on some corpses of the Bronze Age found preserved in peat (see Figs. 122, 123). We are now able with their help to form some conception

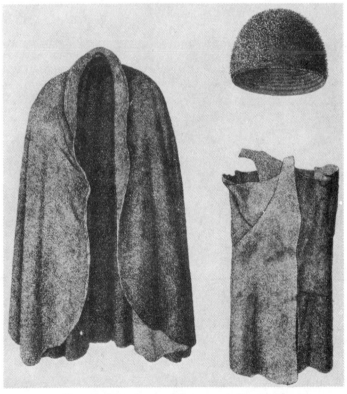

Fig. 122. Skirt, Cap, and Cape of the Bronze Age

of the stage of civilization that succeeded that of the primitive dress of pelts and skins. The costume of these men of the Bronze Age

121

exhibits the same amazing beauty of form which delights us in their dainty bronze brooches. Long ages of evolution must have gone

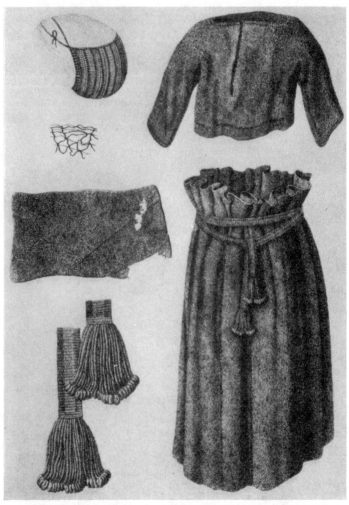

Fig. 123. Skirt, Cap, Bodice, etc., of the Bronze Age

before the attainment of this style of dress and the development of the material which was used.

EARLY TEUTONIC COSTUME—THIRD AND FOURTH CENTURIES A.D.

An equally faithful picture is provided by the numerous discoveries of later corpses belonging to the third and fourth centuries A.D. in peat in North-west Germany, Holland, and Denmark, and we have now a fairly complete idea of the dress current in these countries at the beginning of the early historical period. The men of the Teutonic

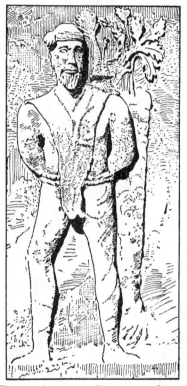

Fig. 124. One of the Basternæ in Chains

tribes to which these corpses belonged wore short breeches, a smock with or without sleeves, a large plaid which served as a cloak, leg-bandages round the knee and shin-bone, and leather footwear like sandals, fastened with laces. (See Figs. 125–127.) The hair above the forehead was kept short, and the same practice was followed with the hair at the back of the head, the moustache, the beard, and the whiskers. The hair seems to have been ruddy-fair in colour.

123

The material used for the garments was presumably dressed hide and leather, and at a later time patterned material made of wool,

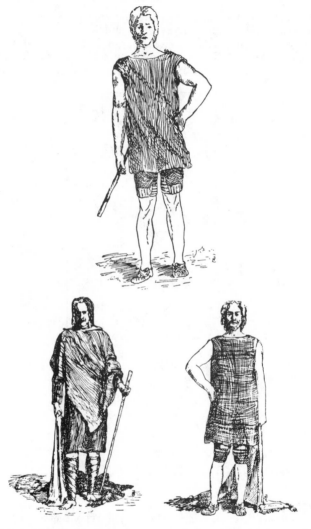

Figs. 125, 126, 127. Reconstructed Clothes of Bodies found in the Peat at Marx-Etzel, Bernuthsfeld, and Obenaltendorf

bast, ticking, and twill cloth, as well as frieze, felt, and, among the Goths, linen. The smocks were plain or striped, and trimmed with braid made from dyed thread. These shirt-like smocks had an opening at the breast, and came as low as the knee. They were either slipped on over the head or were sewn at one shoulder and fastened at the other with a brooch or clasp. Smocks with long sleeves do not appear till later. The sleeves were sometimes made of other

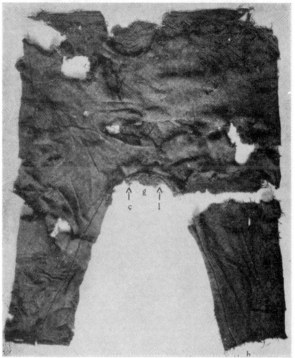

Fig. 128. Knee-breeches from the Body found in the Peat at Marx-Etzel

material than that of the body of the garment, and were trimmed with coloured braid. With the smock from the second century onward a shirt was worn—first of wool, afterward of linen. The smock was worn either over or under the hose, and in the former case was kept in place by a buckled girdle. The Teutons wore hose of some kind as far back as the Bronze Age. At first they were long trousers, then knee-breeches and ankle-length breeches, and later still ankle-length breeches with bands which fastened below the knee. Foot-coverings were worn with the knee-breeches.

As garters the Teutons used woollen strings or strips of hide (Fig. 126). Loops were attached to the top of the breeches to hold the girdle in place.

The following are the measurements of breeches from Damendorf : length, 1·15 m. ; width, 85 cm. ; width of legs at the foot, 28 cm.

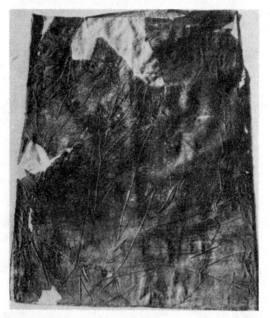

Fig. 129. TRUNK GARMENT OF THE BODY FOUND IN THE PEAT AT OBENALTENDORF

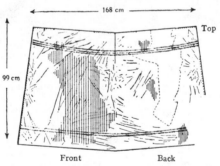

Fig. 130. CUTTING-OUT PATTERN FOR FIG. 129

Those from Thorsberg measured 1·20 m. in length and 1·05 m. in width.

In South-west and Central Germany from the first to the fourth

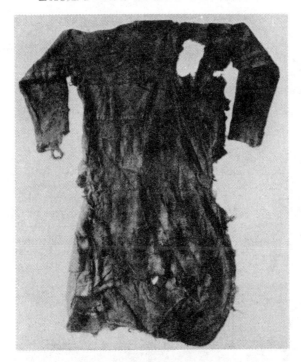

Fig. 131. SLEEVED FROCK OF A BODY FOUND IN THE PEAT AT
BERNUTHSFELD

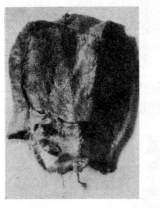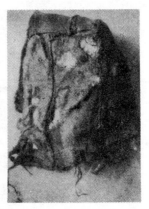

Figs. 132, 133. HOOD FROM A BODY FOUND IN THE PEAT AT
BERNUTHSFELD

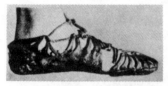
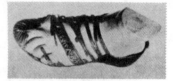

Figs. 134, 135. THE LEFT SHOE OF THE BODY FOUND IN THE PEAT AT
OBENALTENDORF

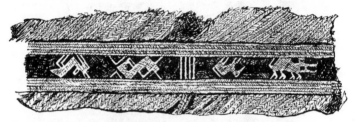

Fig. 136. PATTERNED WOVEN CLOTH FROM NORWAY

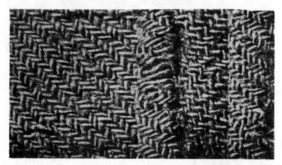

Fig. 137. REMNANT OF WOVEN MATERIAL FROM THE BODY FOUND AT
MARX-ETZEL

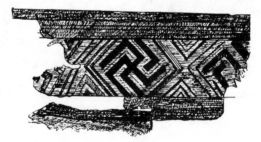

Fig. 138. PIECE OF WOVEN MATERIAL FROM NORWAY

128

century ankle-length breeches were worn.   They were made of leather or woollen material—more rarely of ticking.

Over these garments was worn a cloak of fur without sleeves, or a woollen cloak closed at the breast.   The woollen cloak was usually oval or rectangular, and at a later time square.   There were also hooded cloaks, or cloaks with openings for the head like the rough woollen coats of the hill-peasants of Bavaria.

The Teutonic footgear even in early times was specially handsome (Figs. 134, 135), with its numerous latchets and delicate lattice ornamentation.

In the period that immediately followed the migration of nations came the intermingling of the ancient Teutonic civilization with those of the Roman and Byzantine Empires.   An ever-increasing fondness for rich-coloured materials grew up, especially among the Angles and Saxons, and beautiful trimmings, gay braid, and fringes came into fashion.   The treatment of fur became more skilful, and the art of weaving made great progress.   The fastening of garments was now done with the aid of clasps, buckles, ribbons, straps, and girdles. From the earliest times great care was taken with the hair, as is proved by the discovery of razors, combs, and scissors.   It was a favourite practice to dye the hair bright red.   The Western Teutons wore the hair in a knot at the right side of the head, with the ends hanging down or stiffened so as to project like horns.   Among the Northern and Eastern Teutons the hair hung down loose, while the Saxons cut it short.   There was no uniform fashion regarding the beard, but the moustache was rare.

Teutonic women wore a linen garment like a sleeveless shirt, fastened at the shoulder with a brooch and held in by a buckled girdle.   A pocket was fastened to the girdle.

We possess little accurate information regarding the dress of Teutonic women.   Roman works of art, most of which are purely imaginative and therefore unreliable, are our only sources of information.   Most of these garments were made of linen, and this material cannot withstand like wool the effects of burial in bog or earth.   The only reliable information we have concerns their jewellery.   We possess a large number of beautiful brooches and buckles of gold and silver set with coloured stones.   Dainty hair-combs, necklets, armlets, and finger-rings bear witness to the characteristic Teutonic fondness for bright metal ornaments, of which the ancient songs and legends say so much.   The expert maker of such objects was held in high respect by these peoples—witness the story of Wayland the Smith. It is only toward the close of the early historic period that we come upon coloured garments, made presumably of textile materials or coloured braids such as were used for men's dress.   The sixth century A.D. brought for the women too the improved wardrobe that was introduced under Roman and Byzantine influence and developed into lavish luxuriousness under the Merovingians.

The cloak was not often worn by women. It was a large wrap, or shawl, drawn over the head and fastened, like the under-garment, by means of a brooch or a clasp. Unmarried women wore the hair loose or encircled by a hoop ; married women gathered it up with the help of combs and hairpins. The southern tribes, Franks and Alemanni, plaited it with ribbons or even with gold thread. Women's shoes, like the men's, were of the finest leather-work.

THE MIDDLE AGES

ELEVENTH TO THIRTEENTH CENTURIES

THE costumes worn in the Middle Ages were based on the types that had been evolved about the middle of the first millennium from the intermingling of native fashions with those of later antiquity. In the first centuries after the migration of the nations (A.D. 600) there was little difference between the styles of dress current

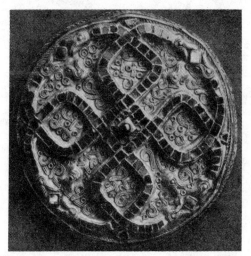

Fig. 139. CIRCULAR BROOCH FROM WITTISLINGEN
Seventh to eighth century A.D.

among the various nations of the West. Then ensued a period of separate development, each nation following its own tastes, and this lasted until the Crusades brought all the peoples of Europe into close touch with each other and reintroduced a greater measure of uniformity. This uniformity, however, was greatly enriched by the fruitful influences of ancient Oriental civilization, particularly in respect of material and ornamentation.

There is a very close connexion between the styles of the early Middle Ages and those of ecclesiastical dress. The latter has retained down to our own day survivals which enable us to form a clear conception of the costume of the Middle Ages (Fig. 191). Unfortunately, we possess very few original garments belonging to this long period. One of them is the white silk dalmatica that belonged to the Emperor Henry II (Fig. 168) which is among the treasures of Bamberg Cathedral. Samples of material and inwoven patterns are

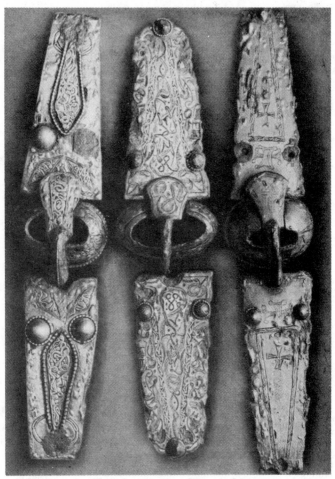

Fig. 140. SILVER BUCKLES FROM FÉTIGNY, SWITZERLAND
Seventh to eighth century A.D.

more numerous. It helps our imagination when we look at the minia-tures in ancient manuscripts and the tombs that still exist. And in quite recent days the discoveries made at Herjolfsnes, the ancient Norse colony, have brought to light a number of garments that reveal the dress of the later Middle Ages. These are so perfect that they constitute a source of inestimable value for the history of European dress, even although these Norse settlers were limited in their choice of material by the remoteness of their situation. (See Figs. 187 and 190.)

Equally interesting is the golden dress of Margaret of Denmark, belonging to the second half of the fourteenth century, with the extraordinary length of the front of the skirt and the extreme shortness of the bodice, which was fastened at the back (Fig. 193). The

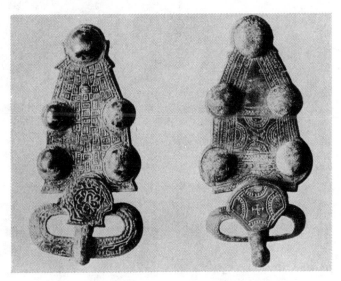

Fig. 141. Bronze Buckles, Engraved
Early period of the migration of nations.

beautiful material—cloth of gold shot through with a dark red-violet colour—helps us to imagine the rare splendour and beauty of the royal robes of that time.

To the period between fifty and seventy-five years later we must ascribe the coat of carmine red satin (Fig. 199) which is said to be part of the spoil from the battle of Granson in 1476, and is now in the Museum of Bern. It looks like an under-garment meant to be worn beneath the *robe*—an over-garment of heavy, rich material. It is said to have belonged to Charles the Bold of Burgundy, whose Court was one of the most brilliant of his time and powerfully affected the development of contemporary fashions.

To complete our conception of the dress of the Middle Ages we must add the jewellery. It was both beautiful and valuable, and fortunately numerous specimens still exist. Especially charming are the

133

examples of the goldsmith's art which belong to the zenith of the Middle Ages—the time of the Ottos and the Henrys (Figs. 165, 166,

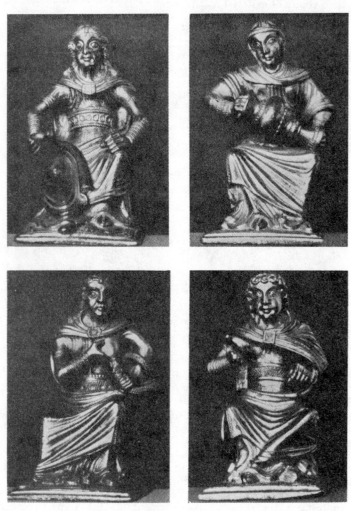

Figs. 142–145. THE FOUR ELEMENTS
Bronze statuettes from Lower Lorraine. End of the twelfth century.

and 167). Their high perfection of technique is a constant delight. The breast-ornaments of the Empress Gisela, which belong to the year 1000, together with her earrings and clasps, bear eloquent testimony to the outstanding skill of the craftsmen and the cultivated taste of those who employed them. The jewels combine the strength of the Carolingian genius for design with the delicacy of Byzantine technique, and they are among the finest things of the kind in existence. The ancient Teutonic fondness for gold and precious stones, which had already been shown in the brooches and clasps of an earlier day, finds eloquent expression in these jewels.

GERMANY

At this period men were wearing a fairly wide tunic of varying length, girdled at the waist, and having sleeves that covered the whole arm down to the wrist. It was no longer unusual, although it was still far from being the universal practice, to wear beneath this tunic (which was generally made of wool, but frequently of silk) a linen shirt. This was worn next the skin. Over the tunic was worn a cloak, usually oblong in shape, which was thrown over the left shoulder and gathered on the right by means of a clasp (agraffe)

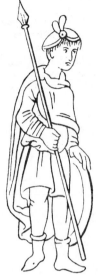

Fig. 146. MEN'S DRESS ABOUT THE YEAR 1000

(Fig. 146). Finally, men also wore leg-garments of varying length, and over these was drawn the footwear, mostly of eather and reaching up to the calf.

The cut of all these garments was still in all essentials the same as it had been for centuries (see Fig. 147)—that is to say, the coat consisted of two similar pieces, back and front, sewn together down the sides and on the shoulders. The sleeves were straight, with only one seam, and narrowed gradually from the shoulder to the wrist. The opening for the neck was fairly wide, sometimes rounded, sometimes square, and was cut in the front piece. The coat was usually made of bright-coloured material, and wide strips of braid or other stuff were sewn round the foot, the neck, and the wrists.

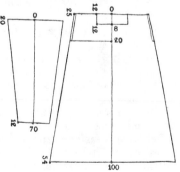

Fig. 147. SHAPE OF MEN'S SLEEVED COAT OF ABOUT A.D. 1000

The shirt was shaped like the coat, but it was usually wider, and always much longer, often reaching as low as the ankles.

The cut of the cloak was rectangular, the length of the narrow sides being equal to the distance from the wearer's neck to the middle of the lower leg, and about a third less than that of the long sides, which made the width of the cloak.

The leg-garments were long stockings, made of two pieces shaped like a leg and sewn together at the front and back. The lower part of the shirt was tucked into these; they were attached to a girdle (worn under the coat) by means of tapes sewn on the outside of them, and were thus held in position. Beneath these stockings many men wore long, wide under-hose of linen, somewhat like two bags sewn

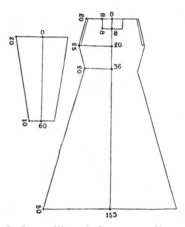

Fig. 148. Cut of Women's Coat in the Year 1000

together in the upper part. Footwear consisted either of ankle-high shoes or boots that came up to the middle of the calf.

The usual female dress consisted of a long chemise of linen or hemp, with a low neck and short sleeves. Over it came the coat, or tunic, which had the same shape as the chemise, and reached from neck to feet. (See Fig. 148.) It had long, tight sleeves. These coats, like those of the men, were trimmed with wide strips of coloured braid at the neck and wrists and round the foot. Over the coat women wore either a cloak fastened at the middle of the breast with a clasp or a garment similar to that underneath, but shorter and with shorter sleeves. This over-garment was usually worn ungirt, but many women, if they were wearing only one garment, gathered it round them with a girdle.

The only difference between these coats, or tunics, for the two sexes was that those of the women were longer and not quite so full. Further, apart from slight variations, such as the low neck of the chemise and the short sleeves of the garment worn over it, all the items in the woman's wardrobe were of the same shape.

On the whole, women's garments were made in the primitive way. The front piece was joined to the back piece (which was narrower at

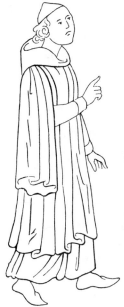

the height of the breast) by seams on the shoulders and at the sides. The sleeves were straight, and had but one seam. The cut for the neck was invariably made in the front piece.

From the middle of the thirteenth century onward some changes appeared in the fashion of men's clothes. To the coat was added a hood which could be pulled over the head in rough weather. This hood, which was more or less pointed, was cut in one piece with the rest of the coat and sewn at both sides. An oblique cut in front not only left the face clear, but served to let the head through when the hood was thrown back. Again, the opening for the neck began to be made considerably smaller; a slit at the breast was introduced, and so arranged that it could be fastened with buttons or hooks.

About this same time—the middle of the thirteenth century—actual over-coats began to come in. They resembled the ordinary coats, but were fuller and shorter (Figs. 149 and 150). The chief difference lay in the great width and length of the sleeves, through which an opening was made to allow the passage of the arms. These over-coats were usually provided with a hood.

Fig. 149. GERMAN MALE COSTUME OF THE THIRTEENTH CENTURY

The thirteenth century saw little change in the garments for the leg, except that the stockings were made longer and fastened more firmly to the waist-belt that held them up.

In the eleventh century women's dress had altered but slightly from the fashions that had formerly prevailed. The chief variation affected the upper garment of the higher classes. It gradually became shorter, while the sleeves were much longer and fuller (Figs. 151 and 152). They came at least half-way down the forearm, and frequently to the

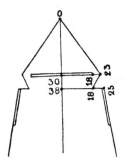

Fig. 150. PART OF PATTERN FOR A MAN'S COAT, SHOWING THE HOOD

wrist or even further. They were widest at the lower end; at the upper end they were no wider than the thickness of the arm required see Fig. 152). One kind of sleeve widened gradually from top to

137

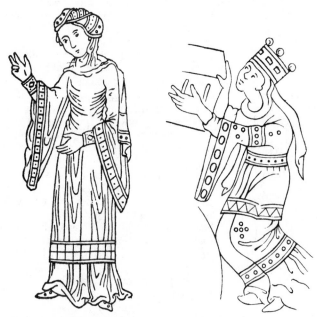

Figs. 151, 152. German Women's Dress of the Eleventh Century

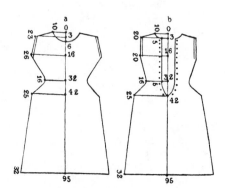

Fig. 153. Cut of Women's Upper Garment of the
Eleventh Century
(a) Front piece ; (b) back piece

bottom ; another widened suddenly down near the hand. (See Figs. 154 and 155.)

The seam in the sleeve was no longer on the under side, as before, but was shifted a little toward the back, so that if two seams were necessary—as was the case when the material was narrow—the top seam was a little toward the front and the under seam toward the back. At the same time the under part of the sleeve was shortened at the top. In other respects the over-garments (two of which were often worn together, in which case the outer one was shorter than the other, and the second only had the sleeves very wide at the

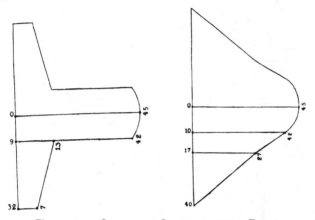

Figs. 154, 155. Sleeves for Garment shown in Fig. 153

lower arm) followed the fashion that had previously been current, except that they were now considerably tighter than before.

About the middle of the eleventh century clothes began to be made so close-fitting that they followed the lines of the body from shoulders to hips like a glove (Fig. 151). In order to achieve this result the back piece of the garment was divided from the neck to the fork, and the edges of this cut so arranged that they could be tightly laced. Further, the front and back pieces were both shaped to fit the body. These garments were usually worn ungirdled, but they were ornamented with strips of braid round the foot, at the wrists, and sometimes at the neck.

The under-garment had retained its earlier form, except that it was now so long that it trailed on the ground ; while the sleeves were still trimmed at the wrists, the foot of the garment was now left plain.

In the twelfth century women continued to wear the same style of under-garment. The over-garment, which was now much worn by middle-class women, as well as by those of higher standing, was much longer, and frequently trailed on the ground. Sleeves were now longer, and the width at the wrists had increased ; the upper part of the garment was now even more close-fitting than before. Over- and under-garment were occasionally of the same colour, but as a rule they were made of different or at least differently coloured material. Trimming on the over-garment was rare save at the wrists and half-way up the upper arm. The foot of the skirt was now hardly ever trimmed. The sleeves of the under-garment usually had coloured braid at the wrists. When the under-garment alone was worn, as in the case of the lower and working classes, its lower edge continued to be trimmed, and occasionally also a wide strip of braid was sewn down the front from the girdle to the foot.

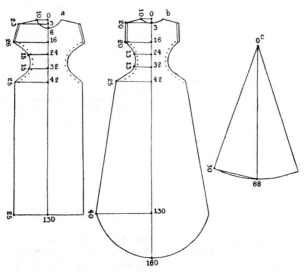

Fig. 156. WOMEN'S UPPER GARMENT IN THE TWELFTH CENTURY
(a) Front ; (b) back ; (c) gusset.

On the other hand, the fashion of the over-garment had considerably changed. Owing to the tightness at the waist, the great width at the foot could be retained only by inserting at both sides a large gusset between the front and back pieces (see Fig. 156). The upper part was made as close-fitting as it could possibly be, and was arranged for lacing either at the back or down both sides from armpits to hips. The under-garment was exposed—usually at the sides. Further, in order to emphasize the outline of the breasts the front of the over-garment was made in two pieces, the lower one being cut away each side, so that a peak ran up between the breasts (Fig. 157). At the top was sewn a piece of material longer and broader than the excisions, and this fell from the neck to the breasts. By sewing together these two pieces from the peak toward both sides, bag- or purse-shaped

140

enlargements for the breasts were produced. The fashion for the sleeves continued as in the eleventh century, except that they were now made very much wider at the wrists.

The under-garment remained as it had been for centuries, except that the neck was lower and sleeve-holes were cut.

The over-garment was now usually worn without a girdle, but the under one was still girdled, especially when the wearer had no other on. The lower classes made the under-garment of wool or linen ; the

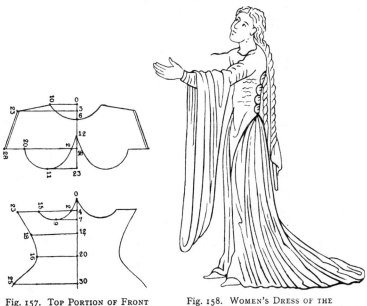

Fig. 157. Top Portion of Front of Women's Upper Garment, Twelfth Century

Fig. 158. Women's Dress of the Twelfth Century

upper classes usually used silk. It was the dress for indoors, and when no other garment was worn it was usually supplemented by a neckerchief. The low neck rendered this almost necessary.

The thirteenth century brought in extensive alterations in women's dress. Not only were the items in the wardrobe made lower at the neck, but in other respects also there were considerable changes in their shape.

The most striking of these affected, as before, the over-garment. The coat style was almost entirely abandoned, and a simple wrap was substituted. The first step toward this revolutionary change was taken when sleeves were discontinued, for this occasioned various other alterations in the cut of the whole garment. The new fashions for the sleeveless dress—called *Suckenie*, or *Sukni*—can be reduced to three main types, which were followed concurrently for a considerable time. First there was the very long dress, closed all round, and growing gradually wider from the top downward. It was pleated at the neck, but in other respects was of simple cut. Front and back were shaped alike, except that the top of the back was slightly narrower. The second style was very wide over the shoulders (Fig. 159), so that it fell to the middle of the upper arm. It was much

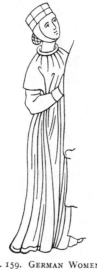

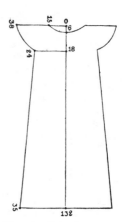

Fig. 159. German Women's Dress, Thirteenth Century

Fig. 160. Pattern of the Garment shown in Fig. 159

tighter across the breast, widening toward the foot. (See Fig. 160.) Front and back were sewn together only at the shoulders, so that the sides were quite open. The neck had a wide hem, and through this was passed a ribbon, by means of which the neck could be adjusted to the liking of the wearer. The third style was principally worn by girls and unmarried women. It combined features taken from the other two ; the sides were open as far as the hips, but closed below that point. These over-dresses, *cotellæ*, or *cotelettes*, as they were called (see Figs. 161 and 162), were very popular at the close of the thirteenth century. Like the two styles already described, they were always worn without a girdle. In this third style also the back and front pieces were shaped alike.

The under-garment of the thirteenth century retained the shape it had had at the end of the twelfth. It was very long, fairly close-fitting from the shoulders to the hips, and increased in width down to the foot. The sleeves were long and tight. Round the neck and

142

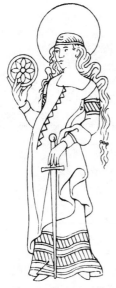

Fig. 161. Dress of Un-
married German Woman,
Thirteenth Century

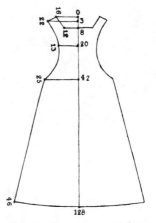

Fig. 162. Pattern of the Outer
Garment shown in Fig. 161

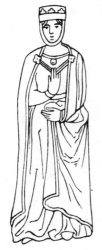

Fig. 163. Women's Dress,
Thirteenth Century

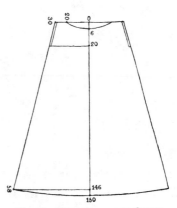

Fig. 164. Pattern of the Outer
Garment shown in Fig. 163

143

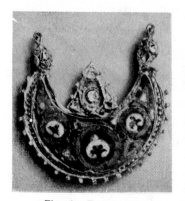
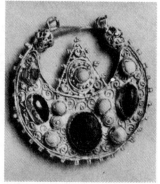

Fig. 165. Earrings that belonged to the Empress Gisela
About A.D. 1000.

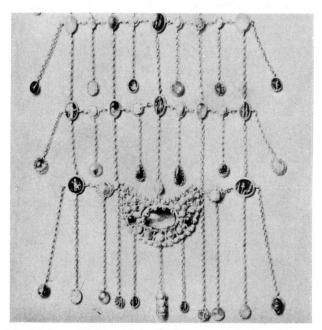

Fig. 166. Lower Part of Necklace (Loron) of the Empress Gisela,
with Stones, Goldwork, and Pearls
About A.D. 1000.

the ends of the sleeves coloured braid or threads of gold were sewn. Sometimes a girdle was worn with it and sometimes not. Women of the upper classes often wore an agraffe, or clasp, at the breast. Most of these garments were of material in one colour only, but some women, especially of the servant class, had them made of several pieces of different material and of different colours. The colour, however, was not a matter of arbitrary choice. It indicated the colours of the coat of arms of the wearer's mistress. Toward the end of the century it became the fashion for the mistresses themselves to

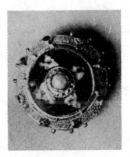

Fig. 167. BROOCH OF THE EMPRESS GISELA
About A.D. 1000.

dress in the colours of their coats of arms or to have these embroidered on their clothing.

During the thirteenth century there was little change in the cloak. The shape continued to be semicircular or nearly so, and it was put on as before (see Fig. 163). To keep it more securely on the shoulders, however, a single or double string crossed the breast, and was fastened to the cloak at both sides by means of clasps. This string was not drawn taut, but was allowed to hang loose in an ornamental way, and ladies frequently held a finger or fingers on it to tighten it.

The thirteenth century found women still wearing their hair loose in the ancient Teutonic fashion. Occasionally they parted it into separate strands and tied each with ribbon. The veil-like kerchief which had been worn on the head in the Carolingian period was discontinued, and was replaced by a garland of flowers or a circlet set with precious stones. This circlet was soon exchanged for other forms, such as a crown or a coronet. The young girl wore flowers in her loose, flowing hair. Matrons wore a cap that fitted tightly round the head and was fastened under the chin.

GERMAN ROYAL COSTUME

The robes with which the German kings were invested at their coronation in Aachen (Aix-la-Chapelle), and from 1711 onward in Frankfort-on-the-Main, and which, together with crown, sceptre, and orb, etc., composed the Imperial regalia (Fig. 169), are as follows :

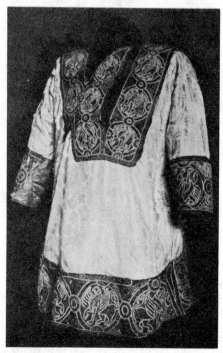

Fig. 168. Coat of the Emperor Henry II, Eleventh Century

(1) The *dalmatica* (Fig. 170), a magnificent under-garment of violet-coloured material, closed all round and reaching to the knees. The neck has a border of braid, and can be made lower by means of a gold cord that passes round it. The sleeves are long, and cut very narrow in front ; they are embroidered with leaf devices in gold and pearls. The hem has similar ornamentation.

(2) The *alba* (Fig. 171), worn over the dalmatica. It takes its name from its colour. It is of white silk material, a kind of thick taffeta of good quality. It is like a chorister's surplice, and very wide at the foot. The sleeves are slightly pointed, and ornamented with broad stripes of gold and pearls on the shoulders, at the wrists, and in front at the neck, where there are two gold cords. At the foot is a

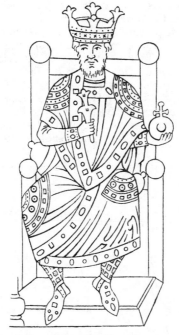

Fig. 169. GERMAN ROYAL COSTUME, BEGINNING OF THE
ELEVENTH CENTURY

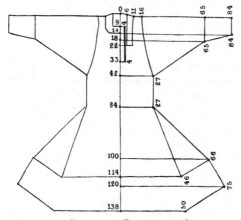

Fig. 170. CUT OF THE DALMATICA, PART OF THE CORONATION ROBES
OF THE GERMAN EMPERORS

very wide hem divided into five horizontal stripes. The first and fourth of these stripes have various lines, which look like *moiré*. In the second and the lowest of the stripes is a Latin inscription, and in the middle stripe (the broadest) there is ornamental embroidery. From the inscription it appears that this robe was made in Palermo in the year 1181, in the fifteenth year of the reign of William II, King of Sicily, the son of King William I. Presumably it came to be part of the German Imperial treasures through the Emperor Henry VI, who married an aunt of William II, or through Henry's son, Frederick II, who had become heir to the kingdom of Sicily.

(3) The *stola*, a long, narrow strip of violet silk richly studded with pearls and precious stones. From both ends depend three long tassels

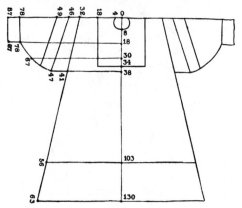

Fig. 171. Cut of the Alba, Part of the Coronation Robes of the German Emperors

of gold. The king who was to be crowned had this stola put round his neck over the alba in the vestry. It was crossed over the breast and fastened with a girdle.

(4) The *pluviale*, or *pallium*, is a mantle reaching to the feet, open in front, having at the top a golden clasp ; it has a sash studded with stones and kept in place by a pin thrust through it. The mantle is made of red silk lined with taffeta. A tree-like decoration edged with diamonds divides it longitudinally into two halves. On each half is embroidered in pearls and gold a large lion, with a camel beneath it. The neck of the mantle is low, and has a hem of gold braid. The garment is so made that it has to be put on over the head. The braid, edged with stones and pearls, goes round the neck and down the front on both sides to the foot. In the angles formed by the braid at each side of the neck a rose is embroidered in small stones and surrounded by pearls. Along the foot of the mantle, between two double rows of pearls, an Arabic inscription is embroidered in gold lettering.

Probably this mantle was part of the spoil brought from the Holy Land by the Emperor Frederick I, or by his son Frederick, Duke of Swabia, afterward finding its way among the Sicilian royal treasures through the Emperor Henry VI, who in 1186 married Constantia, sister of William I, King of Sicily, and finally being added to the German treasures through the Emperor Frederick II, son of Henry VI. A large part of these treasures was lost in the year 1248, when the Parmese conquered the city of Vittoria.

(5) The *gloves* are knitted in purple silk and decorated with pearls and precious stones.

(6) The *stockings* are of red silk, with a fairly broad stripe braided with gold at the top.

(7) The *shoes* are of dull satin, cornelian red, and embroidered with

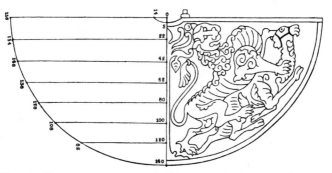

Fig. 172. Mantle belonging to the Coronation Robes of the German Emperors

gold and pearls. The soles, inside and out, are covered with red saffian.

(8) Two *girdles*, which were used to lift the robes from the ground. One is of spun silk, cornelian red, made like galloon braid, with lettering in gold thread. The ends of this girdle are decorated with lion-heads stamped out of sheet gold and with five gold buttons hanging from five triple strings. Each of the lions has a pearl in his maw. The other girdle is made of silver-gilt thread, and has a buckle of gold.

FRANCE

In France, as in Germany, the dress of the eleventh century was a development from the fashions of previous periods, though here the change was accomplished more quickly. This was already so evident at the opening of the thirteenth century that from that time onward French fashions became the standard for the upper classes among al the peoples of Central Europe.

In the eleventh century the style of the men's long, tight-sleeved tunics and of their leg-wear was exactly the same as that prevailing in Germany.   In France, as in Germany, the dress of the upper classes was distinguished from that of the lower orders by a superior quality of material (silk), by the length of the garments, and by richness of trimming.

During the twelfth century women's dress remained for a considerable time without change.   Women were wearing at that time a long, fairly wide over-garment, the *cotte hardie*, held by a girdle. Men wore the same garment.   It was high at the neck, and could be tightened by means of a draw-string.   Over this was worn another similar garment or a cloak.   The headdress was a kerchief.   The men

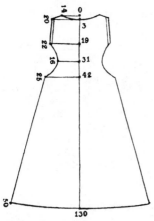

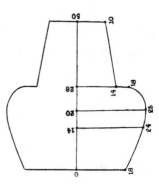

Fig. 173. PATTERN OF WOMEN'S DRESS IN FRANCE IN THE TWELFTH CENTURY

Fig. 174. SLEEVE BELONGING TO FIG. 173

also wore a long-sleeved tunic reaching to the knees, tight hose fastened by tapes to a waist-belt, and a cloak fastened by a buckle or brooch.   The footwear consisted of ankle-shoes or high boots.   All these were similar to those worn in Germany.

Women's dress, however, gradually underwent so many slight alterations that it finally took on another character.

The coat no longer showed a gradual increase in width from the shoulders to the foot.   It was now made to fit tightly under the bust (Fig. 173), the fullness beginning at the hips.   In order to secure this tight fit both front and back pieces were shaped from the bust to the hips ; the waist was made with a broad band, through which ran strings which could be tied behind as the wearer thought fit.

The other great change from previous fashion was in the sleeves. These were much wider at the top, but as tight as before at the wrists, where they were now buttoned.   Another style of sleeve (Fig. 176) fashionable at this time for over-garments was very tight from the top to a point more than half-way down the forearm, where it suddenly became extremely wide. This wide portion was a separate piece sewn to the sleeve proper as a cross-piece, so that its length made the width of the sleeve.

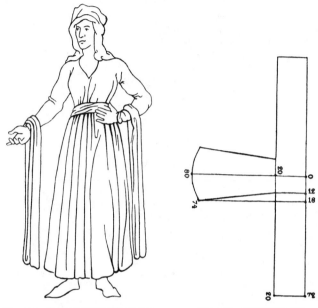

Fig. 175. FRENCH WOMEN'S DRESS, TWELFTH CENTURY

Fig. 176. SLEEVE IN THE TWELFTH CENTURY

In the twelfth century the cloak was rarely worn by Frenchwomen. It had been almost entirely supplanted by the ordinary over-dress.

The headdress at this time was either the kerchief as before or an actual cap. Women's footwear was still exactly the same as that worn by the men.

MEN'S DRESS IN THE THIRTEENTH CENTURY

In the thirteenth century the style of long over- and under-garments remained unchanged, except that the sleeves were now very long and wide or omitted altogether. But when these clothes ceased to be the ordinary wear and were used only on ceremonial occasions it became the fashion to wear only one coat.

This coat, *le pourpoint*, was made in various styles, which differed in the material, the trimming, or the cut. It continued to be made ever shorter and closer-fitting, till toward the end of the century it had become a garment for the upper part of the body only, and was very tight-fitting (Fig. 177).

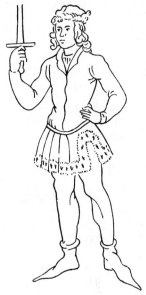

Fig. 177. FRENCH MEN'S DRESS, THIRTEENTH CENTURY

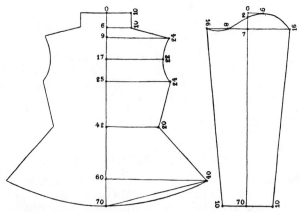

Fig. 178. PATTERN FOR POURPOINT, THIRTEENTH CENTURY

Various changes were also made in the cut. The coat still consisted of two pieces, back and front, but the latter was now partly or wholly open, and was fastened with hooks and eyes. To obtain as close a fit

152

as possible both pieces were shaped at the sides, as were also the sleeve-holes, which were now either round or oval. The result was a sleeve which was greatly improved, because it now had to be of the proper width in order to be comfortable both above and below the shoulder. Therefore, although the sleeve had still only one seam, it was now cut sharply convex above the shoulder and concave underneath. When the sleeve was sewn into the garment, the concave part was exactly at the armpit. The seam ran down the front.

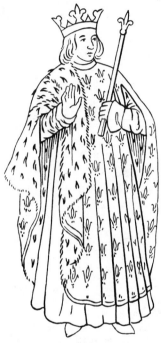

Fig. 179. FRENCH ROYAL COSTUME

Speaking generally, the tunic worn by the knights retained the shape it had had in the twelfth century, although it too was now closer-fitting and shorter. The chief difference was a considerable increase of trimming.

This period saw a great improvement in the dress for the lower limbs, called *les chausses*. Till now the hose had always been separate, but about this time it became the fashion to join them at the top, thus making actual trousers, which covered not only the legs, but also the lower part of the trunk. This new practice, however, was attended by great difficulties. The inelastic materials hitherto employed impeded the free movement of the limbs and made it almost impossible for the wearer to sit down. And even although an attempt had been made at the end of the previous century to meet this difficulty by using elastic materials, tailors had not yet completely succeeded in preventing the strain at the seat. Once, however, the fashion had been started of joining the separate hose into one garment by running a seam from back to front between the legs, the authorities, both ecclesiastical and secular, used every endeavour to bring the new

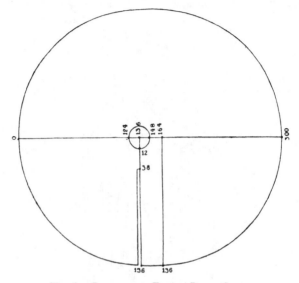

Fig. 180. PATTERN FOR FRENCH ROYAL CLOAK

style into universal use. They condemned the previous fashion as indecent, and so the new practice of wearing trousers tied round the waist with a belt made rapid headway.

These trousers, entirely closed at the top, were made of wool, linen, or silk of the brightest colours available. Indeed, the legs were frequently of different colours. This fashion was especially popular with the knights, who were thus able to reproduce their own colours in their trousers, and with the militia of the cities when they took the field, for they could thus wear the city colours. The cloak, *le manteau*, almost entirely ceased to be worn during the thirteenth century. When it was still worn it was so much shorter that it came only a little below the hips. The shape too was greatly altered. It was no longer segment-shaped, but sector-shaped (mostly two-thirds of a circle), so that the top of the cloak was not now a straight, but a broken line. By and by the sides, where the cloak was pulled up by the shoulders, were cut longer than the back and front; the cloak was also taken in above the shoulders at both sides. It thus not only

154

fitted better at the neck, but lay better and more securely at the shoulders ; there was also less strain. (See Fig. 183.)

The headdress of this period was a cap resembling a cowl, called

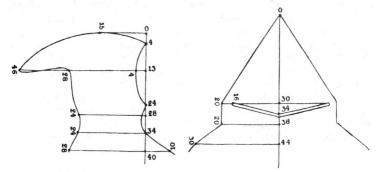

Figs. 181, 182. SHAPE OF HOOD IN THE THIRTEENTH CENTURY

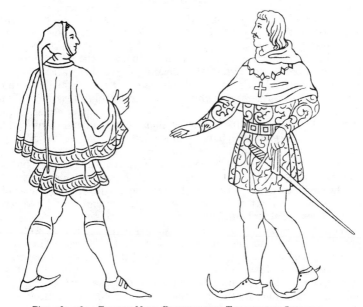

Figs. 183, 184. FRENCH MALE DRESS IN THE THIRTEENTH CENTURY

a *chapel*, worn with its lower edge turned outward, and a hood called *le capuchon*. This latter was much worn, either under or over the cap, or even by itself. It varied in shape according to the manner in which it was to be worn ; it was made either of a front and a back piece or of two side-pieces. (See Figs. 181, 182.) The former type,

155

which was often attached to the cloak or made long enough to serve
as a cape, was closed all round except for an opening for the face. It
was fairly wide, and could easily be brought over the head, seeing
that it did not fit closely at the neck. This form was called *la chape*,
and was worn in rough weather over some other headdress in order
to protect it, or on the occasion of some late revel in order to conceal
the face. At ordinary times it was flung back and lay round the neck
like a wide ruffle (Fig. 184).

The second type of hood, *l'aumusse*, which was also frequently
worn as sole headdress, fitted somewhat closely round the head and
neck, and was therefore quite open in front, but it had strings or
buttons by means of which it could be closed. It sometimes came
down only as far as the shoulders, but was often long enough to serve
as a cape, coming half-way down the upper arm.

ENGLAND

Even in the twelfth century dress in England exhibited many
innovations, thereby proving very clearly how quickly even in that
early time new fashions could gain currency. The differences between
Norman and Saxon styles were disappearing, and the descendants of
these two peoples were gradually blending into a new nation.

Men's Dress. Men's dress still consisted of the usual items, but
practically each of these had undergone considerable alteration. This
was especially the case with the long robes of the upper classes ; the
lower orders still continued to wear their former short, comfortable
clothing. The greatest changes concerned the coat—especially the
over one, for many men were now wearing two similar coats, one
above the other. The sleeves were made as tight as possible, but so
long that they came down far beyond the hand, widening in front.
To the cloak was attached a very close-fitting, pointed hood ; the whole
garment was so tight and short that it finally resembled a large cape
falling over shoulders and back.

Women's Dress. The case was similar with regard to women's
dress. Here too the chief alterations were in the sleeves. They were
now very tight half-way down the lower arm—sometimes even to
the wrists—and then suddenly became extremely wide (Fig. 185).
In most cases this widening was in the sleeve itself, which had still
only one seam (on the under side—see Fig. 186), but sometimes it
took the form of a cuff attached to the sleeve (Fig. 185, *b*) ; in this
case the lower end of the sleeve was wider in front. The added piece
was sewn up behind and turned back so that the cuff was closed in
front and open at the back.

Sometimes the sleeves were also so wide toward the wrist that they
trailed on the ground, and had to be fastened up for half their length.

In other respects the coat remained as it had been during the previous century. This is specially true of the under-garment. It was now made exactly as before, with very tight sleeves.

The cloak or mantle was now usually semicircular, but some preferred to have it in the shape of a very much elongated oval, so that it trailed. The oval was divided in the direction of its short diameter. These mantles were made of light material, and were fastened across the breast with a clasp.

Women's headgear had undergone great changes in the twelfth century. The kerchief went out of fashion, and there was a return

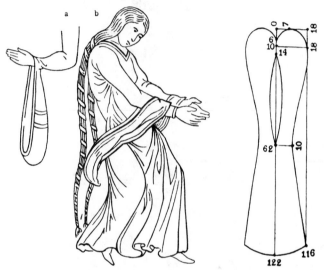

Fig. 185. ENGLISH WOMEN'S DRESS, TWELFTH CENTURY

Fig. 186. PATTERN FOR THE SLEEVE IN FIG. 185

to the primitive style of wearing the hair loose. It was gathered back from the forehead in two strands. Each of these was bound from top to bottom with coloured ribbon, and the two parts hung down the back (Fig. 185, b). Some women wore also a small, closefitting cap trimmed at the edge.

NORSE RELICS DISCOVERED AT HERJOLFSNES, GREENLAND

Valuable information regarding dress from the thirteenth to the fifteenth centuries was supplied by the discoveries made in Norse graves in the south of Greenland. These finds are the earliest specimens we possess of original garments belonging to the Middle Ages, and a fortunate chance has preserved them for later times.

the year 1921 a large number of well-preserved graves were discovered in the burial-ground of a Norse colony in Herjolfsnes. The clothing on the bodies gives accurate indications of the styles of dress and the tailoring art of that age. The make of the clothing is extremely simple ; there is practically no trimming, but along some of the seams there is ornamental back-stitching and cord-edging.

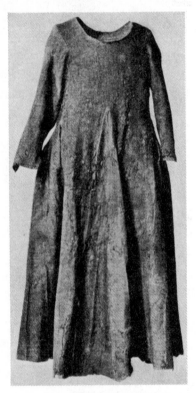

Fig. 187. WOMAN'S DRESS
From the Norse settlement at Herjolfsnes, Greenland. Fourteenth to
fifteenth century.

Although the garments are plainly made, the cut, including that of the sleeves, is good—one might even say stylish. There is no sign of lining, but it is possible that the clothes had been lined—presumably with fur. Numerous hoods, hats, and cowls were found. It is not always possible to distinguish between male and female dress. The shirt-like garment predominates. Only a few are open in front ; these have a row of buttons.

There is very little ornament, and even girdles are rare, but some fragments of coarse cord were found. The woollen material was between black and brown in colour, but probably among the clothes

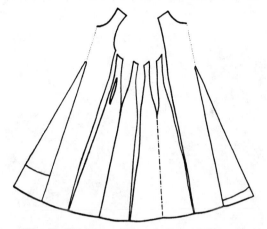

Fig. 188. Pᴀᴛᴛᴇʀɴ ᴏꜰ Wᴏᴍᴀɴ's Gᴏᴡɴ ɪɴ Fɪɢ. 187

were coloured garments, although the colour has faded during the centuries of interment.

The clothes of men and women were alike. Front and back were sewn together at the shoulders. At each side were from one to four

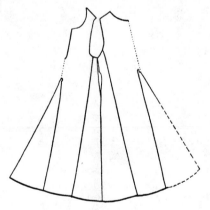

Fig. 189. Cᴜᴛ ᴏꜰ Mᴇɴ's Cᴏᴀᴛs ꜰʀᴏᴍ Hᴇʀᴊᴏʟꜰsɴᴇs, Gʀᴇᴇɴʟᴀɴᴅ

gussets, in the front and back pieces six gussets, so that some garments consisted of sixteen pieces (see Figs. 188 and 189). The side-gussets are very narrow at the waist, and become much wider from the hips downward. The greatest width at the foot amounts to

4·25 metres ; the average width is 3·50 metres. The gussets in the front and back pieces begin at the hips ; the side ones run up to where the sleeve joins the garment. The neck is higher at the back than

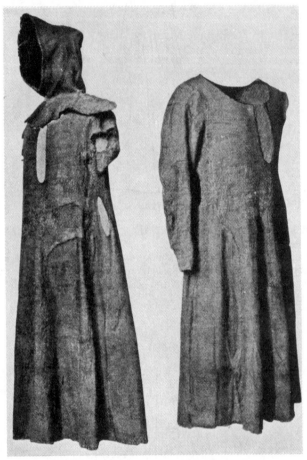

Fig. 190. MAN'S COAT WITH HOOD
Found at Herjolfsnes, Greenland, a Norse settlement. Fourteenth to fifteenth century.

in front. It is usually round, but sometimes square, and there is often a slit, which was fastened with buttons, strings, or a clasp. Most of the sleeves are in one piece ; a few are in two ; all have a gusset at the shoulder. Some are short ; some reach to the wrist, where they are wide. One specimen has buttons at the wrist.

A few female garments have all round the waist, between breast and hips, very narrow perpendicular pleats, 3 mm. wide and 26 cm. long. This fashion is exactly like that prevailing at that time in the rest of Europe, if we are to judge from the works of art that have come down to us. A sort of waistcoat (bolero) may have been worn with the dress. There are also dresses without any side-gussets, and some in which gussets are found only in the front and back pieces.

The date of the gowns is determined by the cut of the hoods, because hoods and gowns belong together. The same holds good for the leg-wear, which consisted of stockings both long and short.

FOURTEENTH AND FIFTEENTH CENTURIES

FRANCE

Men's Dress. In the course of the thirteenth century French dress had continued to develop into more and more attractive forms, and had gradually taken the lead in fashion for ornament and style for Western and Central Europe. Various national peculiarities of course persisted. French influence was most felt in England ; Germany, Italy, and Spain were more independent. For a time there was not much change in cut, but the employment of splendid silk stuffs and beautiful trimmings opened up new possibilities of attractive clothes not only for the upper classes, but also for the citizens of the towns. The girdled coat grew tighter and shorter, and although the over-garment was still long, it too was now closer-fitting ; even the mantle became much shorter. Headdress now comprised caps made of velvet, cloth, and silk, as well as stiff hats with broad brims. About the middle of the fourteenth century there came a change in fashion that affected chiefly the coat and the *robe* (the over-garment).

This over-garment now began to develop on two new lines. The *housse* was a long, wide, sleeveless wrap or shawl, open at both sides, and having a slit at the breast made to button. The neck and foot were trimmed with fur. The *houppelande* was a long, wide over-coat with long, wide sleeves. It was open in front, and fastened with a girdle.

The favourite style of coat, especially among the lower classes, was the *jaquette*. It was cut like a tunic. The close-fitting coat (*pourpoint*) continued to be worn, but the skirt of it was shorter. The sleeves were as tight as they could be made, and were buttoned at the wrist. Some men wore the *pourpoint* with long sleeves, but in that case they wore beneath it a garment with tight sleeves.

The neck was made in various fashions—low, high, round, square, in a point at back and in front ; even the erect collar came into fashion.

Up till this time a girdle had been worn over the other clothing, but as coats were now made to be fastened with buttons or tapes or hooks the girdle became unnecessary, and was now worn only with the very long over-coat. The members of the knightly orders retained the girdle as an indication of their rank, but wore it lower down than the ordinary girdle, and fastened it with hooks. The *robe* of rich

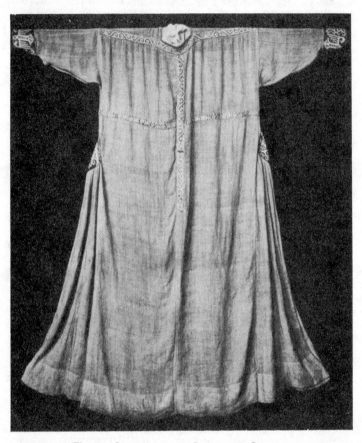

Fig. 191. SURPLICE OF THE FOURTEENTH CENTURY

stuff trimmed with fur and the *soutane* were important items in the wardrobe of the day. The latter consisted of front and back pieces —both long. The side-seams left long openings for the sleeves. Toward the end of the century the seams were discontinued, and the *soutane* was left open at the sides. It was now also less full, and became ere long a mere wrap or plaid.

The mantle retained its old shape, but it now had a train when it was worn as a ceremonial dress. Toward the end of the century the edges of the shorter mantles began to be cut into points or to be fringed with pieces of different material. These mantles were now fastened not at the breast, but at the shoulder, and large buttons were provided for that purpose.

Hose and breeches were made as before, but there were great changes in footwear, both in shape and in trimming. There were high-lows,' low shoes, and ankle-shoes of various kinds. The shoes were slit at the instep and fitted for lacing, or had lappets which were hooked together. All these forms of footwear had pointed toes, which were occasionally of considerable length. The shoes were called *à la poulaine*.

Changes in the headdress were merely variations of the existing fashions. The collar of the hood was lengthened, and trimmed with scallops. The brim of the hat varied in width ; the hat itself was either conical or cylindrical, high or low, and made of felt, velvet, or silk. Gold cord or fringes of gold adorned the brim. A novelty was

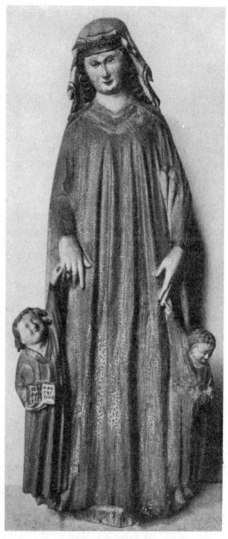

Fig. 192. So-called Grammatica, with the Diligent and the Lazy Child
About 1350.

the *chaperon*, a skull-cap with a brim stuffed into the shape of a roll, with a broad piece of material hanging from one side of it to the shoulder.

The hair was kept moderately short. The chin was shaved till

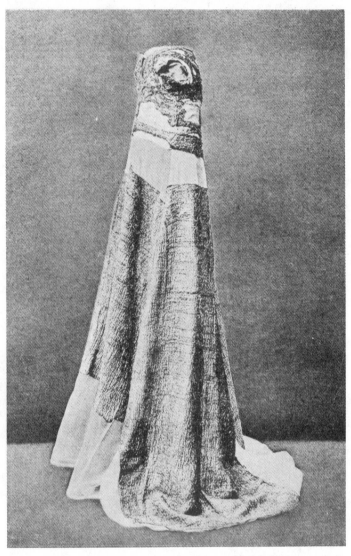

Fig. 193. GOLDEN GOWN OF QUEEN MARGARET OF DENMARK,
SWEDEN, AND NORWAY (b. 1353, d. 1412)

about the middle of the century, but it then became fashionable to wear a beard. The most usual type was pointed. About this time knights again began to wear beards and moustaches.

Women's Dress. Corresponding changes were introduced into women's dress. It too became closer-fitting. The garments were as

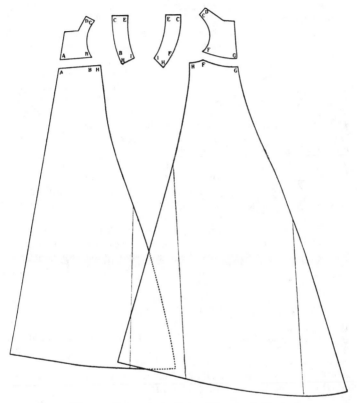

Fig. 194. PATTERN FOR QUEEN MARGARET'S ROBE

tight as possible, and were laced or buttoned at the sides. The sleeves also were tight, and buttoned from elbow to wrist.

The under-dress had a train ; various forms of over-dress, also ending in a train, were worn over it. The sleeves were very short, never reaching below the elbows. Those which came as low as the elbow sometimes had elongations in the shape of broad or narrow strips which fell to the knees and sometimes to the ground.

About the middle of the fourteenth century women's dress began to be divided into two parts—a bodice and a skirt. These were of different colours; the skirt was pleated and sewn to the bodice. The over-coat was still worn, but it was now much tighter round the shoulders. It was often made of fur. Although now unnecessary, the girdle was still retained by many women as an ornament. The mantle, or cloak, was unaltered. Men wore it fastened at the shoulder with some kind of ornamental clasp.

Footwear was the same for both sexes. Unmarried women still wore their hair loose. Married women wore it in plaits wound closely round the head. The side-hair was plaited and arranged round the face, but some women preferred to arrange it in rolls.

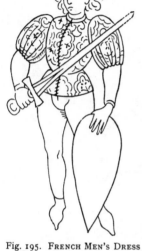

The second half of the fourteenth century saw little change in women's dress. The neck was lower and sleeves were longer, but it was only when the century was drawing to a close that fashions again changed and entirely new modes were adopted.

The *robe* and the *surcot* were now very low-necked, and the sleeves of the dress worn beneath were longer and fuller. The girdle again came into fashion, for a style of over-dress now came in so very low at the neck and so very wide lower down that a girdle became necessary. The bodice of this dress was short, leaving the breast almost bare. The edges had a trimming of fur.

It was in the headdress that the most important changes were made. Two styles enjoyed most favour. One was a skull-cap with two side-pieces rising in a high curve. The other was a pointed cone of silk or velvet, with a veil attached at the top. It was called *le hénin*. The veil was arranged in various ways. The hair was combed back and hidden under the *hénin*.

Fig. 195. FRENCH MEN'S DRESS (POURPOINT), ABOUT 1400

Men's Dress. The fifteenth century brought with it numerous changes. The close-fitting coat, the *pourpoint*, was much shorter than in the fourteenth century; it now came only a little below the hips. It was as tight as it could be, and was padded at the breast, sides, and hips, thus emphasizing the waist-line in extreme fashion (Figs. 195 and 196). The cut of the coat remained in all essentials as it had been. It consisted of an undivided back piece[1] and a front piece, which had now to be much wider in order to allow for the

---

[1] Where the back piece did not fit exactly in the small of the back it was pleated; the pleats were sewn down there and left free above and below this stitching.

padding. The two were joined on the shoulders and down the sides. The front piece was divided at the middle of its length and made to be laced or buttoned. Owing to the padding, it was not cut straight, but with an outward curve, thus leaving room for the convexity at the breast. The sleeve-hole was still oval in form, and a very peculiar outline was given to the sleeves by padding them very heavily at the shoulders. These padded shoulders, which ere long degenerated into all kinds of extravagant forms, were called *mahoîtres* (see Fig. 195).

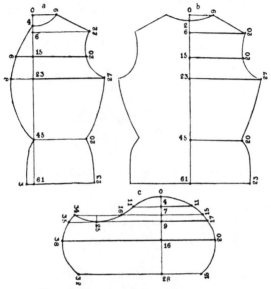

Fig. 196. PATTERN FOR POURPOINT OF 1400

All sleeves came to be padded, so that the upper part had now to be cut far wider than before. This widening of the upper part explains why for a considerable time all sleeves were wider than they had been, tightening more or less toward the hand.

Sometimes, in accordance with earlier practice, a still shorter garment, with long, very tight sleeves, was worn beneath the *pourpoint*. In this case the sleeves of the *pourpoint*, whether short or long, open or fastened at the wrist, or even pendent, were padded at the shoulders.

Over the *pourpoint* was worn the jacket. This still retained the tunic shape it had had in the fourteenth century, but as it was now an over-garment it had no longer pleats round the body, but was fastened round the waist with a girdle or cord. On the whole the cut of the jacket was unchanged, although it was shorter and the sleeves wider and longer. The upper part of the sleeve had to be

wider when the jacket was to be worn over a *pourpoint* with *mahoître*
—*i.e.*, padded shoulders. Sometimes a part of the sleeve-seam which
ran down the front was left open, so that the arm could be thrust
through at that place ; when this was done the rest of the sleeve
was left pendent.

As a rule the jacket was untrimmed, but the lower edge, the neck,
and the wrists had a trimming of fur. The neck, which was usually

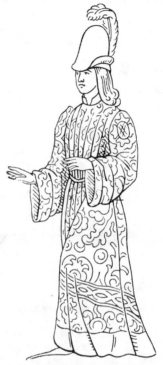

Fig. 197. FRENCH MEN'S DRESS IN THE FIRST HALF OF
THE FIFTEENTH CENTURY

high and fitted with an erect collar, had a short slit in front which
could be hooked at the top. Like the *pourpoint*, the jacket was made
of various materials—velvet, silk, cloth, and even leather.

Along with these short garments the long over-garments maintained
their place. They were again, as before, irrespective of cut or shape,
called by the name of *robe*. This *robe* resembled the garment that had
hitherto borne the name of *houppelande* (see Fig. 197). It extended
from neck to feet, was somewhat wide, and had the front open from
top to foot. The sleeves were always long, but varied in width.
The neck was high, and usually had an erect collar. In make this *robe*,

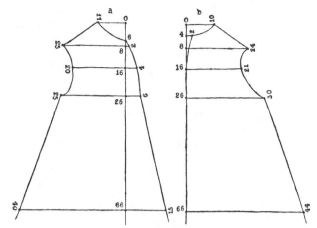

Fig. 198. Pattern of Men's Robe, First Half of the Fifteenth Century
(a) Front ; (b) back.

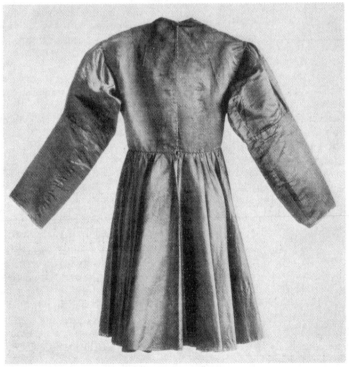

Fig. 199. So-called Satin Coat of Charles the Bold, 1476

which often had a long train, was exactly as it had long been. The sleeves had still only one seam, but the shoulders were wide, in proportion to the amount of padding that was to be used, for the *mahoîtres* were even more universally introduced into the *robe* than into the *pourpoint*. It was fastened with a girdle or cord, the latter being either loose or stitched on. It was an extremely serviceable garment, and was used by all classes either as a comfortable indoor or a convenient outdoor walking dress. It was even worn at Court. The material was accordingly of different kinds, but it was usually both good and expensive.

Well-to-do men found opportunity in this dress to display their luxurious tastes. They not only had it made of silk patterned with gold,[1] but trimmed it with fur at the wrists and along the bottom edge, and even lined it with fur. Originally this *robe* resembled the *houppelande*, and alterations came slowly. The sleeves were the first to change. The wrist-ends were sewn up, making sack sleeves. These were always very long and full, and the opening for the hand, which was usually very small, was either half-way down or near the wrist. This hand-opening, like the lower edge of the *robe*, was trimmed with fur (Fig. 200).

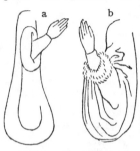

Fig. 200. Sack Sleeves, Fifteenth Century

Women's Dress. During the first half of the fifteenth century women's dress changed less than that of men. Almost the only change was that the *surcot*, which remained practically unaltered, was discarded by many women in favour of the *robe* belted close up to the breast.

The under-garment continued to be as close-fitting as before. The neck was lower and the train longer, to suit the garment worn over it. The over-garments were now much wider from the hips downward, and so the under-garment was also widened when necessary by the insertion of gores at both sides. These gores, however, did not now begin at the hip, but at the waist, extending upward to under the arm. They were about 10 cm. in width all the way. When the *surcot* was to be worn over it, the under-dress was as close-fitting as before from the shoulders to below the hips. It was fastened by lacing—not now at the back, however, but at the front, down to the middle of the abdomen. The best possible material was now used

[1] Silk stuffs of this kind, patterned or plain, threaded with gold, used to be procurable only in the East, but at a later time they were also imported from Spain and Sicily, where they were manufactured by the Arabs. When silk-weaving was introduced into Central and Northern Italy the art of weaving in colour and with gold came with it. This ancient art of gold-weaving has been extinct since the end of the fifteenth century.

for these dresses, because the over-garment was so long that it had to be lifted in front, and this exposed the under-dress.

The *surcot* still retained its place as a fashionable over-dress, and although the cut and make had remained unchanged since the end of the fourteenth century the trimming had undergone considerable changes. The old custom of wearing on the *surcot* a badge with the family coat of arms had disappeared, as well as the old practice of trimming it round the foot with ermine. The ermine was now replaced by a wide border of gold or other braid. Ermine still continued to be used on the upper portion of the long *surcot*. A further change was the disappearance of the long, pendent sleeves. About the year 1430 the front and back piece of the bodice were widened, while the formerly large side-slits were considerably reduced. In the course of the fifteenth century the neck of the *surcot* became lower and lower, almost exposing the shoulders.

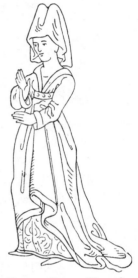

The *robe* brought about a great difference in the appearance of Frenchwomen (Fig. 201), for it had none of the tightness that had been customary. It came high up on the shoulders, and was cut in a low V-shape in front. The width gradually increased from the bust downward. It was very long in front and at the sides, and had a long train. Close under the breast it was caught up by a wide girdle with a metal buckle. The neck had a turn-over collar, broadest at the back and gradually narrowing toward the front till it met the girdle. This collar was always of a different colour from the *robe*, and frequently of another material—sometimes of fur. The sleeves varied in width. Most frequently they were narrow or even tight, but occasionally they were quite wide, sometimes open at the wrist and at other times close-fitting. Some women continued to prefer the sack sleeves (Fig. 200), and still others had the sleeve-seams trimmed with pointed braid.

Fig. 201. FRENCH WOMEN'S DRESS, FIFTEENTH CENTURY

There was nothing in the cut of the *robe* that calls for special mention. The great width of the skirt was attained, as before, by the insertion of gores, which extended up to the armpits. When in the course of the century the fashion of *mi-parti* was introduced into women's dress both front and back were divided longitudinally into two or more sections so that these sections, which were of different colours, gave an equal appearance throughout their length.

The bust exposed by the low, V-shaped neck was covered either by the under-dress or by a bib, according to the fashion of the day. The ermine wraps which had been customary at the end of the fourteenth century were now hardly ever worn.

The cloak, which was now worn only on great occasions, had retained its earlier semicircular form, but it sometimes took the shape of a sector minus the pointed corner (see Fig. 203). This cut-out part, which ran parallel to the lower edge of the cloak, was cut so wide that the garment could be arranged as low on the shoulders as desired. The cloak was now little more than a cape hanging down

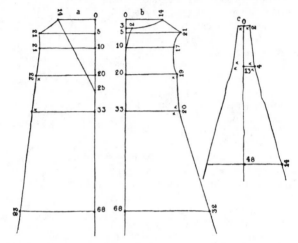

Fig. 202. Pattern of Woman's Robe in the Fifteenth Century
(a) Front ; (b) back ; (c) gusset.

the back. It was fastened with a clasp either on the shoulder or at the breast.

Women's footwear had changed as little as that of the men. They too wore shoes with long, pointed toes and used the same kind of inner shoes as were worn by the men.

No part of women's *toilette* underwent greater changes at the beginning of the fifteenth century than their headdress, although the main types had already appeared at the end of the fourteenth century. The numerous forms of headdress worn at this period can be reduced to two leading styles. (1) The hair-nets arranged on both sides of the face in cylindrical or spherical shape. These were made larger and larger, until they became veritable horns. They were called *atours*. (2) The *hénin*. In this style the tall, pointed cone, like the projecting horns of the *atours*, supported the veil. With the help of various arrangements of wire the veil was disposed over the cone, and hung down to the ground. Sometimes two cones stood up from the head side by side, the veil being draped over these. Some women still preferred a simpler arrangement, and wore merely several kerchiefs laid one over another. The once popular hood completely disappeared during the fifteenth century. Some of these styles of headdress are still in use in various parts of France—the *hénin* style, for example, is to be seen in Normandy. The fifteenth century knew various other types of headdress, perhaps the most popular being a turban-shaped hat adorned with gold and jewels.

Toward the end of the fifteenth century women's dress began to exhibit all the signs of a period of transition. Thus the *robe* assumed various contrasting styles—with very tight sleeves and very wide sleeves, very low-necked and very high-necked. The upper part could be long or short as the wearer desired, but it was always as close-fitting as possible. The train was shorter, and the *robe* itself was often so short that the tips of the toes were visible. These short *robes* were always laced at the back. It now also became the fashion to cut the bodice (*le corsage*) and the skirt (*la jupe*) separately, and to sew them together with double seams. This did not in any way alter the form of the *robe*, because the bodice was made sometimes short and sometimes longer. With a short

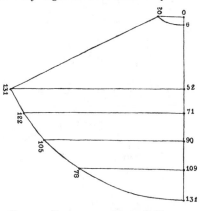

Fig. 203. **Pattern for Woman's Mantle in the Fifteenth Century**
Length in front same as length behind.

bodice an ornamental waistband was worn just as when the *robe* was cut in one piece. It had to lie close up to the breast and hide the junction of the skirt and bodice. The skirt was rarely pleated. Tight sleeves were preferred. Like men's sleeves, they were slashed, or were divided at the elbow, the gap being stuffed with white padding material and then loosely laced.

The *surcot* went quite out of fashion, and the cloak too was less worn, even on ceremonial occasions. When it was worn it retained the semicircular shape, and was fastened with clasps in front of the shoulder. The popular *hénin* either disappeared or lost much of its height. Its place was taken by rolled, turban-like caps adorned with pearls and precious stones and worn with a veil. Some women still wore simple kerchiefs draped in various ways round the head, fastened with pins and covering the entire neck. Those whose position allowed them to wear a coronet added this to their headdress. The new fashion of headdress gave a fresh importance to the hair. It was plaited into pigtails and enclosed in nets of gold thread. Girls and unmarried women began to wear it loose again. The wearing of gloves had meantime become so general that by the end of the fifteenth century they had become an indispensable adjunct for ladies and gentlemen.

ENGLAND

Men's Dress. About the middle of the fifteenth century the items of attire commonly worn in France were brought from the Court of Burgundy into England. These included the *tabard*, wholly or partially open at the sides, and the *robe*, of varying length, closed all round and pleated round the waist. One of the

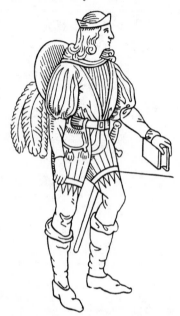

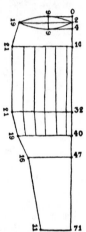

Fig. 204. ENGLISH MEN'S DRESS, END OF THE FIFTEENTH CENTURY

Fig. 205. SLEEVE FOR FIG. 204

chief importations was the fashion of thickly padded shoulders. English fashion also adopted the ' slashed ' style that had gained currency in France during the second half of the century. By all kinds of ornamentation, including embroidery on the breeches, the English imparted to their dress a motley appearance that surpassed that attained by the introduction of *mi-parti*.

Like that of the Frenchmen, the dress of Englishmen took on a different character toward the end of the century. The slashings increased both in number and in size, and the long, wide-sleeved over-garments had broad turned-down collars of fur, which ere long appeared also on the shorter overcoats. These latter had often very long sleeves, which, like those of the longer overcoats, were slashed either longitudinally or across. The close-fitting, low-necked under-coats were shortened and transformed into jackets, and in place of the padded shoulders came large puffs reaching to the elbows. The puffs were likewise slashed.

These puffed sleeves were made as follows. They were cut straight, but were much longer and much wider at the sleeve-hole than the ordinary sleeve. The upper parts of these sleeves were slashed either to the edge of the material or to some little distance from it. (See Figs. 204 and 205.) When the sleeves were sewn in other sleeves were inserted as lining. These were cut wide and slightly padded, and were sewn to the sleeve-hole along with the outer sleeves.

Englishmen's dress was even more gaily coloured than that of Frenchmen, for in addition to wearing over their close-fitting breeches shorter breeches striped in different colours and extending to the middle of the

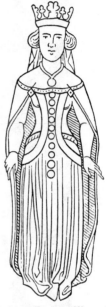

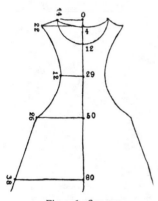

Fig. 206. Surcot

Fig. 207. English Women's
Dress, Beginning of the
Fifteenth Century

thigh, they also wore stockings that came up higher than the calf of the leg (see Fig. 204).

An important part of male attire was a round, wide-brimmed hat, mostly turned up at one side, with a large plume. A small skull-cap was worn beneath it. This was a genuinely French fashion, as were all the other forms of headgear—hats and caps—that came into use in England during this century.

Changes had also taken place in footwear. About the year 1480 the long, pointed shoes disappeared, and boots and shoes became rounder at the toes. About the year 1500 the round toes were replaced by broad ones. Tight-fitting boots, knee-high, and turned over at the top, were at this time as popular in England as the over-stockings already mentioned.

175

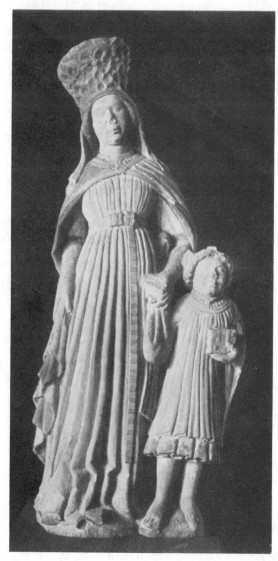

Fig. 208. PRINCESS AND CHILD
About 1450.

Women's Dress. The usual over-garment for women at the beginning of the fifteenth century was the *surcot*. In the main it had retained its earlier shape, but was now longer and fuller. The difference between the English and French forms of this coat was that the Englishwomen's *surcot* was seldom made of fur, but was only trimmed

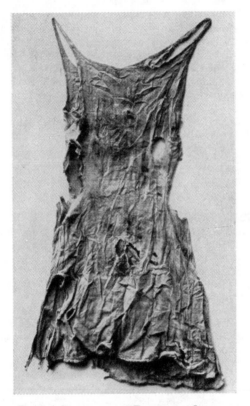

Fig. 209. CHEMISE OF THE FOURTEENTH CENTURY

with fur at the sides, so that the material of the coat came up to the neck both at back and in front between the fur trimmings. It was still the fashion also to have a row of large buttons from the neck down the front. The neck was now much lower than it had been. In the main the cut of the *surcot*, both in England and in France, had all along remained the same. In France the upper portion was always entirely made of fur. The width of the skirt varied from time to time, but was always dependent on the size of the gores. The *robe* as worn by Englishwomen had a peculiar shape. It was intermediate between the earlier *cotte hardie* and the French *robe* of the beginning of the fifteenth century. The English *robe* was high at the neck, was made to lace at the back, fitted close to the bust, and widened downward. When very wide it was arranged in regular pleats and girdled close up to the breast. Otherwise it was worn without a girdle, as it fitted close from the bust down to the hips. Both types of the *robe* had wide sleeves long enough to reach the ground. The cut of the sleeves was the same as that of men's sleeves at the time. When the material was not wide enough there had to be two seams. The *robe* itself was cut exactly as it had always been. A front and a back piece were sewn together at the shoulders and at the sides, and the needful width below was secured by the insertion of gussets of the size required. The sleeve-hole was now cut partly in the back and partly in the front piece and was in shape an upright oval.

With these *robes* the under-dress was always high at the neck, and sometimes had a small erect collar, open in front. The under-dress, too, had extremely long sleeves, very full in front, hanging down over the hands.

GERMANY

Men's Dress. During the fourteenth century the war dress of the knightly orders in Germany underwent the same transformation as in France. The German knights, like the French, began to have their tunics made shorter and closer-fitting, as well as open in front, and sometimes also at the sides almost up to the hips. The material of these tunics, which reached to the knees, was in most cases cloth, but they were frequently made of velvet or silk or other material, lined with fur, and embroidered with the coat of arms of the wearer. The tunic was held in place by a richly ornamented waist-belt, which was buckled loosely. This belt also served to hold the knight's sword on the right side and on the left side his dagger. These were attached to the belt by special thongs. In the second half of the century the tunic had become still shorter and closer-fitting, until finally it was very tight and hardly covered the trunk ; the belt encircled the body below the hips. These tight tunics were called *Lendener*. They were made of very thick but pliant leather, and were sometimes sleeveless. Usually, however, they had short sleeves, which were laced or buttoned in front or at the side or behind. The *Lendener* was magnificently trimmed. It was usually dyed the colour of the wearer's scutcheon. His crest was painted on it, or it was covered with dyed velvet on which the crest was embroidered. The breast of the tunic was decorated with metal rosettes from which gilt chains depended. To these were attached the knight's helmet, sword, and dagger, so that they could not be lost in the field. Beneath the tunic the knight wore a suit of chain mail that covered the whole person ; it was strengthened at the arms and legs by leather straps and joint-pieces of iron. The knight's chief defensive armour was his thick, padded coat of leather worn beneath the mail shirt.

This leather coat, the *Wammes*,[1] in England called gambeson, and by the French *gambesson*, was the knight's indoor dress. (See Fig. 210.) It resembled the usual male coat of the day as well as the *Lendener*, except that, as already mentioned, this last was either sleeveless or had very short sleeves and, as it was worn above the *Wams* (or, in later English, doublet) and the mail, was much wider. The *Wams* had always long, tight sleeves. It was open all down the front, and could either be laced or buttoned (Fig. 211). It was also open at the sides from the hips downward, and there too it

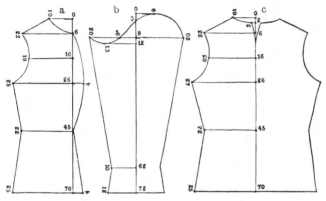

Fig. 210. PATTERN OF THE WAMS IN THE FOURTEENTH CENTURY
(*a*) Front piece ; (*b*) sleeve ; (*c*) back piece.

could be buttoned. If it was to be used merely as an indoor dress, it was longer than when it was to be worn under mail. In that case, too, it was padded only slightly or not at all.

The material of which this doublet (*Wams*) was made varied greatly. It was mostly of leather or of coarse or fine cloth, but sometimes it was of silk or velvet. It was never trimmed or embroidered in any way.

Over the doublet a longish over-garment was often put on. This was worn, however, only during the first decade of the fourteenth century ; it was worn with the usual long, wide under-clothes. Later, like the *Wams*, it became much tighter and shorter. About the middle of the fourteenth century this over-garment had lost so much of its earlier fullness that it differed from the *Wams* only in its greater length and its shorter sleeves. This greater length made

[1] The name *Wammes* instead of *Rock* (coat) was used by the Germans long before the fourteenth century, and it is quite possible that the French and the English borrowed from the Germans their almost homonymous names for the leather coat worn beneath armour.

inevitable, of course, a much greater width below, because the width gradually increased from the hips down. The garment was closed in front. The equally tight sleeves of a similar over-garment did not come quite down to the elbow in front, but a considerable piece of the sleeve hung down behind the elbow. This pendent piece was sometimes extremely long, and was frequently lined with silk or fur.

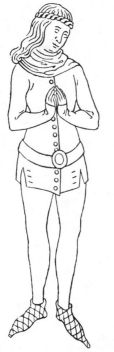

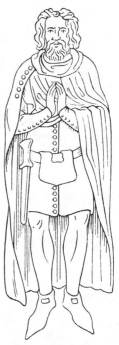

Fig. 211. GERMAN MEN'S DRESS OF THE FOURTEENTH CENTURY

Fig. 212. GERMAN MEN'S DRESS, SECOND HALF OF THE FOURTEENTH CENTURY

The cloak, *Heuke* or *Henke*, was not so often worn as in the fourteenth century. It still retained its earlier semicircular shape, and was gathered at the shoulder and fixed at first with a clasp and later by several buttons. (See Fig. 212.) It was no longer worn with the centre over the nape of the neck, but was put on so as to hang lower on the left side than on the right. It could be shortened by being raised with the left arm.

Besides these open cloaks, cloaks closed all round were worn, as well as cloaks which could be buttoned from top to bottom in front. These varied in length. They were called *Glocken* (bells), and were almost circular in cut.

The commonest form of leg-wear in the fourteenth century was still long hose. Like long stockings, they had feet, and covered the whole of the leg (Fig. 213). They were kept up by being attached at the top to a belt which was buckled round the body beneath the coat. These hose were as tight as possible ; they were sometimes of leather and sometimes of elastic material like wool. Those made of cloth had either one or two seams. The material was cut exactly in the shape of the leg, and was sewn either up the back only or at both back and front. The legs were often of different colours.

Toward the end of the fourteenth century tailors began to make hose of elastic material,[1] and to sew them together so that the combined hose made a garment that covered not only the legs, but the lower body. If the hose were made of inelastic material, the side-flaps with which the hose were fastened to the waist-belt were as broad as the material allowed, so as to cover the body completely front and back. If the hose were joined only at the back, the feet were made separately and attached afterward.

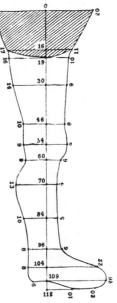

Fig. 213. Pattern of the Hose of the Fourteenth Century

The most usual form of headdress was the hood, variously called *Gugel*, *Kogel*, or *Kugel*, but it was worn only in rough weather. At other times it was allowed to hang down the back. These hoods varied greatly both in size and shape. Some were made with one seam in the front ; some with two seams, back and front. Sometimes the *Gugel* fitted closely round the head ; sometimes it was looser, and sometimes it reached down to the shoulders or encircled the body collar-wise, coming down almost to the elbows. It was either closed all round or made to be buttoned in front. These were the so-called *geknäuften Kogeln* (buttoned hoods). The hood had tips of varying length ; toward the end of the century it was often so long that it hung down as far as the calf of the leg, like a thin, stuffed tail. About the same time the edge of the *Gugel* was cut into points or trimmed with material of a different colour.

These hoods were made of cloth or of soft, pliant leather, often

[1] A material of this kind was *Scharlach* (scarlet), made of the finest wool, which was in great favour both with knights and rich citizens and which, owing to its great elasticity, was a more suitable material for hose than any other. The commonest colours of *Scharlach* were red and brown, but it was also obtainable in green, blue, or white. Probably the name of the material was afterward transferred to its colour.

dyed. They were lined with fur, adorned with erect plumes, and trimmed round the edge with numerous small pendent metal bugles.

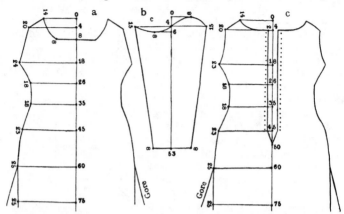

Fig. 214. Pattern of Woman's Dress in the Fourteenth Century
(*a*) Back ; (*b*) sleeve ; (*c*) front.

The usual footwear consisted of ankle-shoes enclosing the entire foot, but low shoes with long, pointed toes were also worn. These were fastened over the instep by clasps. In addition to these a tall kind of boot was worn. During the second half of the fourteenth century boots and shoes were often dispensed with, being replaced by leather soles on the hose.

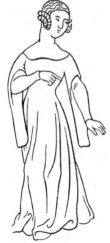

Fig. 215. German Women's Dress of the Fourteenth Century

Women's Dress. Changes in women's dress were chiefly at the neck and hips and sleeves. The under-dress was now somewhat low. It was laced in front or at the side—more rarely at the back—and fitted very closely all the way from the shoulders to far below the hips. From the hip-joint down it was gradually widened by the insertion of gussets at the back and side seams. It was of the same length all round, and was so long that the wearer had to raise it in front in order to be able to walk. The sleeves were tight from sleeve-hole to wrist, and were trimmed with small buttons at the back and from the wrist to the elbow. The sleeves were sometimes so long that they came half-way down the hand. Both dress and sleeves were still made in the old way—*i.e.*, back and front were sewn together only on the shoulders and down the sides, while the sleeves were straight and had only one seam, down the back. (See Fig. 214.)

The over-dress had the same shape as the one worn beneath it, and, except that it was made of more expensive material, differed from it only by having shorter sleeves (Fig. 215). These short sleeves were also as tight as possible ; in front they came only to the elbow, whereas the back of the sleeve fell in a long strip to the knee. The width of this strip was usually half that of the sleeve.

Another over-dress popular in Germany was the *Sorket*. It had no sleeves, and was cut away at both sides from shoulders to hips.

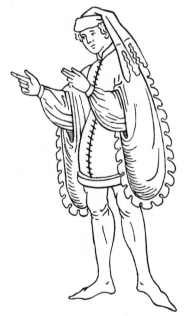

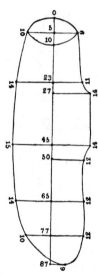

Fig. 216. German Men's Dress of the First Half of the Fifteenth Century

Fig. 217. Sack Sleeve of Fig. 216

Its name clearly betrays its French origin, and it exactly resembled its prototype the French *surcot* (Figs. 206 and 207).

This dress, which went entirely out of fashion during the second half of the century, was trimmed in accordance with English ideas. The *Limburger Chronik* tells us : " The over-dress was called *Sorket*. At both sides and at the foot it was slashed and trimmed, in winter with fur and in summer with silk, so that it was suitable for any lady at any time." If German women, like Frenchwomen, had had the upper part of the *Sorket* made entirely of fur the *Chronik* would certainly have mentioned it, or some mention of the fact would be found in the literature of the subject.

Men's Dress. Men's dress at the beginning of the fifteenth century

183

was in all essentials similar to that which they had worn at the end of the previous century, but the character of the separate items had undergone considerable change owing to incongruous combinations and degenerations in shape. An Austrian chronicler of this period says : " Every one dressed as he pleased. Some wore coats made of two kinds of material. Some had the left sleeve much wider than the right—wider even than the length of the whole coat—while others

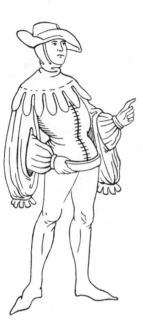

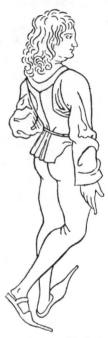

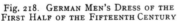

Fig. 218. German Men's Dress of the First Half of the Fifteenth Century

Fig. 219. German Men's Dress, Fifteenth Century

wore sleeves of equal width. Some again embroidered the left sleeve in various ways, with ribbons of all colours or with silver bugles threaded on silk strings. Some wore on the breast a kerchief of various colours embroidered with letters in silver and silk. Still others wore pictures on the left breast. Some had their clothes made so long that they could not dress or undress without assistance, or without undoing a multitude of small buttons dispersed all over the sleeve, the breast, and the abdomen. Some added to their clothes hems of cloth of a different colour ; others replaced these hems by numerous points and scallops. Every one wore hoods, until the former headdress of men had disappeared. Cloaks were hardly long enough to reach the hips."

In spite of all these differences the cut of the chief garment, the *Wams* (now called *Scheckenrock*, or *Schecke*, after the English ' jacket '), remained essentially as it had been. The sleeves exhibited some peculiarities of shape. They were now more or less wide, and took the form of sack sleeves (Figs. 216 and 217). These were either actual sacks closed at the end, or were left open and loosely tied, but provided with an opening higher up to let the arms through (Fig. 218). In the former case the sleeves were made in two parts, the only difference between them being that the lower part was cut away at the top while the other was not. In the other case—*i.e.*, when the sack sleeves were tied at the foot—they were made in one piece, cut quite. straight, and sewn up back or front. If the arms were to be completely covered these sack sleeves had to be supplemented by a second pair, which were either attached to the jacket with the first pair or belonged to an under-jacket. There were also jackets with sleeves equally wide all the way down. These wide sleeves were usually tied with a ribbon at the wrist so as to form a sort of ruffle. Sleeves were often so long that they extended far beyond the hand ; if the wearer wished to use his hands freely he had to turn the sleeves back. These elongations were called *Pieschen*.

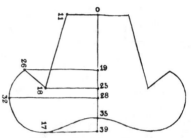

Fig. 220. SLEEVE OF FIG. 219

The *Wams*, or doublet, underwent other changes. By being considerably shortened it was transformed into a jacket. This usually had a small erect collar and a slit at the back or at both sides from the bottom hem to the hips. The back piece was sometimes made wider than necessary, and then gathered as tightly as possible in two pleats at the waist. The front was also cut very wide, but instead of being gathered in pleats it was heavily padded.

Toward the middle of the century the sleeve-holes of the jacket were very wide (Fig. 219), and the sleeves, which were not very wide, were cut to fit these wide sleeve-holes (Fig. 220). When such a sleeve was sewn up, its wide upper part formed a flat piece projecting all round ; when it was sewn into the jacket (the seam being on the under-side) the sleeve more than filled the sleeve-hole, the sleeve-hole being smaller than the flat piece. The sleeve was pushed through from inside and sewn in inside the jacket.

Another over-dress was the *Tappert*, also called *Trappers* or *Trapphart*. It had been evolved from a garment that was closed all round, but it had sleeves, often edged with fur. In course of time the *Tappert* assumed various forms. A very long and wide style of it, with sleeves, was a dress for high occasions, while a shorter type, equipped with a hood and open at the sides, served as an overall. The *Tappert* ousted the cloak almost completely.

Various other articles of dress besides the *Tappert* were in general use, but these were less for protection than for ornament. It was toward the end of the century that they came into use. Some were short and others were long, but all were fairly wide.

One was a kind of short tunic (Fig. 221) with low neck and long sleeves open on the upper side for almost their whole length. This

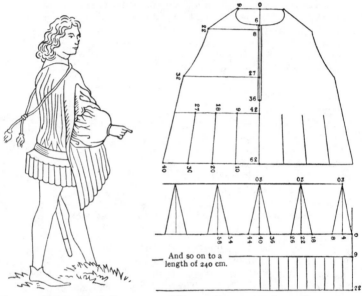

Fig. 221. GERMAN MEN'S DRESS, SECOND HALF OF THE FIFTEENTH CENTURY

Fig. 222. PATTERN OF OUTER GARMENT IN FIG. 221

tunic was open from the neck downward, and was fastened by means of buttons. The edge was stiffened and hung down like a series of tubes set closely side by side, the pleated tunic being stretched over these. This peculiar style of edge, closed all round, was obtained as follows. The bottom edge of the tunic (which was tighter at the top than lower down, though the front and back pieces were cut alike) was cut into peaks (Fig. 222) ; then a strip was sewn on whose upper edge was cut into the same number of peaks as there were in the tunic. These peaked edges were fitted into each other.

The stiffening of the edge was done thus : out of parchment or stiff leather, casings were made, 3–4 cm. in diameter, and 15–18 cm. long. A sufficient number of these were taken to give a total diameter equal to half the width of the edge that was to be stiffened. These casings, or tubes, were cut longitudinally into halves and sewn close together into the bottom band of the tunic trimming. The work was begun in the middle of the back. A deep pleat was made, and sewn down between two tubes at top and bottom. Then another tube was put at each side ; the material was drawn taut over the first tubes and sewn again to these and the next tubes at top and bottom. The material was then pulled over the second pair of tubes, and the third pair put in place, the material again being sewn between the tubes. And so on. It was of great importance that the tubes should hang perpendicularly and be quite close together. Finally, this band was strengthened by an inside lining of coarse linen, which was stitched down between each pair of tubes.

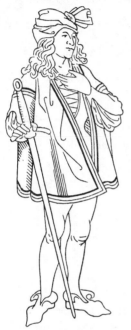

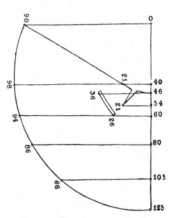

Fig. 223. German Men's Dress, Second Half of the Fifteenth Century

Fig. 224. Pattern for Outer Garment in Fig. 223

In the sleeves of this short tunic the seam was, as usual, on the under-side. It was hidden by the lining, because the upper side of the sleeve was slashed from near the shoulder.

Another form of over-garment was close-fitting at the top, but was widened from the waist down by gores to such an extent that large folds were produced at the foot. This was a short coat, with short sleeves ; it was open in front from neck to waist. The breast was padded. It is worthy of notice that the sleeve-seam was on the under-side and that the sleeve was pleated when it was sewn in at the sleeve-hole. The lower end of the sleeve was made to suit the taste of the wearer.

There was still another kind of tunic, reaching to the knee, with the upper part somewhat close-fitting. The width at the foot was considerable, and a girdle was always worn with it. In some cases it could be buttoned in front ; in others it was cut in a low V-shape down to the girdle, having a turn-over collar broad at the top and narrowing to a point. The sleeves were either long and wide or open and pendent. These tunics were made of rich material, sometimes

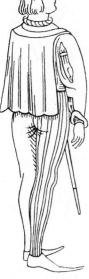

of different colours, and were often trimmed with fur or a wide border of gold. Some were quite plain.

In addition to these tunics there was also a kind of plaid, cut almost like a cloak, with very short sleeves, or merely with armholes (Figs. 223 and 224).

Toward the end of the century the upper classes were wearing the long, wide *robe* which was at the time fashionable in France. It was open in front, and a girdle was worn with it above the waist. This *robe* was usually made of finest damask, and had wide (or very tight)

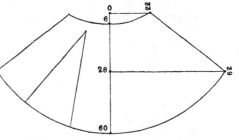

Fig. 225. German Men's Dress, Second Half of the Fifteenth Century

Fig. 226. Pattern of Cloak of Fig. 225

sleeves slashed at the elbows, and very often a fur collar, although some men wore it without the collar.

The cloak became again fashionable in the second half of the fifteenth century, but its shape had entirely changed. The large semicircular cape was now worn only on great occasions. The usual cloak of this period was small. It was made of cloth, velvet, or silk, thin felt, or even of fine, soft leather. It was rarely long enough to reach to the hips. Its shape was still semicircular, but it was much shorter than it had formerly been. It was usually shaped so as to lie closely on the left shoulder and to fasten on the right shoulder with strings or a small clasp.

There was another form of cloak, shaped like part of a sector. It was held in place by a cord across the breast. It covered only the back. (See Figs. 225 and 226.)

There were still other styles of cloak. They were worn loosely over the shoulders, and required no fastening, because they retained their position by their weight, which fell forward. They were mostly very wide, but much shorter at the back than at the corners.

Hose and breeches presented a motley appearance owing to the variegated colours and designs of the trimmings. Toward the end of the century the Germans began to wear the 'shorts' that were already in general use in France and England. They were put on over the long hose.

Footwear had not greatly changed, but the top-boots were now considerably longer. The legs of these boots were somewhat wide, and were slashed in front. Toward the end of the century the pointed toes gradually became shorter, and finally disappeared. The shoes

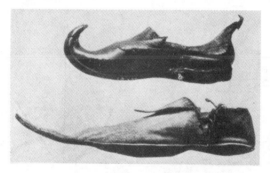

Fig. 227. Shoes with Pointed Toes, Fifteenth Century

were now round at the toes, and about 1492 they began to be very broad. In 1480 the pointed shoes had attained such a length that special wooden under-shoes had to be worn in order to preserve the shape and maintain the fit of the long shoes while on the foot.

The most important item of headdress was now the hat. It was made in all shapes and colours, and of various materials, including fur. Caps of different kinds were also worn, and coloured bandeaus were still fashionable. The hair was allowed to grow long, and was curled. The beard was shaved.

Women's Dress. The fashions that prevailed at the end of the fourteenth century were still in vogue at the beginning of the fifteenth. The bodices were still as close-fitting as ever, and long sleeves were still the rule.

The extravagantly expensive materials and trimmings, including points and bells, called forth various prohibitions from the ruling powers, but these were all in vain. Women as well as men trimmed their clothes with long peaks and points. Waist-belts, necks, and the points of the peaks were hung with little bells.

The under-dress continued without much change during nearly the whole of the fifteenth century. It fitted closely from the shoulders to below the hips, and was widened from that point downward by the insertion of gussets on both sides. It was made to fit still more closely by being laced in front (Fig. 229). It came only a little higher than the shoulders, and was very wide at the top, being cut in a very low V-shape at the back and in front.

The sleeves were tight, and came down to the hands. Short sleeves were worn only when the over-dress had long, very tight sleeves. The under-dress was the usual indoor wear, and was long enough to hide the feet. Some parts of this dress, especially the sleeves and the

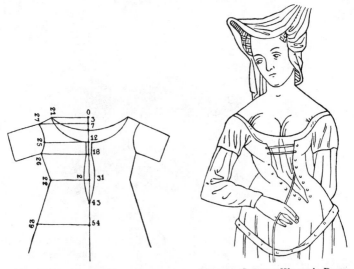

Fig. 228. WOMAN'S DRESS IN THE FIFTEENTH CENTURY

Fig. 229. GERMAN WOMAN'S DRESS (UNDER-ROBE), FIFTEENTH CENTURY

band round the foot, which were not covered by the over-dress, were made of the best and finest material available. If only a cloak was worn over it, the under-dress was fitted with sleeves like those of an over-dress both in shape and length (Fig. 230).

The over-dress was like the under-dress, except that it was laced at the back. It was very long (and became longer about the middle of the century), and was low-necked, although at the beginning of the century the neck had been high. The width varied. Like the under-dress, it sometimes fitted very closely from the shoulders to below the hips; sometimes the widening began at the bust. In the latter case the waist-belt came close up to the breast. The greatest change was in the sleeves. These were mostly long and pendent, but sack sleeves and long, open, wing-shaped sleeves with or without points were also fashionable. These points appeared not only at the edges, but also along the sleeve-seam. The shape of women's sleeves was similar to that of the sleeves of men's coats.

The cloak still served as a gown for special occasions. It was worn then, however, only by women of the upper classes (Fig. 230), who were distinguished by the simple cut and tasteful colour of their clothing from the middle classes, who were still fond of garish dress. The cloak was still the long-established semicircular one, and was still

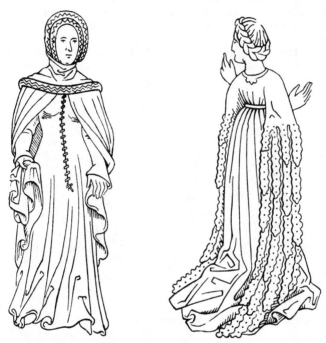

Figs. 230, 231. German Women's Costumes, First Half of the
Fifteenth Century

fastened with one clasp. The cloak for great occasions, however, was sector-shaped, and was fastened with clasps on both shoulders.

During the first half of the fifteenth century various cap-shaped forms of headdress were worn by women, both married and unmarried, but women of the upper classes wore nothing but the coif (*Haube, Hulle, Kruseler*), trimmed with several close rows of ribbon (Figs. 230 and 232). Over the back of this *Haube* was drawn, as in the fourteenth century, a white *Gugel* (hood), the lower edge of which was also trimmed with several close rows of ribbon. Frequently, also, women wore over this a long kerchief, of no great breadth, which was folded in two longitudinally and then rolled loosely and bunched into cap-shape.

This kerchief was in most cases white. The long ends were allowed to fall down behind.

The ordinary footwear consisted of low shoes with long, pointed toes.

Most of the attire described above underwent a complete change during the second half of the fifteenth century. Dresses became lower and lower at the neck and trains became longer. At the same time the preference for *mi-parti* and for points and bells as trimming went so far that the authorities did all they could to discourage the use of rich material, expensive trimming, and extravagant ornamentation.

While the under-dress remained as it was, the changes in the over-dress were extensive. The fashion now was to have the dress

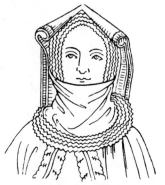

Fig. 232. HEADDRESS WORN BY GERMAN WOMEN, FIRST HALF OF THE FIFTEENTH CENTURY

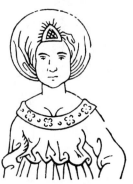

Fig. 233. GERMAN WOMEN'S DRESS, MIDDLE OF THE FIFTEENTH CENTURY

close-fitting to below the bust, even without a waist-belt, and as wide as possible from that point down. Nearly all the changes that were made in it were intended to achieve this end.

With that purpose in view the over-dress, which was open at the back to below the shoulder-blades, and arranged for lacing, was now made close-fitting to below the breast, then quickly widening downward. The waist-belt was first put on low down ; later waist-belt and dress were pulled up so that a loose mass of folds was made at breast-height all round (Fig. 233). Dresses that were tight all the way down to below the hips were widened in another way. A strip was cut out of the front of the dress from the foot up to below the breast, then replaced by a much wider one (see Figs. 234–236). Before it was sewn in the top of this wider strip was folded or pleated so that it fitted exactly into the place of the excised strip ; then its upper edge was sewn in with a double seam. The folds of the inserted strip were stitched to a distance of 14 cm. or a little more from the top,

and then allowed to fall loose. Finally the sides of the whole strip
were sewn in. The dress was thus made much wider below, but
close-fitting from the top to the point where the folds were stitched.
These folds or pleats were frequently padded. If still more width
were desired additional gussets were inserted at the sides and at the
back. These reached up to the hips. Dresses of this kind were

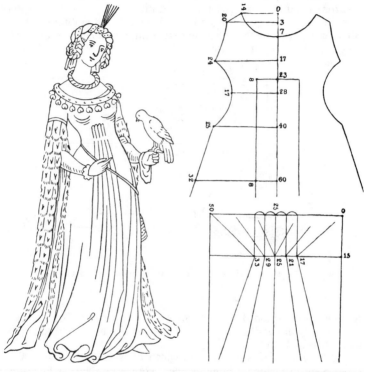

Fig. 234. GERMAN WOMEN'S DRESS,
FIFTEENTH CENTURY

Figs. 235, 236. PATTERN FOR FIG. 234
WITH INSERTED STRIP

usually open at the back down to the hips, and were fastened by
lacing.

The most important improvement in women's dress, however, took
place at the end of the fifteenth century. The bodice was then
divided entirely from the skirt. The two were cut separately, and
then sewn together by a double seam. The tailor was now able to
make the dress of any desired shape, to make the bodice long or short,
loose or tight, and to pleat the skirt in any way that was desired. This
improvement brought with it a far greater variety of cut, but it was
a considerable time before the new style was universally adopted.

The greatest possible variety characterized the shape and width of the neck and the sleeves in women's attire during the second half of the fifteenth century.

The neck was as low as possible ; various styles were current. The shoulders were sometimes completely exposed, or if they were covered, most of the back and breast was bare. In the latter case women covered the bust with a dainty wimple embroidered with gold. A chronicler of the day describes this fashion thus : "Girls and women wore beautiful wimples, with a broad hem in front, embroidered with silk, pearls, or tinsel, and their underclothing had pouches into which they put their breasts. Nothing like it had ever been seen before."

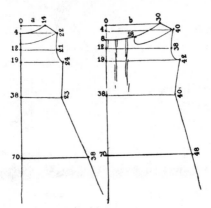

Fig. 237   Over-dress of German Women, End of the
Fifteenth Century
(a) Back ; (b) front.

At the same period, however, some dresses were by no means so low-cut. Some of them were quite high at the neck, and some even had fairly high collars.

Similar variety was seen in the width of women's dresses. Many types were in fashion. Some women wore waist-belts, while others dispensed with their use. The favourite style was a dress that fitted closely from the neck to the hips. As a rule dresses were immoderately long, and ladies of the upper classes frequently wore trains (*Schleppen*, or *Schweifen*) so long that they had to be carried.

Toward the close of the fifteenth century women began to wear very long, wide dresses, with long, wide sleeves. These fitted closely only over the breast and shoulders, hanging loose all round from the waist down. These dresses, which were cut like wide tunics, were made still fuller by the insertion of gussets. Some of them were closed all round ; others were open all down the front.

In the former case the dresses were very low across the shoulders (Fig. 237). The front was gathered at the bust in several large pleats

Plate III

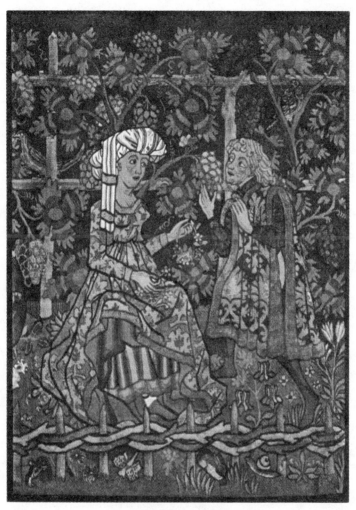

PAIR OF LOVERS
From a Swiss tapestry of the fifteenth century

194

and fastened with a clasp (Fig. 238). In the other style, although it was quite open in front, the dress was very close-fitting to below the breast ; this was achieved by gathering the material into a clasp (Fig. 239). This not only fastened the front parts of the dress together, but also raised them a little.

Toward the middle of the century the long, pendent sack sleeves went quite out of fashion, except those with the hand-opening near the wrist. More popular than these, however, were the long, open,

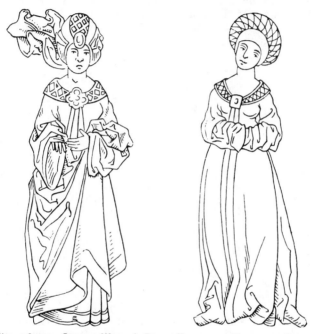

Figs. 238, 239. German Women's Dress, End of the Fifteenth Century

hanging sleeves called *Flügel*. Frequently so long that they trailed on the ground, they were splendidly finished with fur and points. Near the end of the century appeared sleeves that extended beyond the hand. They were rather tight at the top, but so wide lower down that the width at the foot was nearly equal to their length. At the same period slashed sleeves came more and more into favour. Some were slashed the whole length at the back, and tied with cords drawn not quite taut over the dainty, puffed white under-sleeves. Some sleeves were so long that they extended beyond the hands and had to be turned back when the hands were to be used.

All these sleeves were cut straight, and, except the very wide ones, had only one seam. According to taste this seam ran in front or at the back, or even under the sleeve. The sleeve-hole was usually as small as possible, and shaped either like an egg with the small end up or like an upright oval.

The sleeves of the under-dress, which were visible through the open sleeves of the over-dress, were now wide, now tight ; in some cases they were so long that they came beyond the hands and in others so short that they hardly reached the middle of the forearm.

Now that wide over-dresses were fashionable the cloak was used only for protection in rough weather. It was either semicircular or shaped like a sector or like an arc, and was gathered into numerous close pleats. It had a broad, smooth, turn-over collar, sometimes

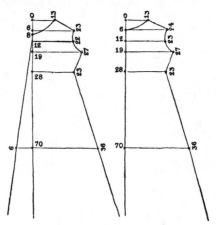

Fig. 240. Women's Over-dress, End of the Fifteenth Century

stiffened, and was usually more than knee-length. Only married women wore it. Girls did not wear it till they became brides.

The cloak still continued to be worn at the various royal Courts as the dress for occasions of great ceremony. It was shaped like a sector of a circle, covered only the back, and was held in position by a braided strap that passed across the breast. This cloak had a train, and its length was in proportion to the rank of the wearer.

The *Tappert* continued to be worn till about the year 1480, but it was mostly used as an over-coat, and therefore always had a hood. The most popular type of it was open down both sides.

During the second half of the fifteenth century the headdress exhibited great diversity of appearance. There were hair-nets made of gold thread, in which the hair was so disposed that it formed large pendent masses at both sides of the face. Over these nets women wore kerchiefs with points at the ends, or cowl-like coifs, also with points. There were also other forms of headdress which did not cover the hair. The hair was then worn in plaits, which either hung down the back or were arranged in various ways round the head. Other women wore circular rolls or pads covered with ribbon or cloth (see Plate III), as well as various kinds of caps, circlets, bandeaus, etc. Ruffled caps (*Kruseler*) had been out of fashion since the middle of the century.

Footwear took the form of pointed shoes. Ladies wore them of such length that special soles had to be attached to keep the long points in position. At the close of the century even women's shoes were much shorter, and the fashion of long, pointed toes ultimately disappeared.

Gloves of silk material or of soft leather were at first worn only by ladies of high standing. The fashion quickly spread, however, and by the end of the century gloves were looked upon as indispensable by prosperous middle-class people.

ITALY

In the fifteenth century Italian dress exhibited the same variety as that of France, England, and Germany. Still, in spite of foreign influences, it preserved its own peculiar national character, and was distinguished from German dress by far more lavish adornment and by the richness of the materials used. In Italy, as in other countries, numerous enactments were promulgated with the object of restraining the ever-increasing luxury in attire, but these were just as unsuccessful in Italy as elsewhere.

Men's Dress. For the short over-dress the styles that prevailed in the fourteenth century continued into the fifteenth. These were either close-fitting all the way down, or widened from the shoulders down, but changes in shape and finish greatly altered their appearance. Fur trimming was still in favour, and was displaced only for a brief period by points, which appealed to Italian taste also. The greatest change was in the sleeves. Fashion prescribed no special styles, and every one was left free to follow his own taste.

The first changes in the shape of the coat that the fifteenth century saw were unimportant. The coat was much shorter. Although the high neck remained fashionable for a time, the neck was now mostly low, cut in a deep V-shape both back and front, allowing the under-dress to be seen. Thus the slit at the breast, which came down to the waist, and could be buttoned, became unnecessary. During the first half of the fifteenth century close-fitting coats went entirely out of fashion. Coats were cut away above the hips and a pleated skirt sewn on, the seam being hidden by a girdle buckled over it. Even with the coats that widened gradually the girdle was now worn higher up, to keep in place the pleats of the coat. In most cases, however, these pleats were sewn down when the coat was made. This last style of coat, the sleeves of which were long and full, or tight and half-length, or long, wide, and pendent, was mostly open at both sides from the foot to the hips, and had all the edges trimmed with fur.

These coats (Fig. 241), widening downward, were made to fit the body closely ; the skirt was sewn on in such a manner that the pleats in it reached into the upper part in the shape of thick, pointed scallops (Fig. 242). The skirt was sewn to the body of the coat as

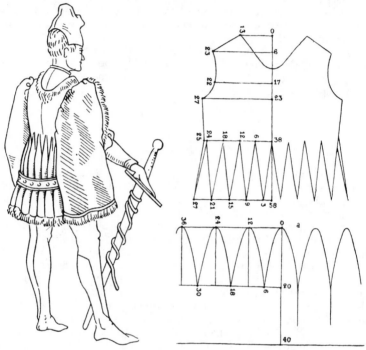

Fig. 241. Italian Men's Dress,
Fifteenth Century

Fig. 242. Extension of Skirt
for Fig. 241
(a) The skirt to be added.

follows. In the bottom edge of the upper part was cut a long, narrow gusset for each pointed scallop. The upper edge of the skirt, which was straight and wide, was shaped into an equal number of scallops, as long as the gussets, but much broader. These were sewn to the top of the skirt so that each formed a roll that increased in width downward. Each of these rolls represented a pleat whose size varied with the shape of the scallops. The coat was then arranged for buttoning down to the abdomen.

Besides these somewhat long coats, the Italians also wore the short, close-fitting German jacket, but with wide, slashed sleeves.

In ceremonial dress or dress indicating distinction the long over-

198

garments continued almost exactly as they had been in the fourteenth century. They were, if anything, even longer, and open all down the front. The increase in width began only at the breast, and if twice or four times the width of the material was not enough, the necessary width was obtained by sufficiently large gussets at the sides.

The sleeves of the long over-coats were of all kinds. They were mostly long and, especially in front, very wide. Sack sleeves were

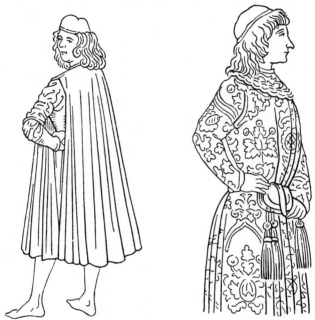

Figs. 243, 244. ITALIAN MEN'S DRESS, FIFTEENTH CENTURY

also worn, the opening for the hand being at the wrist and as tight as possible. Fur trimming continued in the fifteenth century.

When, during the second half of the fifteenth century, long, wide over-coats again became the universal fashion in Italy, as elsewhere, they showed a great variety of shape, due more to small changes of detail than to any great change of general cut. The cut of the tunic was, strictly speaking, the same as before. Usually it reached to the feet, sometimes to the ankles, and sometimes only half-way down the calf. The width showed similar variation, but the coats were never so tight that the wearing of a girdle did not cause numerous folds round the body. A girdle was not always worn, but when it was used it was a richly ornamented leather belt worn obliquely, or a thick cord, or a long shot silk sash. Sometimes the coat was fitted with a small strap, through which the cord or belt was passed and tied according to taste.

There were other changes in these long over-garments. They were either closed all down the front or had merely a long opening at the breast. The neck was high or low, round, oval, or square, and the coat was fitted either with an erect collar or with a hood. Toward the end of the century the practice came in of omitting sleeves altogether (Fig. 243) or of making them like those of the German *Tappert*—i.e., open down both sides from the shoulder—or they were more or less tight instead of wide as hitherto.

When the fashion of tight sleeves for the long coats came in the cut of the coat also was slightly changed. Instead of gradually widening from the breast down, it fitted closely down to the hips, the widening beginning there. This style usually had a long opening at the breast, which could be buttoned, but it was sometimes preferred to have it open all down the front, with a drawstring by means of which it could be open or closed at will.

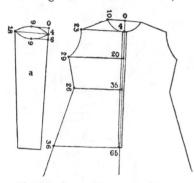

Fig. 245. OUTER GARMENT OF FIG. 244
(a) Sleeve.

Beneath this long over-garment was worn either a long or a short coat, or even a kind of jacket. The trimming was usually a narrow edging of fur or coloured material; very often the entire jacket was lined in the same way. This jacket was wide and open in front, and both sides of the front were very wide, so that they could be thrown back. This extra width at the front was often made like a wrap by being continued round the neck as a fall-over collar.

Mi-parti was sometimes introduced into the long overcoats.

The under-coat usually worn beneath the overcoat was of the same shape, except that it was much shorter and tighter, and in particular had short sleeves. Speaking generally, the under-coats were close-fitting, the skirt gradually widening from the hips down. The neck was in most cases high rather than low, and usually had a low, upright collar. The breast was made to button.

Hose were still close-fitting. They were not very different from what they had been at the end of the fourteenth century. Made of elastic material, the hose (which now had feet) came up to the hips and were sewn together both between the legs and down back and front, so that they completely covered the lower part of the body all round. They were fastened either with a belt or with a cord drawn through the top hem, or were connected with the foot of the jacket by strings or buttons. Hose made of less elastic material could not be joined in this fashion unless they were first widened greatly at the seat, for the wearer could neither have stooped nor sat down in them. At the end of the fourteenth century a beginning had already been made with this widening—*i.e.*, the wearer's seat was covered by a broad gore. This was not, however, sewn to the hose. During the second half of the fifteenth century a better method was found—the gore and the hose were cut much wider, even some-

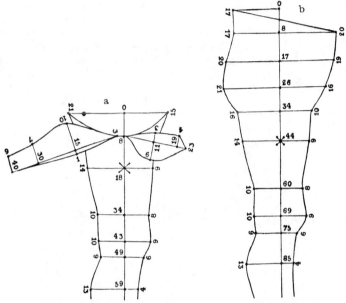

Figs. 246, 247. Pattern of Hose, Second Half of the Fifteenth Century
(*a*) Inner half ; (*b*) outer half.

what convex. When the hose were sewn together there was produced an enlargement which prevented actual strain, but still left an uncomfortable tightness. In front the hose were joined, as in former times, by a pouch-shaped flap which closed them. These hose, made of coarse material, were fastened at the top in exactly the same way as the elastic variety, except that no cord was needed, as they were made to fit better above the hips than those made of elastic material and were not so likely to slip down. (See Figs. 246–248.)

The cloak, the long, wide cape over back and shoulders, without either sleeves or armholes, went entirely out of fashion in Italy in the first half of the fifteenth century. On the other hand, the coat-shaped, wide plaids were in general use in rough weather. Some of them were more like a cloak than a coat. They were simply square pieces of material hanging over both shoulders down to the knees,

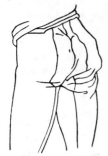

with elongated armholes at the sides. They could be worn either like a Roman toga or down the back like a cloak. The voluminous folds gave them a handsome appearance.

There was another kind of wrap, which, although similar to that just described, was really more like the sleeveless over-coats, only much wider (Fig. 249). These were mostly of dark material, lined with brighter stuff. They were semicircular, and had armholes. The great width across the breast was disposed of by being turned back and outward at both sides. Some-times flaps of this kind were added to wraps of a different shape ; they were connected by means of a collar that reached some way down the back.

Fig. 248. Back Part of Hose, Second Half of the Fifteenth Century

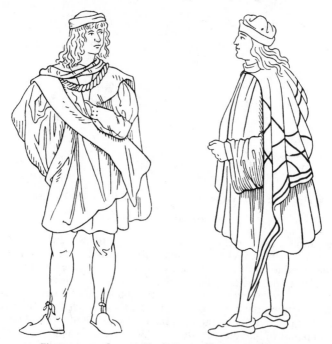

Figs. 249, 250. Italian Men's Dress, Fifteenth Century

To wraps of this kind a shoulder-collar (or real cape) was added, completely hiding the armholes. This garment was something like a close-fitting tunic across the breast, but was much wider behind. These collars were variously shaped, and many of them were very peculiar. (See Figs. 250 and 251.)

Not content with these wraps, dandies sometimes decked themselves out in the various short and close-fitting shoulder-capes then current

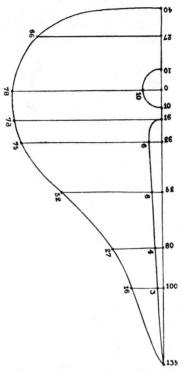

Fig. 251. COLLAR OF WRAP OF FIG. 250

in France and Germany. The *toghe*, a shoulder-cape reaching to the feet and gathered at the breast, was worn during the fifteenth century only as part of ceremonial dress.

Footwear underwent little change during the fifteenth century, and only the tops, shape, and trimming of shoes were altered. Of all the various styles of shoes, the wide, ankle-high variety was the most popular. These were made of some soft leather, and ornamented with a broad strap, usually white. Low-cut shoes of this kind were usually kept in position by means of a strap across the instep.

Women's Dress. Women's over-dresses underwent some very important alterations during the second half of the fifteenth century

The first change affected those garments which began to widen from the bust down. These were made still more voluminous by the insertion of larger and more numerous gores or gussets. The height or lowness at the neck continued to be a matter of individual choice. Older ladies wore high-necked dresses, and younger ones favoured a low neck or an open, V-shaped front. The sleeves lost their amplitude, and were either quite close-fitting or of a moderate and equal width throughout, but they were now so long that they extended beyond the hands and had to be thrown back. These dresses were usually worn without a girdle, but one was sometimes

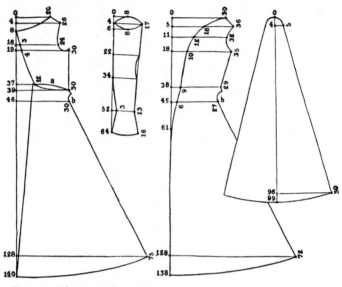

Size of cut at hip at *a* according to hip
measurement.

Fig. 252. PATTERN OF CLOSE-FITTING BROCADED DRESS OF ITALIAN
WOMEN, FIFTEENTH CENTURY

worn to assist in tucking up the dress and thus to correct its extreme length. Something quite new was the use of thick patterned silks and velvets, interwoven at times with silver or gold. As these materials were very heavy, and could be draped only in large folds, the cut of the dress had to be altered so that the stiffness of the material should not unduly interfere with freedom of movement. Previous to any change in the cut, however, the long train was abandoned with these stiff dresses. Trains were worn only on great occasions, and were then borne by attendants.

On the whole, the dresses were of the same shape as before. They were either close-fitting or wide all the way down. But both styles suffered some change in cut.

The style that was close-fitting down to the hips was made open down the whole front ; the two front wings were laced across the breast. The dress was usually left open from the waist down, although buttons and buttonholes were provided. The sleeves were as tight as possible, but very long—down to the tips of the fingers— and slashed longitudinally or across at the elbows, revealing a puff

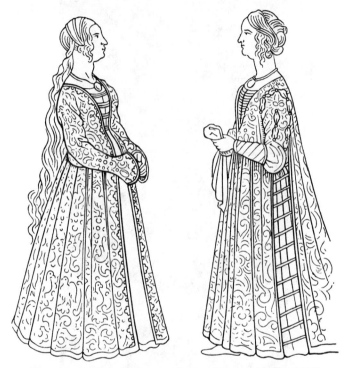

Figs. 253, 254. ITALIAN DRESSES, SECOND HALF OF THE FIFTEENTH CENTURY

made of some delicate tissue disposed in folds. There was also a change in the back. It was divided longitudinally, and shaped at the waist somewhat after the manner that had previously been restricted to the sides. The two edges were then sewn together, a perfectly close fit being thus produced. The gussets at the sides extended up to the hips ; they were not now pointed at the top, but were blunted or rounded.

In order to secure a perfectly close fit at the back, the back was separated from the skirt. Both were shaped to some extent at the sides and again sewn together. The longitudinal folds that appeared in the dresses made of stiff material were ironed in with a warm

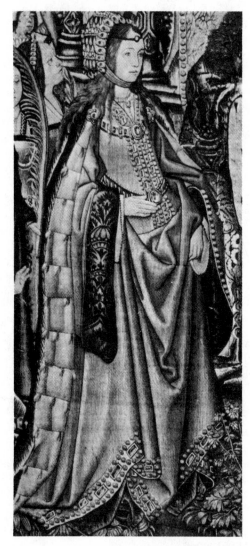

Fig. 255. SECTION OF A SO-CALLED MAXIMILIAN GOBELIN
End of the fifteenth century.

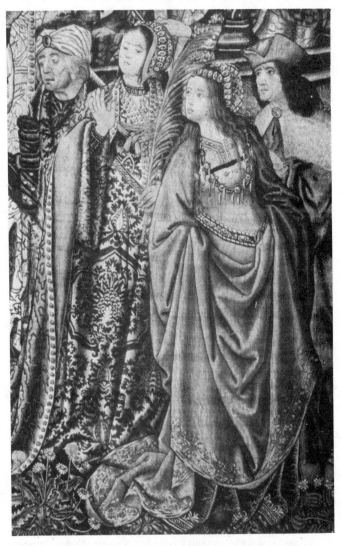

Fig. 256. SECTION OF A SO-CALLED MAXIMILIAN GOBELIN
End of the fifteenth century.

rounded iron. Dresses that were wide from the shoulders down were
cut in the same way as those made of thinner materials, but in their
case the neck was low and the front slit extended to below the breast
(Fig. 254). Other differences were due to the manner of making
rather than to the cut. The back and front (each being made of

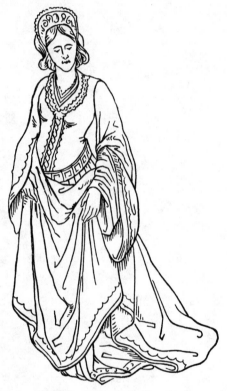

Fig. 257. ITALIAN WOMEN'S DRESS, SECOND HALF OF THE
FIFTEENTH CENTURY

suitable width by the insertion of gussets) were sewn together only
on the shoulders. The sides were left open, either all the way or at
least from the hips down. In both cases the unjoined parts were
loosely laced together. If the dress was open from the armpit only
the top half of the sleeves could be sewn to the dress. This, however,
was not always done with a continuous seam—the sleeves were sometimes attached to the dress by small buttons sewn on short distances
apart, so as to reveal puffs of delicate tissue disposed in folds. The
same delicate material peeped out from all the slashes—at the elbows,
at the back of the upper arm and forearm, and sometimes also at the

front of the upper sleeve. These slashes were held in place by small buttons or by loose lacing. The sleeves were close-fitting on the forearm and gradually widened from the elbow to the shoulder.

Sometimes, too, these dresses were worn with short sleeves reaching only to the elbows, and occasionally they had no sleeves at all. In both cases the similarly slashed sleeves of the dress worn beneath were visible. In these under-dresses the bodice and the skirt and sometimes even the sleeves were not infrequently made of different materials.

SPAIN

Men's Dress. Even after the downfall of the Moorish dominion the influence of Oriental styles of dress long continued to be felt in Spain, and was only gradually ousted by French fashions. The latter were adopted by the upper classes, and especially by the knights (the chief opponents of the Moors), long before they became current among the lower classes of the people.

By the middle of the fourteenth century French fashions had been completely adopted by the aristocratic classes in Spain, but the Spaniards had retained far more of their own national peculiarities than the English or the Germans had done. Like Italian dress, that of Spain developed in a genuinely national way on lines borrowed from France, and after it had attained its highest development, in the sixteenth century, it became in turn the model for French costume.

To begin with, the Spaniards imitated the tightness and shortness that were such outstanding features of French dress. As a result, their coats in front and their sleeves were made to button. The waist-belt of the knight was fastened low down round the hips, and the nether-garments were made as tight as possible. The cut of these clothes was the same in Spain as in France, Germany, and elsewhere. Along with this costume was worn a semicircular cloak which reached only to the hips, and was fastened with a few large buttons from neck to breast.

Besides this close-fitting clothing, the Spaniards wore long, wide clothing like that of the same period in France. Occasionally both were worn together.

Of these wide coats two were usually worn at the same time, one over the other. The inner one fitted closely round the shoulders, the width gradually increasing from that point down. It was as a rule closed all round, and had a short opening at the breast and long, very tight sleeves that buttoned from wrist to elbow (Fig. 258). The over-garment was always open down the front, and had buttons down to the knee. These were used or not in accordance with individual taste. The sleeves (if they could be so called, for they were more like flaps covering the armholes, and did not quite reach the elbow) were semicircular, and quite open on the under side. Their edges were sewn to the edges of the armslits or armholes. The military uniform of the knights was also modelled on the French style, although it retained features that betrayed Moorish influence. It was distinguished by truly Oriental splendour. In contrast to those of other nations, the Spanish military coats always had sleeves. These coats, worn over the chain mail, were till the fourteenth century long and wide. That is to say, they rather resembled the Moorish caftan—all the more so as they were made of richly patterned Arabian stuffs.

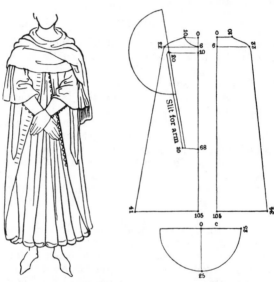

Fig. 258. SPANISH MEN'S DRESS, FOURTEENTH CENTURY

Fig. 259. CUT OF FIG. 258

During the first decade of the fourteenth century these military coats were open all down the front, and held in position by a girdle or a coloured sash. Later they were buttoned, and were much tighter and shorter, while the sleeves were also smaller. As nothing but silk or fine woollen stuffs with coloured patterns was used for these military coats, they retained a great deal of their Oriental character. They were cut in the manner usual among the knights of other countries at that time. They fitted smoothly across the chest (Fig. 260), becoming gradually wider lower down. The only differences were in the sleeves, which came above the elbow, in the erect collar, and in the open front, which was buttoned at the breast. The front skirts of the coat increased in width downward, so that they overlapped a little. The sleeves of the military coat were cut straight, widening a little only at the elbows, and gradually narrowing toward the hand. Toward the middle of the fourteenth century these military coats became ever tighter and shorter. They were then made of material of one colour, embroidered with the scutcheon of the wearer, so that during the second half of the century the only difference between them and those of other countries lay in the peculiarly Spanish style of the sleeves. (See Fig. 262.) At a later time the sleeves were cut open longitudinally in front and made into pendent sleeves, or they were considerably lengthened and divided into six or eight or more stripes with pointed edges.

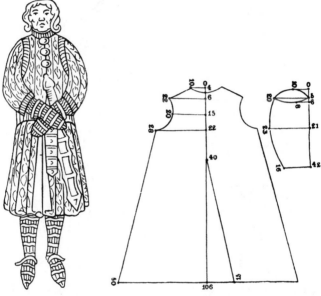

Fig. 260. Spanish Men's Dress, Fourteenth Century

Fig. 261. Cut of Fig. 260

In the course of the fifteenth century the introduction of iron armour made this military coat out of date here as elsewhere, and with it disappeared in Spain, as in other countries, the richly ornamented girdle buckled low down round the hips.

The commonest headdress was the hood. The lower edge was very frequently extended so as to form a capacious cape, reaching half-way down the upper arm and ending in a cord-like tip. The hood buttoned down the front ; the edges were trimmed with braid or shaped into points. The simplest style was the most favoured one.

The Spaniards also wore a kind of turban. It was simply a close-fitting, stiff cap, with a band made of numerous folds of other material round it.

Their footwear consisted of high ankle-shoes of leather or other hard-wearing material, or of soft, pliant boots reaching to the calf. In both cases the French fashion of long, pointed toes was adopted.

Women's Dress. From the middle of the fourteenth century Spanish women too began to adopt French styles of dress, after having retained for long a costume that had developed out of the ancient Roman dress. This costume consisted of a tunic with long, tight

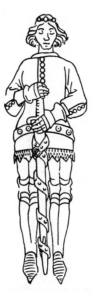

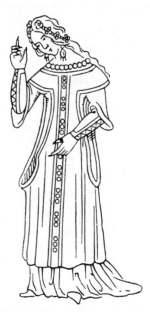

Fig. 262. SPANISH MEN'S DRESS,
FOURTEENTH CENTURY

Fig. 263. SPANISH WOMEN'S DRESS,
FOURTEENTH CENTURY

sleeves, a similar tunic with wide sleeves, worn over the first, and an oblong, cloak-like over-garment. Moorish influence had affected women's dress but slightly, and was evident more in the trimming than in the cut.

From the middle of the fourteenth century onward the principal garment of Spanish women was the dress. It no longer enclosed the body in voluminous folds, but was somewhat close-fitting. It was mostly very long, and had a long train. No girdle was worn with it. (See Fig. 263.) It had very tight sleeves, and was buttoned or laced at the back. The sleeves were so narrow that they did not quite enclose the arms, but allowed the dainty white sleeves of the chemise to be seen.

These dresses fitted closely down to the hips, but were wider from that point down. This widening was produced by the insertion of gussets at the side-seams which connected the back and front pieces of the dress. When this dress was worn alone it was opened all down the front and buttoned. When a second dress was worn above it, this second dress was buttoned down the front, but the under-dress was open down to the middle and laced. When the two were worn together the under one was shorter than the other, while the sleeves of the upper were much wider than those of the under-dress, but did not come below the elbows. In addition to these, Spanish ladies of the upper classes wore various kinds of wraps, chief among them being a large, semicircular, embroidered, lined cloak, low at the neck. The

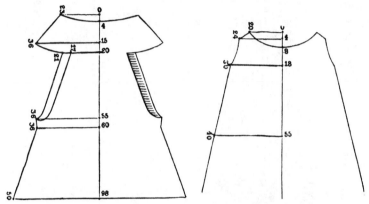

Fig. 264. Wrap of Spanish Women   Fig. 265. Spanish Women's Dress, Fourteenth Century

cloak was fastened with a clasp at the breast or on the right shoulder. In the latter case the neck was high, and the cloak was oblong in shape.

Another style of cloak resembled the *surcot* worn by Frenchwomen in the thirteenth century. The cloak of the Spanish women, however, had much less ornamentation. It was made of material of one colour, and the only trimming was one row of buttons down the front. The side-openings were remarkably long, and the back piece from the shoulder-blades down to the middle of the thigh was much wider than the front.

Toward the end of the fourteenth century the close-fitting dresses were displaced by others which were tight only at the bust, gradually widening lower down. These had a quite different appearance according as they were worn with or without a girdle (see Figs. 266 and 267). Even the sleeves were different. Sometimes they were wider and longer than before, or were tight at the top as before ; sometimes they were very wide at the forearm and very long. This last style of sleeve had the edge cut into points, while the former styles of sleeves (as well as the cut at the neck) were trimmed with a broad edging of braid. (See Figs. 266 and 267.) The neck was not

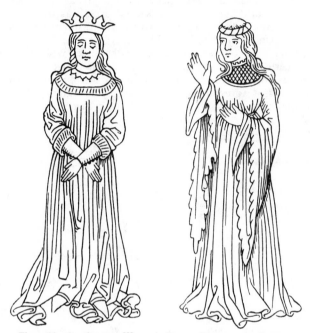

Figs. 266, 267. SPANISH WOMEN'S DRESS, FOURTEENTH CENTURY

so low, and the bareness of the neck was covered by a chemise of fine embroidered material with a frill at the top.

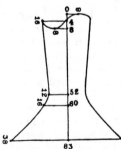

Fig. 268. SLEEVE OF UNDER-DRESS OF SPANISH WOMEN

While the over-dress passed through all these changes, the under-dress retained its earlier form, except that the tight sleeves were so long that they extended beyond the hand, widening greatly beyond the wrist. The cut of the sleeves was the usual one for tight sleeves, but enough length and width were left in front to suit the new shape (Fig. 268). The sleeve-seam was at the back.

Spanish women were specially fond of loose wraps, and by combining the roomy cloak with the more comfortable *surcot* they produced a quite peculiar over-garment (Fig. 269). It came only to the knee. In cut it was little more than a semicircle ; it was open at the sides from about the middle of the upper arm to the foot. (See Fig. 270.) A wide, stiff, erect collar surrounded the neck. The upper edge of this collar was made to turn slightly outward by having a few narrow pieces cut out of it.

All the edges of these garments were cut into points or bordered with fur.

In colour the clothes of Spanish women were bright and attractive. White, red, pale blue, pink, light violet, and sea-green were favourite colours.

The shape of the women's foot-coverings resembled that of the men's. They were, of course, daintier and more delicately made, and were frequently adorned with embroidery and gold braid. They were usually of leather or some hard-wearing coloured material.

Spanish women wore no headdress till the end of the fourteenth century. They used a kerchief of moderate size. It lay on the head, and was kept in position by a bandeau which passed across the forehead (Fig. 269). This peculiar kerchief had, of course, been employed at an earlier period as a protection against rough weather, and seems to have been of Moorish origin. The hair was worn hanging loose, or held together by a string of pearls, a wreath, or a roll of coloured material. At the end of the fourteenth century women began to enclose it, loose or plaited, in large hair-nets.

In the fourteenth century it was considered fashionable for Spanish ladies to grow their fingernails to what would now be thought an inordinate length, but although they were not pared they were tended with great care.

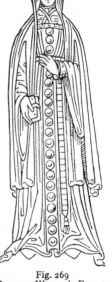

Fig. 269
SPANISH WOMEN'S DRESS,
FOURTEENTH CENTURY

The love of finery that prevailed in Spain during the fourteenth century continued to increase to such an extent, in spite of all the edicts of the authorities, that in the fifteenth century all attempts to control it were finally given up as useless.

Men's Dress. Dress was made more or less closely in accordance with French models, but it was the men who imitated these fashions most faithfully, retaining only a few national features.

As in France, two styles of dress were worn in Spain : a long, wide coat girdled at the waist and the short, close-fitting doublet. The former was worn by the upper classes. It was not only the usual ceremonial dress, but also the prescribed garb of the numerous knightly orders, who held a prominent place in Spanish life.

The cut of these long, wide coats was that of the ancient tunic.

Any changes were merely in the method of fastening, and this followed the French model.   At this period French fashions also governed the styles for the sleeves of these long, wide coats.   Straight sleeves, sleeves tight at the top and very wide lower down, the various styles of sack sleeves, the numerous types of pendent sleeves—all were imitated.   Over these long, wide coats was worn a cloak—especially by the knightly orders—which was either semicircular or oblong, the latter passing in thick folds round the neck.   The cloak, which usually had a small, erect collar, was fastened in front by a cord attached to the top edge of the collar.   It was also worn as a protection

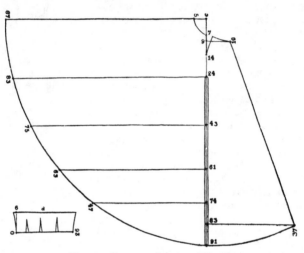

Fig. 270. Shape of Cloak in Fig. 269

against inclement weather, but in that case it was merely a large oblong or semicircular piece of cloth thrown over the shoulders according to individual taste.

About the middle of the fifteenth century padded shoulders, *mahoîtres*, became fashionable, and were worn especially with these long coats.   At the same time long, padded bodices came in, and the folds of the wide coats were drawn tightly from the shoulders toward the waist and sewn firmly down.

The close-fitting clothing which up to the middle of the fifteenth century was worn almost exclusively by the middle classes, and which about that time became the universal dress in Spain, was also a faithful imitation of the French fashion.

Owing to the connexion with Naples which Alphonso V of Aragon had acquired in 1435, the more comfortable Italian dress became increasingly worn in Spain in the second half of the fifteenth century ; by the end of the century it had entirely ousted the French styles.

216

In footwear and headdress too the Spaniards imitated first French
and afterward Italian fashion.   It was only in the matter of headdress

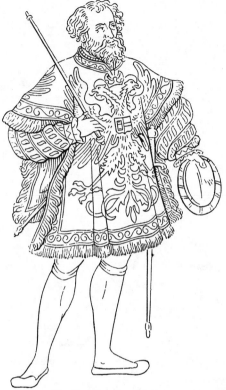

Fig. 271. IMPERIAL HERALD

that the old preference for Moorish styles was still shown, for right
through the century the turban-like caps continued to be worn, even
by the upper classes.

THE SIXTEENTH CENTURY

SPAIN

THE early years of the sixteenth century brought little change in **men's dress** in Spain. Italian fashions continued to prevail —long, close-fitting hose, over these slashed breeches reaching nearly to the knee, a slashed doublet not too tight, over-garments of various kinds, a cowl-shaped cap, and low shoes rounded at the toes.

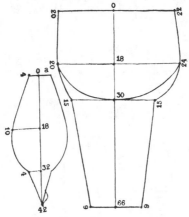

Fig. 272. SPANISH BREECHES, BEGINNING OF THE
SIXTEENTH CENTURY

The first alteration was an increase of the slashes in the breeches and in the sleeves of the doublet. The breeches themselves were cut on lines similar to those of previous years, except that they were now a little easier fitting, and were lined with thin material cut much wider than the breeches themselves and forming puffs visible through the slashing. This lining, which had already begun to be worn at the end of the fifteenth century with breeches, was sewn to the latter at the top and foot and at the edges of the front opening. The front flap was not now a flat pouch, but a protuberance which was often slashed and padded. (See Figs. 272 and 273.) The hose with feet worn underneath the breeches were open both in front and at the back. Many men, however, still wore the two separate long leg-coverings fastened to the waist-belt which had been usual at the end of the fourteenth century.

Toward the middle of the sixteenth century the breeches were

218

shorter, but wider, especially at the foot. The slashings were left unlaced, thus showing more of the lining, and the puffs of the breeches were ornamented with numerous small oblique lines of coloured slashings. The breeches were supported by being hooked either to the underclothing or to the inside of the doublet.

These wider breeches, of course, required more padding, and ultimately the whole garment was lined with some cheap material. The

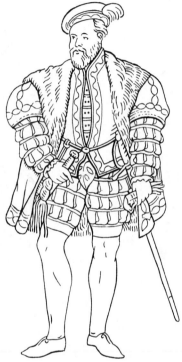

Fig. 273. SPANISH MEN'S DRESS, FIRST HALF OF THE
SIXTEENTH CENTURY

lining fitted closely to the leg, but was slightly shorter than the outer material, so that the lower edge of the material to which it was sewn was pulled slightly upward and inward. This made the breeches baggy ; the spaces between the puffs varied in size according to the shortness of the lining.

The material used for the puffs or padding between the breeches and the lining was usually of the best available quality. At first the padding was slight, but in course of time it was greatly increased, so that the puffs on the breeches lay smooth and tight over it.

The projecting, capsule-shaped front flap continued to be worn throughout the sixteenth century with all styles of breeches.

The practice of dividing leg-wear at the knee (which came in about the middle of the sixteenth century) and the introduction of stockings proper (*i.e.*, a separate garment for upper and lower leg) soon led to a complete change in the style of men's nether garments. The lining (which was always of good material) was now carried down to the

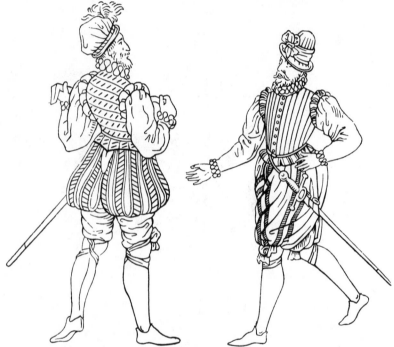

Figs. 274, 275. SPANISH MEN'S DRESS, SECOND HALF OF THE SIXTEENTH CENTURY

knee and fastened to the stockings by means of ribbons (Fig. 274). In the case of very wide, baggy breeches two styles were followed, involving two different methods of making them. If the breeches were thickly padded lower down only, and were tighter toward the top, the puffs of the breeches were laid over the padding close together where the breeches were widest, and therefore met at the top. But if the padding were thickest in the middle of the breeches, the puffs were fewer, and were arranged so as to cover the bulky lining material, and were sewn to the lining at top and bottom.

If the padding consisted of material like tow or straw, the lining had to be cut very accurately so as to avoid folds.

For short breeches, which were never in general use in Spain, the lining was always silk or some similar fine, soft material; for the slashed breeches, which were more commonly worn, velvet or cloth was used.

These, the only true " Spanish " breeches, remained in fashion among the upper classes of almost every cultured nation till well into the seventeenth century. Another style, which came in during the second half of the sixteenth century, was worn at first only by soldiers and by the middle classes, but after a few decades became universal.

The padded lining of course widened the slashes in the breeches, and therefore these openings now became more important. The

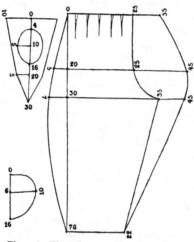

Fig. 276. WIDE SPANISH KNEE-BREECHES

breeches consisted usually of four separate strips covering the thickly padded lining, which now came to be a feature of the garment. The strips of the breeches became narrower and narrower, and finally disappeared altogether. These intermediate styles were specially common in France and Germany, where all kinds of breeches were worn at the same time. Only the final, definitive style was adopted in Spain—viz., baggy breeches, with moderately thick padding, reaching to the knee, where they were fastened with the stocking (Fig. 275).

The cut of these breeches was of course a development of the cut of the original style. They had gradually become wider, and were now lengthened to below the knee. This produced the new type. The bagginess was inevitable when the breeches were tied above the knees. (See Fig. 276.) The new style differed from the earlier close-fitting breeches in another respect. The legs were now no longer sewn at the back and front, but on the outer side and, in the case of narrow material, on the inner side also. These breeches were now so roomy that there was no possibility of strain, and so no special measures were needed to obviate that discomfort. The breeches were now, as it were, two parallel bags narrowing toward the foot, each having a draw-string there for fastening.

These roomy breeches were kept at full stretch by the thickly padded lining, which was shorter and close-fitting, and sewn at all its edges. The outer part of the lining corresponded exactly to the breeches worn over it ; the inner part still closely resembled the narrow hose worn about the year 1500. The lining was sewn to the breeches in front. The front flap both of breeches and lining was pouch-shaped as before, but was now stiffened or padded. The lining at the back was either left quite open or was closed by a gusset. To this close-fitting lining was sewn the padding—tow, calf's hair, swansdown, hay, or bran. It was usually so thick that the breeches showed very little wrinkling.

Stockings, which had in England as far back as the fifteenth century been pulled over the breeches, did not appear on the Continent till about the middle of the sixteenth century, but they were at once universally adopted. At first they were worn, as in England, merely as a warm protection for the legs against cold and wet, but ere long their use suggested the idea of lengthening the breeches down to or beyond the knees and of covering the leg below the knee with the stockings alone. (See Fig. 274.) Both breeches and stockings were fastened by tapes round the knees. The material of the stockings varied with the purpose for which they were worn. Usually of wool or silk—from the second half of the fifteenth century they were *knitted*—they were also made of thin buckskin when they were to be worn over the usual breeches. When so worn the stockings were sometimes so long that they reached half-way up the thigh. They were neatly quilted, and fitted for buttoning or lacing. Buckskin stockings were sewn only at the back, rarely both at back and front.

The doublet too was little changed at the beginning of the sixteenth century. It was still short and somewhat close-fitting, as it had been at the end of the fifteenth century. A doublet high at the neck, with an erect collar, came to be preferred to one with a low neck ; the upper edge of the shirt with a frill was shown above the collar. Similar frills began to be worn at the wrists.

The doublet still retained its slashes and puffs, and these were brought into keeping with those of the nether garments. The breast and back were left entire—the slashes being now confined to the sleeves—and the doublet was now variously trimmed and braided. Occasionally, however, rows of parallel slashes were made, through which a differently coloured lining could be seen. There was no great change in the cut of the doublet, except that the skirt was now made separately and sewn on to the upper part, which came to the hips. The length of the skirt varied according to individual taste and the fashion of the moment. Till the middle of the century the usual length was 8–15 cm., during the second half 12–30 cm. The Spanish

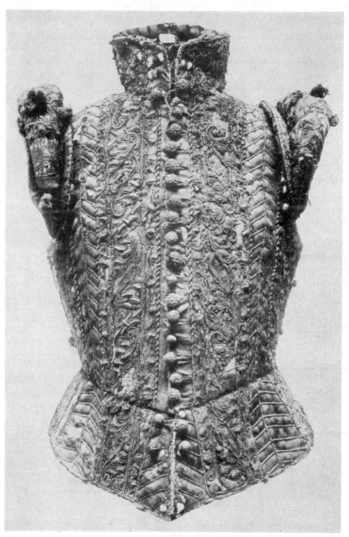

Fig. 277. SPANISH DOUBLET, ABOUT 1570

doublet was always buttoned down the front. About the middle of the sixteenth century it was sleeveless, or had only " false sleeves," which hung down behind. The real sleeves belonged to a short jacket worn beneath the doublet, and were mostly of a different colour. The sleeves were either quite plain or ornamented merely with numerous small slashes at regular intervals. The sleeve-hole was

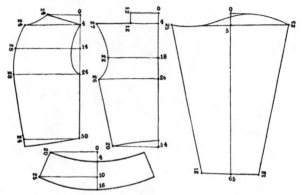

Fig. 278. SPANISH DOUBLET

encircled by a number of bows made of the same material as the doublet and set close together. From about the year 1560 the doublet was much longer in front than behind. The front was padded, and the collar was not so high. The former narrow frill above the collar

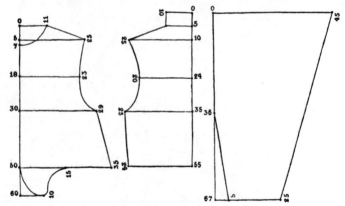

Fig. 279. DOUBLET WITH GANSBAUCH

was replaced by a broad, pleated frill, which continued to increase in size, till toward the end of the century it surrounded the head like a wheel. Simultaneously with the increase in the ruff (the *lechugilla*), which was worn by all classes, the breast padding increased in thickness, and was no longer equally distributed over the whole chest, but was concentrated at the centre. Its usual shape was a ridge running down the middle of the breast. It was pointed at the foot, and was a little flatter from that point upward. Toward the end of the century the padding was so disposed that it formed a pendent sharp point at the lower end. This style was developed in the Netherlands, and the Germans called it *Gansbauch*, or " goose-belly."

The doublet itself, however, was not invariably padded in the manner just described. It was often unlined, and was merely shaped so as to allow for the padding in the sleeved jacket worn beneath the sleeveless doublet. Owing to the padding, this jacket had a double front—one shaped to fit the body, the other to suit the intended outline of the breast of the doublet. Between the two was put the padding of tow or calf's hair. It began at the side and was pushed tight toward the centre. Each of the two fronts, which were made to be hooked or laced, was fastened down the centre of the breast by a triangular piece that connected the inside and outside of the jacket. This piece of material helped greatly to produce the ridge down the middle of the breast. The padding had to be firmest at this part, and had to be sewn in down both sides of the ridge. The padding diminished toward the top and sides. It was quilted down to prevent it from shifting.

The cloak—the real national wrap of the Spaniard—varied not only in length and colour and trimming, but also in the material of which it was made. The occupation, rank, financial circumstances, and personal taste of the wearer, as well as local differences, all had a share in determining the style of cloak a man wore. For example, Spaniards of the upper classes, especially those about the royal Court, wore very short cloaks of silk or velvet (see Fig. 280) ; the middle classes in the towns wore much longer cloaks made of cloth. The cloaks worn by country people reached to the ankles, and were made of some coarse material. But they were all alike in cut—three-fourths of a circle— and they all had a long hood, rounded or pointed at the lower end, with a row of buttons or tassels down the centre. The top edge of the hood was cut exactly to fit the neck of the cloak to which it was sewn. From the neck the hood extended in two strips, which were sewn to the front of the cloak and formed lapels. The hood consisted either of two pieces sewn together at the sides or of one pentagonal piece, two corners of which were folded outward and sewn together.

Cowl-shaped caps were still the usual headdress at the beginning of the sixteenth century. Country people wore broad-brimmed hats or, as in the southern provinces, a sort of turban. Of the various kinds of caps, made of felt, velvet, or silk, those with a low crown soon became most popular. The widening of the crown gave rise to a new style, the *biretta*.

At first this was low in the crown, of moderate diameter, and narrow-brimmed. Toward the middle of the century this new head-dress, mostly of silk or velvet, became so broad that it resembled a

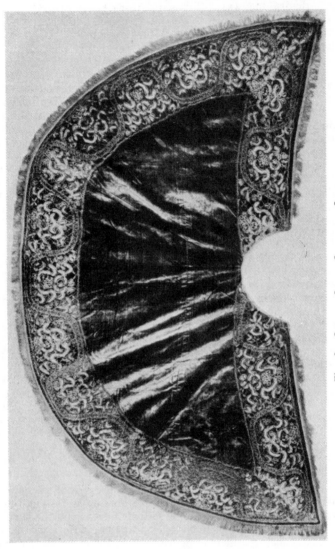

Fig. 280. Spanish Cloak, Sixteenth Century

plate, but ere long the shape was fundamentally altered. The crown was raised and supported by a wire frame.

In spite of this change the *biretta* was still round. The alteration required only a larger piece of material. The make was simple. A piece of material of the requisite size was taken and gathered all round. Then the brim was made by turning in half the breadth of the amount allowed for the purpose and sewing it down. If the amount of folding thus produced was considered excessive, a few gussets were cut out of the edge. Sometimes the brim was made separately and sewn on, instead of being made in the way described. This method was followed when a smooth, uncrumpled surface was desired. (See Fig. 275.)

These *birettas* were usually black, and ornamented with a band of gold braid round the foot of the crown or with a short feather.

During the second half of the sixteenth century the *birettas*, supported by a frame of wire, became higher, and pointed at the top. This gave them an appearance similar to that of a hat with a narrow brim, and about the year 1570 they actually became identical with that type of headdress. This change of shape, however, caused no alteration in the material employed or in the method of manufacture, and hats still continued to be made of velvet or silk, or, to speak more accurately, the framework of wire continued to be covered with one or other of these materials. Toward the end of the century hats of this kind began to be made of felt.

Spanish footwear altered little during the sixteenth century. The prevailing fashion continued to be a shaped shoe covering the whole front of the foot, and cut more or less low at the sides. About the year 1500 the practice came in of slashing the shoe and lining the slashes with material of another colour. This continued till nearly the end of the century. The usual material was *cordouan*, a soft, blackened leather. Slashed shoes were as a rule made of black or coloured velvet.

Women's Dress. From the end of the fifteenth century onward the long, voluminous dress worn by women was no longer made in one piece. It now consisted of a bodice and a skirt made separately. The neck of the bodice was low, leaving visible an embroidered chemise that reached almost to the neck. The bodice was short at the waist and very tight, and was laced at the back. It was usually made of the same material as the skirt, and trimmed with the stuff with which the skirt was trimmed. The sleeves, which were usually gathered at several places and tied with coloured ribbons, were of fine linen. At this time trains were also shortened, but, on the other hand, very thick under-garments were worn. These usually had no bodice, but were held up by tapes passing over the shoulders. The strict etiquette that prevailed at the Court of Charles I of Spain gave rise to new fashions. Ladies, especially ladies of the Court, were no longer allowed to appear with bare breasts. At first this edict was met by the wearing of a plain or pleated chemise of fine material which covered the bosom. From the year 1525 onward these chemises became higher and higher. They were liberally embroidered with gold and pearls, and came at first close up to the neck ; ere long, however, they entirely surrounded the neck in the form of a broad gold-embroidered band, above which appeared a narrow, evenly goffered ruffle. The bodice continued to be low at the neck. It was made longer, especially in front, and was stiffly padded in order to make it free from wrinkles. This padding completely concealed the bust, without, however, compressing it. The skirt was stretched over a framework of hoops and tapes so that it too showed no wrinkles.

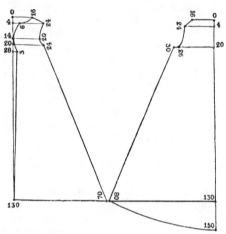

Fig. 281. OPEN OVER-DRESS OF SPANISH WOMEN

Only the wide sleeves of the bodice were wrinkled. The under-sleeves were tight, with a dainty ruffle of linen at the wrists. The puffs which had formerly surrounded the top of the sleeves of the dress were now replaced by a row of loops of varying size made of the same material as the bodice or by iron rings placed side by side. The waist was enclosed by a handsome girdle, one end of which hung down nearly to the feet. The beautifully trimmed skirt was left open from the waist down in order to show the under-skirt. In this case the bodice was permanently laced at the back (the skirt had a slit at the side). The lining of this bodice was laced in front and concealed by the material of the bodice, which was then closed at the side by hooks and eyes.

About the middle of the century the opening of the bodice (which was now closed in front) became higher, till it came close up to the neck. An erect collar was worn, and a ruff, even broader than that worn before, peeped out above the collar. These bodices, stiffened

Plate IV

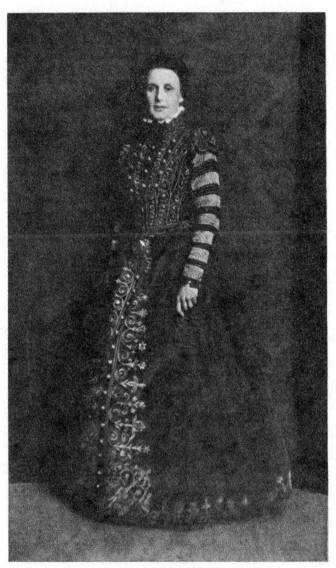

GOWN OF GREEN MOIRÉ SILK 228
Latter half of the sixteenth century

and padded here and there, fitted close to the person.[1] The skirt
when sewn on to the bodice showed few or no folds, and was stretched
from the hips down by means of a bell-shaped hooped petticoat or
farthingale.   There was practically no train with these dresses.   The
sleeves, usually, but not always, of the same material as the dress,
were now made wider, especially at the shoulder.   A trimming of gold
braid ran down the front (and only) seam of the sleeves.   It was a
common practice, also, to have horizontal trimmings of this gold
braid.   As before, the sleeves were cut straight, and had only one
seam.   The top of the sleeve was sometimes wide, sometimes narrow,
sometimes smooth, sometimes pleated, more or less fully.   Unless
they were very close-fitting the sleeves were stiffened by being slightly
padded or lined.   The sleeve-hole was surmounted as before by a

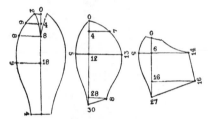

Fig. 282. SLEEVES OF OVER-DRESS

single or double row of rings or of bows of the same material as the
bodice.   Round the wrists were narrow frills of fine linen.
    With an over-dress of this kind the garment worn underneath was
usually a petticoat—*i.e.*, a skirt from the hips to the feet—but
occasionally it was a complete dress like the one over it.   This was
almost always the case when the over-dress was open all down the
front.
    Dresses like these were worn by women of both the upper and lower
classes.   (See Fig. 283.)   The bodice was not separate—the garment
was all in one piece.   The dresses were close-fitting round bust and
shoulders, gradually widening downward, and frequently ending in a
train.   They were usually sleeveless, allowing the bows at the
shoulders of the under-bodice to be seen, but in many cases the over-
dress had either long hanging sleeves (Fig. 284) or sleeves that were
meant to be buttoned on.   In the former case the sleeve-hole of the
over-dress had bows, while the under-dress had none.   In the case
of sleeves that were meant to be pulled on separately and buttoned,
these bows were not put on, because the shape of the sleeves rendered
them unnecessary.   The top of the sleeve was made extra wide, and

[1] In order to have the bodice as smooth and free from wrinkles as possible,
and to secure a slim figure, Spanish ladies wore a sort of corset of thin laths,
about 2 inches wide, held together by tapes passed through them.

stiffened so as to project above the shoulders (see Fig. 283). Sleeves of this kind, which were usually only elbow-length, were made of several pieces, the seams being concealed by braid.

At first the erect collar of the bodice was sometimes altogether, sometimes only in front, less high than before, but the ruff was much fuller and deeper. Toward the end of the century the collar was again broader, and, in order not to crumple the ruff, it was

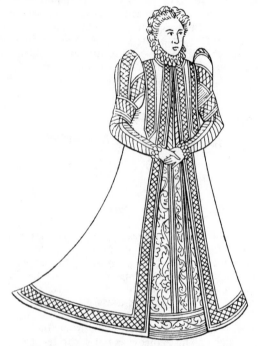

Fig. 283. SPANISH WOMEN'S DRESS, SECOND HALF OF THE SIXTEENTH CENTURY

not only left open in front, but the upper edge was bent outward. In other respects the bodice was made as before, except that it was shorter, and at the shoulders broader. This latter change was soon followed by the omission of the shoulder-bows, their place being taken either by an ornamentation of strips with scalloped edges or by a thick roll-pad. (See Fig. 284.)

An extensive change was made in the sleeves of the over-dress. Hanging sleeves were still fashionable, but they were so made that they needed only to be closed at the hands in order to form real sleeves. They were very wide, but three-fourths of the way down they suddenly became very tight. As such sleeves were always cut straight at their open front part, this contraction in width could be attained only by shaping them to the arm at the back and sewing them there.

There were other styles of sleeves besides these. These were very wide at the top, and only a little less wide at the wrist. They were sometimes made in the manner just described, but mostly they had no seam, but were made by simply folding the material. They were,

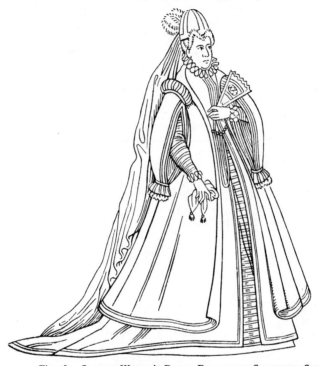

Fig. 284. Spanish Women's Dress, End of the Sixteenth Century

of course, open in front. At the wrist they were tied loosely, and fitted with projecting cuffs.

The skirt of the over-dress fitted almost without a wrinkle to the bodice. According to the fashion of the time the lower edge of the bodice had a narrow trimming. The skirt was much longer at the back than in front, for the farthingale was no longer bell-shaped. It now stood out at the back low down—a change which was due to the reappearance of the train, and which soon ceased with the speedy disappearance of the latter. The over-dress was still open in the front from the waist down, but it was now on the whole shorter, so that the under-dress was visible in front or even all round.

231

When two over-dresses were worn at the same time the outer one had hanging sleeves and the inner one had none. The arms were covered by the tight sleeves of the under-dress. Toward the end of the sixteenth century these sleeves began to be made of two pieces, with a seam down the front and back. This change produced better-shaped sleeves, and also made them more comfortable, by giving room for the elbows. The practice of slightly padding the sleeves all the way down was continued with the two-seam style of sleeve.

There were also other over-dresses which had no separate bodice, but were made in one piece. These were open in front, but they were quite different in shape from their earlier form. (See Fig. 284.) The chief change was that the dress was folded back at the neck, forming a turn-over collar and showing the lining down the front. To make them fit closer at the waist narrow diamond-shaped pieces were cut out there, the openings being sewn up.

Women's headdress was copied from that of the men. Low *birettas* and small hats were worn. Both were ornamented with gold cord and feathers and pinned to the hair. Middle-class women wore out of doors low, broad-brimmed hats put on above the veil or the hood.

Women also wore the same kind of shoes as men, but theirs were daintier and more liberally trimmed. For going out women still put on the thick-soled under-shoes which had long been used in some districts in Spain. These were decorated with strips of coloured leather, gilt buttons, and other ornaments.

FRANCE

Men's Dress. In France too at the beginning of the sixteenth century dress differed little from that of the fifteenth, and therefore for a time various Spanish fashions were retained.

The wraps used by the nobles and young men were roomy, shawl-like garments either with sleeves or with armholes only. Some were more like a coat, others rather resembled a cloak. The former type, which was very like the German *Schaube*, remained nearly all through the century the ordinary dress of the middle class, whereas the nobles preferred the lighter shawls at first, soon exchanging these for the sleeveless Spanish cloak. Although the latter was very fashionable during the reigns of Francis I and Henry II, sleeved cloaks were still frequently worn down to the time of Charles IX (died 1574), and were of the ordinary shapes—either like coats or like cloaks. (See Figs. 285 and 286.) These cloaks were made in two ways. Either the upper part was cut to fit closely and sewn on to a pleated skirt, or the garment was made like a cloak and gathered in pleats at the waist behind.

The cloak proper was of the Spanish type. It varied in length, but it was always circular in shape. The hood, however, was never so

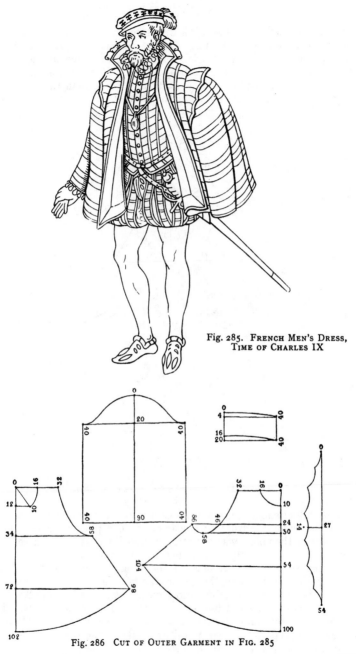

Fig. 285. FRENCH MEN'S DRESS,
TIME OF CHARLES IX

Fig. 286 CUT OF OUTER GARMENT IN FIG. 285

popular in France, and the cloak therefore was usually left bare at the neck except for the trimming. Later the fashionable cloak had a broad stand-up collar (Fig. 287). The lining of the collar was turned outward and slit so as to form broad loops. Bows similar, but made of the same material as the cloak, were used to trim the shoulders. In order to secure a better fit at the shoulders a gusset was cut out

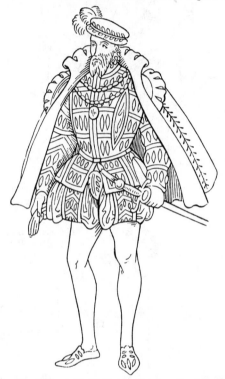

Fig. 287. FRENCH MEN'S DRESS, TIME OF CHARLES IX

of the neck at each side, making a cavity for each shoulder. To keep the collar erect the front of it was cut in one piece with the cloak. The rest of the collar was cut straight and inserted between the two ends of the cloak which formed the front of the collar.

During the reign of Henry III the shoulder-capes became much shorter and tighter, and the collar was very small. Sometimes the collar was omitted altogether, and replaced by a small, round hood.

These short capes did not altogether oust the longer cloaks. The latter were either almost circular or shaped like a sector. Those of the circular type were used as riding cloaks, while the sector-shaped cloaks (called *tabarés*) were used for walking.

The sleeves were wide, narrowing toward the wrists. In most cases they belonged to the under-jacket, the *gilet*, the doublet either being sleeveless or having hanging sleeves. The junction of the sleeves and shoulders was trimmed with rolls or flaps, but occasionally these additions were omitted.

A very popular practice was to ornament both the breast and the sleeves of the doublet with slashes arranged in regular figures. The buttons of the doublet were mostly large, and almost conical in shape, while those of the *gilet* were flat. Both were made of metal.

The reign of Henry III also saw the introduction of considerable changes in the other items of men's attire.

Men's nether garments had already passed through considerable changes between the beginning of the sixteenth century and the

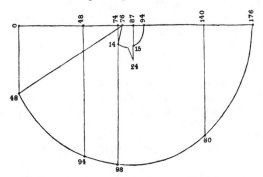

Fig. 288. CUT OF THE CLOAK IN FIG. 287

accession of Henry III. The somewhat tight, slashed over-breeches, the *haut-de-chausses*—only these are meant here, because the long hose, the *bas-de-chausses*, retained their earlier form [1]—were now longer and wider, and ere long were very like the hose worn at the same period in Spain. Slashed breeches of this kind were called *trousses* ; when thickly padded they were called *tonneaux* or *tonnelets*, according to their size. During the reign of Charles IX (1560–74) the latter were the height of fashion.

About the time when the *trousses* were widened into *tonnelets* breeches were made into trousers by being lengthened to the knees or lower and by the omission of slashes and padding. At first these trousers were of the same width all the way down, and were merely gathered at the foot. But ere very long they were made tighter at the knees. This change was accompanied by the disappearance of the padded front flap. Its place was taken by a slit arranged for buttoning.

[1] These long hose were made of various cloths till far on in the second half of the sixteenth century. Later they were knitted. About the middle of the century men of the upper classes began to wear the knitted trousers known as *tricots*.

The broad ruff and the cuffs were still retained, but large, round, embroidered collars were already being worn. These were smooth, and were divided at the front ; the broadest part was at the back. With these were usually worn broad starched cuffs turned back over the sleeves of the doublet and embroidered with designs similar to those on the collar.

These more sensible forms of Court costume pleased the taste of almost every one, and the middle-class citizen also insisted on having his clothes made on the new lines. The only differences between his clothing and that worn by the nobles lay in the material and trimming.

Throughout almost the whole of the sixteenth century the headgear of Frenchmen was the *barrette*. Like the Spanish headdress, this was circular, but, unlike the Spanish style, the brim was stiffened and turned up instead of being soft and hanging down. This meant, of course, that the under part of the brim was shown, and had therefore to be lined. As a rule the lining differed in colour from the rest. The turned-up portion was embroidered or trimmed or slashed or puffed. A feather fixed at the back encircled most of the crown. These *barrettes* varied greatly in size ; about the year 1530 the usual shape was large in circumference, but flat—almost plate-like. By and by this style went gradually out of fashion, and the small Spanish *biretta* again came into favour. In the later style of the Spanish *biretta* the material was stretched over a framework of wire. This identical form was never adopted in France. There the frame was never so high nor the material stretched so tightly over it as in the usual Spanish style.

The reign of Henry III witnessed a great increase in the number of types of headdress. A great many different kinds of hats and caps were worn, as well as the *barrette*. Among these was one much favoured at Court. It was really an item of female attire, the *toque* —a cap with a round crown, mostly made of velvet, and trimmed with gold or silver braid.

Hats proper came into general use only about the middle of the century. The ordinary type was round, with a low crown and broad brim. Down to the time of Henry III styles of hats multiplied so enormously that high hats and low hats, broad-brimmed hats and narrow-brimmed hats, were all fashionable at the same time ; the crown of the hat might be round or cylindrical or conical in shape. There was an equally great variety in colour and material—hats were made of felt or cloth, velvet or silk. The feathers were worn standing straight up either at the front or at the back, and were fastened with a clasp. In the reign of Henry IV the felt hat with broad brim slightly turned up at the side became so much the rage that it soon drove all others out of the field. Hats of this type were usually ornamented with several ostrich feathers. Still another hat, high-crowned and with practically no brim, was adorned with a plume of heron's feathers.

At the beginning of the sixteenth century shoes were very broad at the toe, but in the course of a few decades this type was replaced by a style of shoe more in keeping with the natural outline of the foot and slashed in Spanish fashion. From the middle of the century onward these shoes were higher in the leg, and buttoned over the instep. The material was as before—black or coloured soft leather (*cordouan*), silk, or velvet. Under Henry III slashed shoes went gradually out of fashion, and the practice came in of colouring the edges of the soles red. Thick-soled slippers were also much worn —usually over the ordinary shoes—by people going out of doors. In the time of Henry IV shoes were more blunted at the toes. The heels were higher, and the uppers were adorned with bows or rosettes of coloured ribbon.

Women's Dress. Until about 1530 the dress of Frenchwomen was much the same as it had been at the end of the fifteenth century. It was very slowly that it developed into the so-called Spanish costume which had been adopted in the twenties by the Queen and her ladies. In France, however, an attempt was made to modify the stiffness of this and give it a more tasteful appearance. French ladies could not bring themselves to wear the bodice which was closed all round. The low neck was retained, the bosom being covered with a neckerchief of fine material.

The skirt was gusseted so as to fit round the body almost without a wrinkle, and was kept at full stretch all the way down by the framework of hoops—the *vertugarde*, or farthingale—worn beneath it. To make it possible to put on this skirt, it either had a long slit at the side or was cut down the front and closed with hooks and eyes. Sometimes, however, it was left quite open in order to show the dress beneath it.

The bodice was laced at the back or hooked at the side.[1] Round the body was worn a cord of silk or gold, as thick as a finger, one end of which was tied in a series of knots, with a ball of musk at the extremity, and hung down to the hem of the dress. The chemise of fine material was pleated, and made to button in front, but was often worn open.

At the time of Charles IX (reigned 1560–74) the *vertugarde* increased still further in circumference, and so the dress, which retained the same width as before, and was open from the waist down, was stretched to such a degree that the two edges could not meet. The bodice—beneath which Frenchwomen now wore corsets made of thin, narrow laths—was still the same as before, except that the rolls at the shoulders were omitted. Some Frenchwomen still wore the Spanish bodice, high at the neck and provided with a stand-up collar. Such bodices were exact imitations of the *pourpoint*, the doublet of the men, and the style bore the name of *le saye*.

---

[1] Only the material of the bodice was closed at the side. The lining, which was stiffened with perpendicular strips of cane or wood or steel, was fastened in front, beginning at the foot.

The neck-ruff, worn both with the high-necked and the low-necked bodice, had increased both in thickness and in width. It was exactly the same as the ruff worn by men, both in shape and in the way it was made. Instead of these *fraises*, or ruffs, many women preferred narrower ruffles attached to the reversed top edge of the chemise. (See Fig. 289.) These were worn both with the low-necked bodice

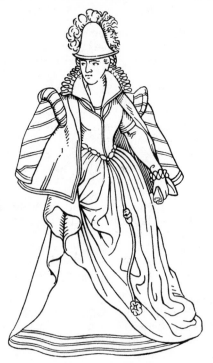

Fig. 289. FRENCH WOMEN'S DRESS, TIME OF CHARLES IX

and with the bodice of the other style, which came up almost to the neck at the back and on the shoulders, but was more or less open in front.

Equally great changes were now made in the over-dress. This had now no train—it was not long enough to have one—but it was so full that, in spite of being worn above very voluminous under-garments, it fell in numerous longitudinal folds. With this dress the farthingale was not worn, and women obtained the girth demanded by fashion by putting on numerous petticoats made of stiff material. The farthingale, however, was still required for Court dress, because it stretched the skirts to their full width and allowed no folds or wrinkles to appear. Such dresses had no train. The style of the over-dress was also determined by the *vertugarde*; it was open in front if the latter was worn with it ; otherwise it was closed.

The chief models for the attire worn in France at this time continued to be the fashions prevalent in Spain, and these were gradually adopted with some changes. The only exception was the high-necked bodice. The very low-necked bodice, which frequently came halfway down the breast, continued to be generally worn. This consisted of a back and a front sewn together at the sides a little in front of the arms. The back was made of two equal pieces either sewn together or, if the bodice was not closed at the sides, laced. Notwithstanding all the changes that were made in the skirt, the bodice retained its former shape, except that it was gradually lengthened in front and brought to a sharp point there. The shape of the sleeves varied. Sometimes they were tight, sometimes wide all the way down or only at the top ; sometimes

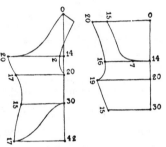

Fig. 290. **Pattern of French Bodice**

they ended at the shoulders, and at others they overtopped them. They were plain or puffed, slashed or unslashed, with or without rolls at the shoulders, and the rolls might be of any kind. A similar variety prevailed with regard to trimming and other ornamentations.

The material and colour of the sleeves might be the same as those of the bodice or those of the overdress or those of the under-dress. If the bodice had hanging sleeves, these were usually of the same material as the bodice, but if shoulder-rolls also were worn, they were of the same material as the bodice, while the hanging sleeves and the over-dress were of another material, the under-sleeves and the under-dress being of a third material. As a matter of fact, the taste of the time preferred considerable variety of material and colour.

The ruffle, with broad, regular pleats, was concealed by a broad stand-up collar.

On short journeys, excursions, and similar occasions Frenchwomen about the middle of the century frequently wore short, close-fitting sleeved cloaks or wide jackets. The cut was very similar to that of the short Spanish cloaks worn by the men.

The *coiffure* and headgear of Frenchwomen developed as independently as the other items of their attire, although here also Spanish influence was clearly perceptible. At the beginning of the sixteenth century the hair was arranged in large or small ringlets all round the head, or the long hair at the back of the head was enclosed in a dainty net, into which were also put the ends of the front hair. The latter was parted, and hung low on the cheeks, either loose or in plaits. But when Spanish fashions spread in France various different kinds of headgear soon appeared. The favourite styles were the *barrette*—at first small and flat, later with a high, stiff crown—and a hat small and narrow-brimmed, and with a pointed crown. These hats and *barrettes* were adorned with a small feather. About the year 1530 women began to wear circlets of gold liberally adorned with jewels.

These fashions of hairdressing and headgear continued until the middle of the century. About this date various kinds of caps came into vogue, and to suit these the front and side hair was slightly raised in tufts. This *coiffure*, called *en bichons*, was very popular at the time of Henry III, and suited the small, soft cap worn on the back of the head and adorned with a small plume. These caps were known as *toques*, and were universally worn at Court. Next to them in popularity came the smaller silk or velvet mutches, called *chaperons*, and various other kinds of caps—some fitting close at the back of the head, with a flat, square piece coming forward to the face, and some with a broad brim bent back, framing the face all round. These. caps, which were usually richly trimmed, had to be made of cloth for women of the middle classes. Only ladies of noble birth were allowed to wear *chaperons*.

Toward the year 1590 the hair was built up still higher, and later it was arranged in conical shape over a wire frame. If necessary, false hair was used to make up for any natural defect. This fashion was modified in accordance with individual caprice, and women's *coiffure* varied both in height and breadth. Ribbons, pearls, or feathers were used to suit the wearer's taste. Both men and women powdered their hair.

This style of *coiffure* forbade anything that could be called a head-dress, and yet small, flat caps or narrow-brimmed, pointed hats were occasionally worn. These were fastened to the hair with pins at the front or sides. Following the fashion that had hitherto prevailed, brides all through this century wore their hair hanging loose.

At the beginning of the century sewn stockings were still in vogue, but toward the end woven stockings from England took their place. With them came garters, and fashion demanded that these should be elegantly adorned. The use of handkerchiefs also dates from the sixteenth century, but rich lace trimming and embroidery made them for a long time an article of luxury.

GERMANY

Men's Dress. In Germany also the old styles of dress continued to be worn into the first decades of the sixteenth century, and it was not till the fifties that changes began to appear.

At first the usual wear was still the tight jacket cut low at the breast and tight trousers, but it became more and more fashionable to wear instead long hose fastened to the waist-belt and over them short breeches that came only to the middle of the thigh. The over-garment was the *Schaube* (cassock), and a small cloak or a short cape with sleeve-holes was also worn. Low shoes with very broad toes and a broad *Barett* with or without feathers were usual. The uncomfortable strain of this close-fitting clothing was remedied by making incisions at the joints and introducing baggy insertions in or under these. Ere long, however, this makeshift was transformed into an embellishment. Slits were cut not only at the joints, but at many other places, and lined with a different material. The open breast was also abandoned. The neck was much higher, but it continued to be somewhat wide till 1520.

The fashion of excessive slashing was introduced by the so-called *Landsknechte,* or mercenary soldiers. These roistering blades delighted in gay clothing, and took every opportunity of indulging their tastes. They were not content merely to slash their garments, but had them made of materials of different colours. They even went so far as to have similar parts of the same garment of different shape ; *e.g.,* the legs of their hose were not only of different colours, but differed also in shape and trimming. They even had one leg quite bare from the knee or middle of the thigh downward, cutting off that part of the garment and either removing it or pushing it down toward the foot.

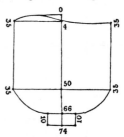

Fig. 291. WIDE SLEEVE OF THE DOUBLET

This peculiar style of slashed nether garments was, after all, not very different from the former fashions. The chief difference was that the breeches varied greatly in length and width, and to some extent also in the slashes and puffs.

Stockings were either of leather or cloth. In the latter case they were of the same colour as the breeches. The tops were slashed longitudinally. The piece of stocking that came above the knee was turned outward, and the knee was surrounded by a circle of bows of varying size. Dandies had a fashion of their own. They often only wore one stocking of this kind, the other leg being clad only in the breeches.

Slashed doublets were now also worn, but the slashes were not nearly so numerous as in the nether garments. Striking effects were produced by bizarre shapes and by variety of colour. The sleeves were wide, and of a colour different from that of the doublet itself. The slashings were at first slight and confined to the breast and sleeves, but ere long they came to be as extensive as in the breeches.

The doublet consisted of a front and a back piece sewn together at the sides. It came down to the hips, and was fastened there to the breeches by means of strings. To secure comfort and freedom of movement these were often undone, a considerable band of shirt being left visible between the doublet and the breeches (see Fig. 292). Various kinds of sleeves were worn ; as a rule they were wide, but were fastened round the wrist. They were either cut in this shape, or were more or less rectangular, and pleated at the sleeve-hole and at

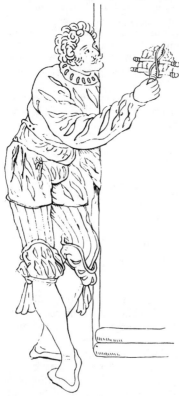

the hand (Fig. 291). In others the same result was achieved by cutting out triangular pieces from the top and bottom of the sleeve. The bagginess of the sleeves was produced by slight padding or by a stiff lining, or simply by making them very long. This last method was followed with tight slashed sleeves, and the slashes were lined with rolled material. This last style came in about 1530. At that time slashed sleeves were very fashionable, but they were on the whole closer-fitting than before. Only the mercenary soldiers retained the old fashion, but their sleeves too were now adorned with numerous slashes of various shapes.

From 1512 onward the doublet was tighter at the neck, and the neck of the shirt higher, so that the shirt-collar could be seen above the doublet. The doublet came close up to the neck, and ended in a broad, slashed, stand-up collar, which was often stuffed into a roll-shape. In other cases the collar was lined with stiff material narrower than the collar. This lining held up the collar, but strips of it were drawn through the slashes

[Fig. 292. GERMAN MEN'S DRESS, FIRST HALF OF THE SIXTEENTH CENTURY

and hung loosely down. Toward the middle of the century the doublet began to be padded and quilted throughout.

Though now higher at the neck, the doublet was in other respects the same as before (see Fig. 292). It was either cut in one piece, or consisted of a back piece sewn in the middle and two front pieces, one of which came right across the breast, while the other was narrower. The fastening—with buttons or hooks or laces—was still at the side. The shirt-collar was also tied or hooked at the side. The size of the sleeve-hole varied according to the width of the sleeves. (See Fig. 293.) By and by, however, the doublet was lengthened, so that it

242

was no longer necessary to loosen the strings attaching it to the breeches in order to be able to move freely.

Similar in cut to the doublet was the coat, which was now worn by people of all classes. Nobles wore it either as a house coat or as a military dress—either over or beneath the armour.

The material and trimming of the coat depended on the occasions on which it was meant to be worn. The house coat was as simple as possible, but the military coat, especially on festive occasions, was distinguished by elaborate trimming. The sleeves of the coat showed the same varieties of slashing and shape as those of the doublet, so that the coat was frequently called a *Schoszwams*—a tailed doublet. The only difference between it and the short doublet was that it had a wide skirt, of varying length. This consisted of a circular piece of material pleated all round and sewn to the doublet either by an

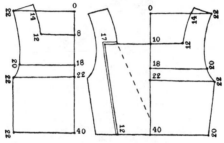

Fig. 293. GERMAN DOUBLET, FIRST HALF OF THE
SIXTEENTH CENTURY

overcast seam or by a seam on the inside. When the garment was to be worn indoors the skirt of the coat was usually closed all round, while the military coat, which was to be worn on horseback, was always open in front, and not rarely behind also. Indeed, the coat varied just as much as the doublet, and the differences extended not only to the trimming and slashing and puffs, but also to the cut. For example, the military coat was hooked sometimes at the side and sometimes in front. The latter style was adopted when it was to be worn above the armour, although even then only the top and bottom hooks were used. Again, these coats had sometimes no collar at all, while at other times there was an erect collar, which might or might not be slashed and puffed. The chief differences, however, were in the width across the shoulders. In some cases the top part of the sleeve-hole was exactly at the shoulder; in others it was about 10 cm. lower down, and the shoulder was cut too wide by that amount.

Ultimately the width of the body of the coat was made easier and a better fit for the figure of the wearer; the length also was more or less increased. It was longest at the beginning of the century, decreasing in length from 1520 onward, until about twenty years later the tails did not come more than half-way down the thigh. When the coat was worn over the short doublet its sleeves were short, widening at the elbows, and it was low at the neck, showing the doublet. In that case the neck, the wrists, the back seam, and the breast were finished with a broad edging of braid.

Kittel (smock) was the name given to a style of coat, worn by almost all classes, which had no skirt or tails, but was cut in one piece, widening gradually from the shoulders down. The smock was

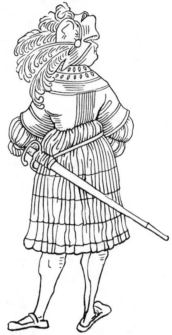

Fig. 294. German Knight's Costume, First Half of the Sixteenth Century

invariably closed all round. In some cases there was a large opening for the head—wider in front—where it could be fastened ; in others the opening was at the side, and the smock was buttoned on one shoulder. A girdle was worn with this garment. The width was occasionally decreased by pleats fastened down at the small of the back. The smock, which was usually quite plain, or at most trimmed with braid at the edges, resembled the coats worn by men in the early part of the Middle Ages. The front and back were exactly alike. Long sleeve-holes were left unsewn at the seams. The sleeves at this time were long, but not wide. The length of the smock varied, but in most cases it reached to the knee or a little below.

The main difference between the smocks of the lower and lowest classes and those of the upper classes was that the former were shorter and less voluminous. (See Fig. 295.) As a rule the coats of poorer people were pleated only at the middle of the back, the rest of the skirt being cut in one piece with the body of the garment or sewn on to it without folds. Another difference was that peasants' smocks opened at the breast, not at the side, and that the skirt was never closed all round. Wagoners and well-to-do peasants also wore short smocks quite open in front, but the skirts were usually thickly pleated. The lower orders were immediately recognizable by the cut of their clothes. These were made for use and comfort, not for

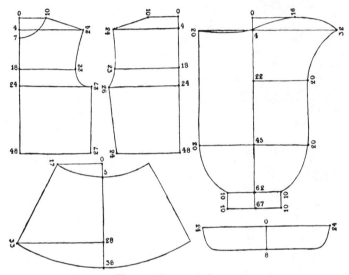

Fig. 295. PEASANT'S SMOCK

show. The sleeve-holes were large, and the sleeves were neither inconveniently tight nor needlessly wide. They were comfortably loose everywhere.

The ordinary shape was departed from only when the clothes were made of leather, for this material had qualities (such as holes or unequal or excessive thickness) which made it impossible to cut the garments in the usual way. For certain purposes almost any article of attire could be, and was, made of leather, even for the use of the upper classes, but leathern doublets were commoner than any other garment. Mercenary soldiers often wore them instead of armour. They were made of a back piece and either one or two front pieces. The doublet that had a one-piece front opened at the side ; the front in two pieces was for a doublet that closed down the centre. Back and front were joined by seams at shoulders and sides.

These leather doublets were always sleeveless. A doublet that

245

closed in front had as a rule to be kept in place by a girdle, because the front pieces were cut obliquely so as to overlap to some extent across the stomach. The lower part of these overlapping front pieces was shaped into a fairly broad strip, which protected the opposite thigh against blows and stabs. The single front piece of the leather doublets which closed at the side was also frequently lengthened to protect the thighs, when it resembled a short apron divided in

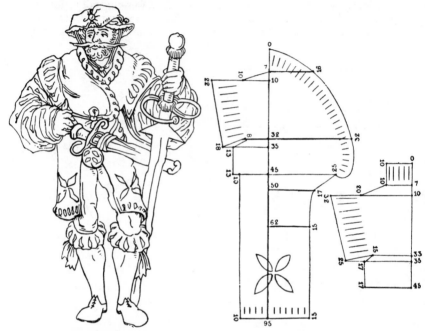

Fig. 296. MERCENARY SOLDIER (LANDSKNECHT), FIRST HALF OF THE SIXTEENTH CENTURY

Fig. 297. LEATHER DOUBLET OF THE MERCENARY SOLDIER

the middle from the abdomen down. (See Figs. 296 and 297.) As the under doublet had wide sleeves, the sleeve-holes of leather doublets were always very large ; the shoulders were very broad, to protect the shoulders and the upper arms. These protective parts were usually made double. The outer part was slashed, and sewn to the inner layer so as to cause the slashed strips to bulge outward. The top edge of the doublet was also slashed and turned outward.[1]

[1] During the sixteenth century it was a very common practice in Germany to slash the upper edges of clothes. It was done as follows. Along the edge, about 2 or 3 cm. from it, equidistant oblique slashes were made of any desired length. At the middle of these cuts the material was bent over outward or inward and sewn down. The broad band thus produced was usually lined with coloured material, which showed through the slashes.

The breast and thighs of the doublet were frequently slashed, or figures might be cut out in them and lined with coloured material.

Toward the end of the fifteenth century the *Schaube*, or mantle, had become so fashionable that it was almost the sole outer garment of German men at the beginning of the sixteenth century. The shape,

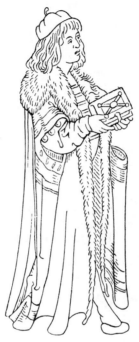

Fig. 298. GERMAN MEN'S DRESS, BEGINNING OF THE SIXTEENTH CENTURY

colour, and material differed greatly according to the standing of the wearer. About the year 1500 the *Schaube* was still ankle-length. It was lined with fur, and the sleeves had an opening high up to allow the passage of the arms. The front edges were turned outward, the part turned over widening upward and forming a collar in the region of the shoulders. The *Schaube*, both in its original long form and in the shorter form that came in about the middle of the sixteenth century, resembled a long-sleeved cloak, except for the wide collar falling over shoulders and back. Other differences were merely in the length and width of the cloak, or in the breadth of the turn-over and of the collar, or (and this was the chief difference) in the shape of the sleeves. The general cut of the *Schaube* was unchanged. The greatest variety was in the sleeves, which had only one feature in common—great length and width. Various kinds of openings were made in the sleeves to allow the arms to pass through, but when the sleeves were very long and very wide these openings were omitted.

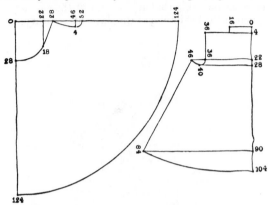

Fig. 299. Cut of the Schaube (Cloak)

The size and shape of the sleeve-holes varied according to the width of the sleeves. As the sleeves were meant to be without folds or wrinkles when they were sewn in, the sleeve-hole was very large. At the back it was angular (Fig. 300). It had a narrow border of fur.

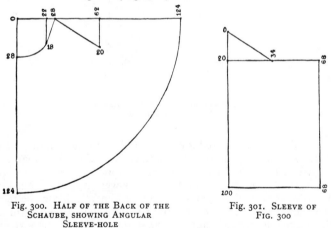

Fig. 300. Half of the Back of the Schaube, showing Angular Sleeve-hole

Fig. 301. Sleeve of Fig. 300

(See Fig. 302.) The top of the sleeve was usually cut straight, but sometimes it had an obliquely cut prolongation. (See Fig 301.) When sleeves of this kind were fitted into small sleeve-holes they were sewn only in front and at the top, so that the long corner hung loosely down.

248

Next to the sleeves, the collar showed the greatest variety. It had a different width from that of the turned-over part in front. For summer wear the collar and turn-over were covered not with fur, but with coloured material, which was slashed. Another style of *Schaube* had no collar at all.

As a rule the *Schaube* was worn hanging loose, with the front open, but it was sometimes girdled with the sword-belt or a sash.

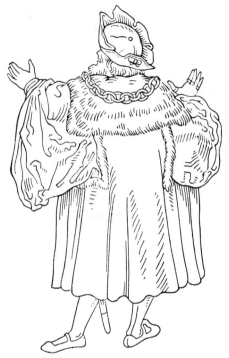

Fig. 302. German Men's Dress, First Half of the Sixteenth Century

Quite different from all the styles hitherto mentioned was the black cloak worn by professional scholars. It lacked the peculiar cloak-like appearance, and had at the top, covering breast, shoulders, and back, a plain, flat piece, called the *Goller*,[1] to which the back and front of the gown were sewn in pleats (Fig. 303). This *Goller* made sleeve-holes unnecessary (see Fig. 304), for it widened the gown over the shoulders and enabled the rest of the voluminous sleeve to be sewn into the seams joining front and back without an undue number of folds. At the beginning of the century the very long sleeves were

[1] Modern German *Koller*.—Translator.

sewn smoothly to the *Goller*, but when the Reformation movement began to spread the ecclesiastical reformers were known by their dress, because the wide sleeves of their gowns were attached to the *Goller* in pleats. Very soon this style of *Schaube*—without fur trimming—became the official dress of all the reforming clergy, and is still worn (with very slight changes) by both Lutheran and Calvinist ministers.

At the beginning of the sixteenth century the light *Barett* had driven out of the field all other hats and caps. At the end of the fifteenth century the low-crowned, broad-

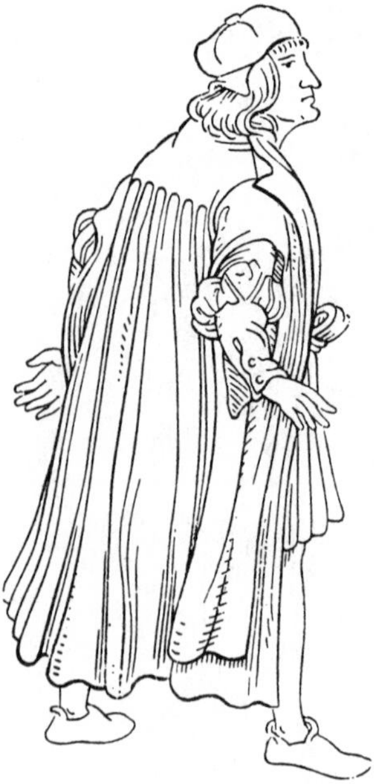

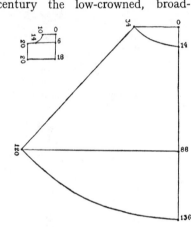

Fig. 303. Scholar's Dress, Sixteenth Century

Fig. 304. Scholar's Schaube

brimmed *Barett* had become more popular than any other, and by the year 1518 it was worn by everybody.

The brim of this *Barett* was rarely cut in one piece with the rest of it ; it was usually sewn on. The straighter the brim was cut, the more nearly perpendicular it hung. But if it were cut more like the shape of the *Barett*, or quite circular, it stood out horizontally. The piece forming the *Barett* proper was always circular ; the edge all round was pleated, or a sufficient number of excisions were made from it to reduce it to the necessary size. The brim of the *Barett* —though it was occasionally made in two pieces—was usually made of doubled material, with stiffening between the two pieces. The outside was slashed, and the ends usually overlapped. *Baretts* of this kind were ornamented by a coloured ribbon which was passed through the incisions in the brim and arranged as a fluted trimming. Crosspieces of material of a colour glaringly different from that of the

Barett were also affixed to the brim. Further, the brim was not merely slashed, but small triangular pieces were cut out of it, the hanging scallops being joined by narrow ribbon so that the brim

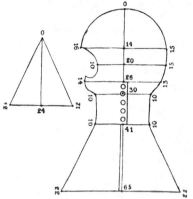

Fig. 305 HOOD, SIXTEENTH CENTURY

assumed an almost perpendicular position. Another way of making the brim was as follows. It was cut nearly double the usual width, then bent outward, and sewn in that shape to the *Barett*. The slashing in the brim was retained, and so the brim now formed a

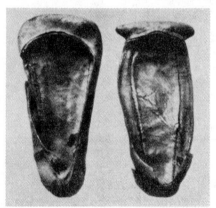

Figs. 306, 307. SO-CALLED KUHMÄULER, OF THE
SIXTEENTH CENTURY

circlet of broad coils of material, the inside of which was lined with material of another colour. This last style of *Barett* was chiefly worn by people of the middle class, whereas knights wore *Baretts* with broad and stiff but unslashed brims. The manufacture of such *Baretts*, which were generally of black stuff, and had feathers hanging

251

round the brim, was a remarkable process. The *Barett* consisted of two circular pieces of the same size sewn together round the outside edge. The hole for the head was cut out of the centre of the under piece, and a thin, flexible support was inserted into the edge to stretch the head hole. On the upper piece was attached a small, low, thinly padded crown, and to this the feathers were fastened. This *Barett* had to be pulled well down over the head, and to fix it still more firmly the opening for the head had attached to it a strip of material, 5 inches wide, which encircled the back of the head. These low-

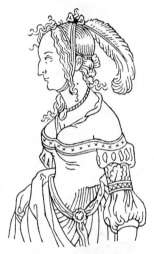

Fig. 308. GERMAN WOMEN'S DRESS, FIRST HALF OF THE SIXTEENTH CENTURY

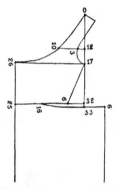

Fig. 309. FRONT OF DRESS IN FIG. 308

crowned *Baretts*, called *Ritterhüte* or *Herrenhüte*, were frequently made of felt covered with velvet or silk.

The headdress adopted when following the chase or when travelling was a cap or a hood worn under the *Barett*. This was worn both by knights and by serving-men, and was made of coarse cloth or soft leather. It consisted of two similar lateral pieces widened at the lower edge by gussets. At the side of the neck the hood had a wide opening which could be buttoned. The length varied with individual taste ; sometimes it reached only to the shoulders, and sometimes it came half-way down the upper arm. The lower edge had a coloured fringe. When worn beneath a helmet these hoods were padded.

Women's Dress. From the beginning of the sixteenth century skirt and bodice were separate items of attire. Even when they formed one garment—though this was now very rarely the case—only the front part of the skirt was cut in one piece with the bodice ; the voluminous back piece was sewn on with an oversewn seam. As the folds of the skirt were meant to come well forward, the front of the skirt was cut much wider than the front of the bodice ; in order to make the two widths equal skirt and bodice were divided at both sides by a cut about 10 cm. in length (see Fig. 309).

The bodice was cut in the same manner as formerly. The back was in two pieces, and was sewn to the front at the shoulders and

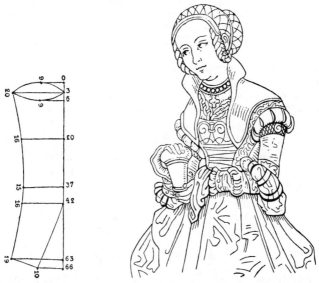

Fig. 310. Sleeve of Women's Dress, Beginning of the Sixteenth Century

Fig. 311. German Women's Dress, First Half of the Sixteenth Century

sides. As efforts were more and more directed to secure a close fit any defects in the cut were remedied by gathering and sewing down the material at the sides and below the bust. The bodice when cut all down the front was fastened by lacing ; otherwise it was fastened at the sides with hooks and eyes. The opening in the skirt was invariably at the side.

The sleeves did not differ so much in cut as their appearance might suggest. The difference really lay in the puffing. Most sleeves were cut straight and sewn with one seam ; they differed merely in length and width. (See Fig. 310.) The tight sleeve fashionable at the beginning of the century is specially noticeable. It was cut in two pieces, and had therefore two seams.

When the bodice was very low at the neck a short *Goller*, or *Koller*, was worn with it (Fig. 311). This was indispensable, as it protected the neck, shoulders, nape of the neck, as well as the exposed part of the bust, against heat and cold. The length and width of the *Goller* varied with individual taste, although much depended on whether it was intended to be merely ornamental or to be also a protection. In the latter case it frequently came down to the shoulders, and was fastened with hooks ; in the former case it was merely a small, light wrap. In cut the *Goller* was approximately circular. The part round the neck was not sewn on separately. (See Fig. 312.) Its erect position was due to the insertion or excision of small double gussets. When the gussets were excised the resultant openings were sewn up again. The stand-up collar was formed by fitting an oblong piece between the ends that extended upward in front.

The *Goller* was either of silk trimmed with velvet or of velvet lined with silk or fur. Some women even wore fur *Gollers*. All were liberally embroidered.

When low necks again went out of fashion *Gollers* still continued to be worn as a luxury, and ladies of high rank had them trimmed

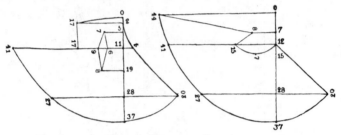

Fig. 312. Cut of the Goller

with gold tissue and ermine. In certain parts of Germany the *Goller* was so popular that it became part of the national dress. In some places, especially on the Rhine, it was worn till well into the seventeenth century.

Soon after the opening of the sixteenth century women's headdress completely changed its character. Almost all the headgear that had been fashionable at the end of the fifteenth century disappeared, especially those types that concealed the hair. The sole survivors were the large caps made of stiffened cloth laid over a framework of wire, and even these were much smaller than those previously worn. About the year 1500 there came in a new style of cap, which rose up at the back of the head like a cone or a slanting comb. It was made of silk richly embroidered with silver or gold. Its shape was due to padding and wire. It gradually fell out of fashion after 1530.

The commonest headdress for women during the first half of the sixteenth century was still the *Barett*. From the year 1510 it was worn by women and girls of all ranks. It was exactly similar to the men's *Barett*, and passed through the same modifications, being trimmed and decorated, slashed and beribboned, feathered and plumed, exactly like that of the men. Like the men, too, the women wore it at an angle on the head. Most women wore beneath it a calotte, or hair-cap, to which it was pinned. Women's *Baretts* were made of light-coloured silk or velvet trimmed with a darker material. Blondes usually wore black *Baretts* with red or yellow trimming.

The calotte was of close network made of gold or silver cord stretched over a cap of gold or silk. Yellow and gold were the commonest colours, but it was also made in red or blue with a gold net over it, or in gold with a net of red or blue silk. Pearls and precious stones, sewn on where the threads of the net crossed each other, were a favourite form of ornamentation with people who could afford it.

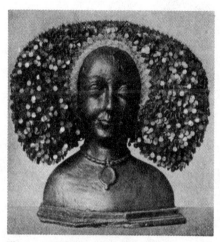

Fig. 313. CAP MADE OF GOLD SEQUINS, AS WORN
IN THE IMPERIAL CITIES
About A.D. 1600.

The year 1530 may be taken as the time when dress reform reached its height. From that time progress ceased. The doublet of the men was now padded. It was close-fitting, and reached up to the neck. The *Barett* lost its *chic* appearance and its plume. It became flatter and stiffer, and finally assumed the shape of a small cap. The hair-cap disappeared, and the hair was cut short all round the head. Shoes became narrower and pointed at the toes. Even the *Schaube* became less voluminous. It disappeared from the wardrobe of the gentleman, and was worn only by the middle classes.

The difference between German and Spanish costume was so great that the transformation could be only gradual. Freedom and limitation opposed each other—on the one hand the puffed, slashed, baggy costume, the *Schaube*, the *Barett* ; on the other hand the close-fitting, padded clothing, the small cape, the stiff hat. And, further, bright, gleaming colours gave way to those that were dark and even gloomy.

255

Men's Dress. In the second half of the sixteenth century the doublet changed very little. The wide, slashed sleeves disappeared in favour of the tight Spanish sleeves which ended in rolls at the shoulders. Doublets with these sleeves were usually padded at the breast, but it was only slowly that this fashion gained ground.

A doublet of this kind, as worn about the year 1570, had very little

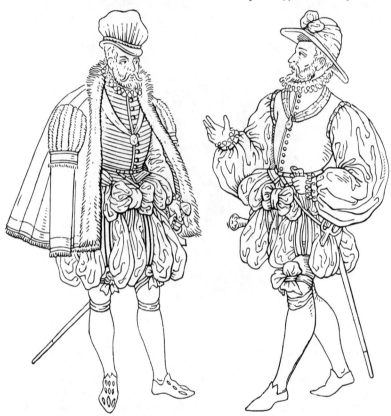

Fig. 314. DRESS OF NOBLEMAN, SECOND HALF OF THE SIXTEENTH CENTURY

Fig. 315. GERMAN MEN'S DRESS, SECOND HALF OF THE SIXTEENTH CENTURY

resemblance to the Spanish style, but the high, stiff collar, with the frill showing above it, and the frills at the wrists were borrowed from the latter.

The doublet was in cut practically as it had been before. It was so made that its appearance could be greatly altered by the addition of tucks and by padding, the cut remaining unchanged. It was only when the *Gansbauch* fashion, which had spread to Germany

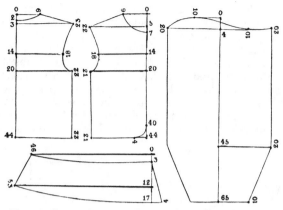

Fig. 316. German Doublet, Second Half of the Sixteenth
Century

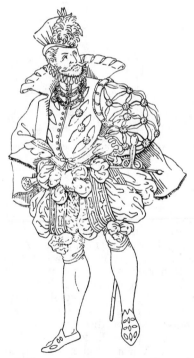

Fig. 317. German Courtier, Second Half of the
Sixteenth Century

257

in the second half of the sixteenth century, was in vogue that the front of the doublet had to be lengthened downward. This style bore the name *Welsch* doublet.

As a rule the tails of the doublet were not longer than 10–14 cm. If they were longer it was called a *Rennröcklein* (racing doublet). This latter style was worn almost exclusively by the nobility as part of the jousting outfit. The long-tailed doublet was very popular with the middle classes during the second half of the sixteenth century.

The cut of the *Schaube* had also altered but little. The new garment was called *Gestaltrock* (form-coat). It could either be put on

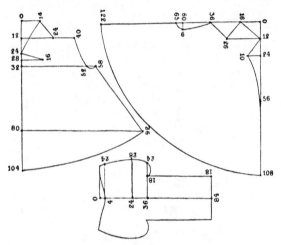

Fig. 318. Gestaltrock, with Hanging Sleeves, Second Half of the Sixteenth Century

like a coat or simply slung round the shoulders. (See Figs. 314 and 318.) It ousted the *Schaube*, and was chiefly worn by noblemen, the *Schaube* becoming exclusively a dress of the middle classes, worn mainly by older citizens, mayors, and councillors. They called it *Ehrrock* (Fig. 319). Almost contemporaneously with the *Gestaltrock* came in the *Harzkappe* (Fig. 320). It was a tighter form of the *Schaube*, and was fashioned in the same manner as the *Gestaltrock*, except that the sleeves were not so long, but short and baggy, not quite reaching the elbow. These baggy sleeves were made of four pieces, two of which were equal in size, one much narrower, and one shorter than the other two. Of these four the narrow piece formed the upper part, the short piece the lower, and the two equal pieces the sides of the sleeve. When the sleeve was fitted into the sleeve-hole the top was disposed on the shoulder with as few pleats as possible.

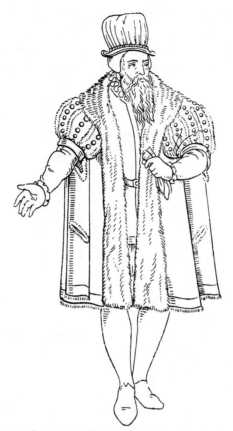

Fig. 319. COUNCILLOR, SECOND HALF OF THE SIXTEENTH CENTURY

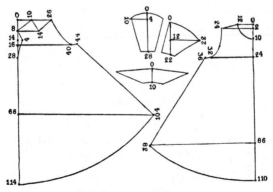

Fig. 320. CUT OF THE HARZKAPPE

About the year 1570 the *Puffjacke*, or puffed jacket, made its first appearance. It was a short coat, either wide or fairly close-fitting, and could be fastened with hooks and eyes from the neck to the waist-belt. About 10 cm. below the waist-belt the coat was cut to

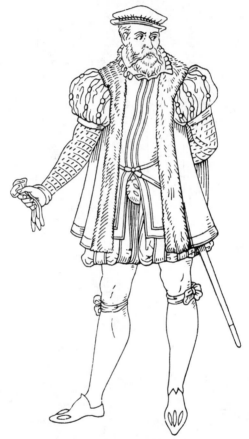

Fig. 321. GERMAN MEN'S DRESS, FIRST HALF OF THE
SIXTEENTH CENTURY

right and left for some distance ; these cuts could be buttoned if desired, or might be allowed to hang down while the wearer was on horseback. These cuts were trimmed. The skirt was sometimes made separately and sewn on, and in that case the two sides did not meet in front. Both sleeves—or in many cases only the right sleeve—had a slash across the middle of the upper arm ; this also was trimmed. In cut the puff jacket closely resembled the

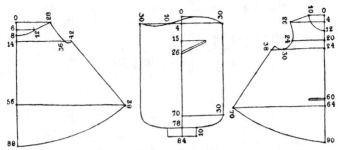

Fig. 322. CUT OF THE PUFF JACKET

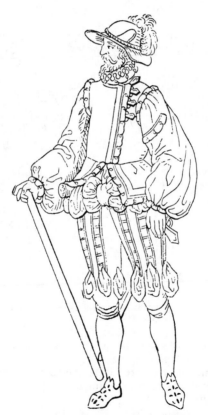

Fig. 323. GERMAN MEN'S DRESS, SECOND HALF OF THE
SIXTEENTH CENTURY

Harzkappe, the main difference being in the sleeves and skirt (see Fig. 322). The puff jackets were really riding dresses, and were often worn over the shoulders like a cloak (Fig. 324). They were therefore also called *Reitröcke* (riding coats), especially when they were long enough to reach the thigh. Any superfluous width was disposed in pleats, and either sewn down or kept in place by a waist-belt.

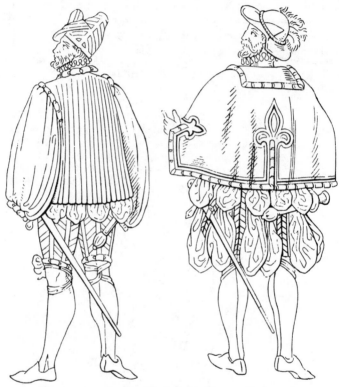

Figs. 324, 325. GERMAN MEN'S DRESS, SECOND HALF OF THE SIXTEENTH CENTURY

Spanish costume was also the model for the short cloak, sometimes called the Spanish cape (Fig. 325). Both in the shape of the collar and in the trimming it differed from the short cloaks and cloak-like wraps worn by young men in Germany during the first half of the sixteenth century.

These cloaks, which were in cut two-thirds or three-fourths of a circle, always had a half-erect collar of varying width, richly trimmed and embroidered in colours. The ridge of the collar and all the edges

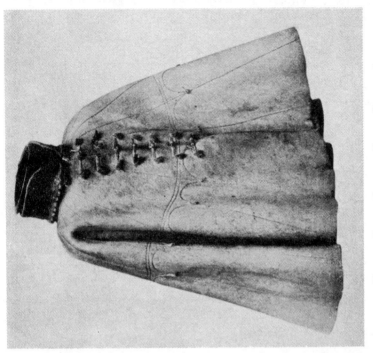

Fig. 327. Pilgrim Cloak of Stefan Praun, 1571

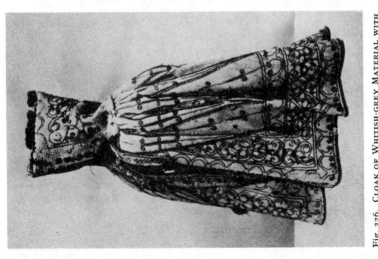

Fig. 326. Cloak of Whitish-grey Material with Black Embroidery, Second Half of the Sixteenth Century

of the cloak were slashed. A peculiar feature of these cloaks was that on both sides in front, about 25 cm. from the bottom hem, was a cut

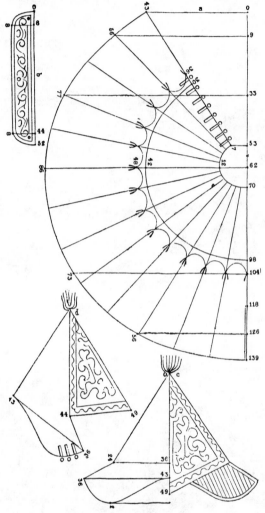

Fig. 328. Spanish Cloak

See Fig. 327. (a) Half of cloak; (b) collar; (c) hood from front; (d) hood from side.

about 20 cm. in length, buttoned and trimmed as in the puff jacket. Cloaks with a hood in the Spanish style were also worn. These hoods were usually so wide that they could be put on over the headdress;

they were very long and pointed, and either trimmed with braid or adorned round the middle with a row of coloured tassels or bows.

Some cloaks were made so that they could be worn either with or without a hood. (See Fig. 328.) These had a small stand-up collar with holes near the lower edge for a cord for fastening the hood.

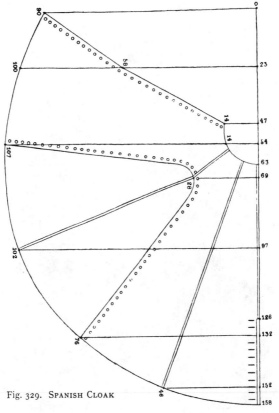

Fig. 329. SPANISH CLOAK

When the cloak was to be worn not merely for show, but as a protection against bad weather, it was made to button. This was specially the case with the longer travelling cloaks. These were, however, not intended merely for protection. They were frequently made to open at the sides so as to ensure better ventilation. For example, the cloak shown in Fig. 329[1] can not only be opened at the

[1] The patterns of these cloaks (Figs. 328 and 329) are taken from garments belonging to the family of Praun in Nürnberg, and now in the Germanisches Museum there. The other patterns of German garments from the sixteenth century are taken from a collection of original drawings which formerly belonged to the Tailors' Guild in Schwabach, and later came into the possession of Carl Köhler.

265

sides, but the side-pieces are buttoned on, and can be removed altogether, leaving the arms completely free. The cloak is then a covering only for breast and back.

Soon after the year 1530 Spanish hose came into fashion with the customary nether garments. Developed into a style of greater length

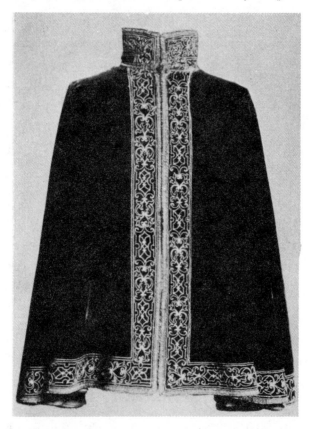

Fig. 330. Dark Red Velvet Cape with Gold Embroidery, about 1570–80

and much greater width, they were adopted by the mercenary soldiers. The make of them was very simple. Like the other nether garments of this period, these baggy breeches (*Pluderhose*) consisted of two garments one inside the other. The outer pair had four to six oblique slashes about 15 cm. wide, filled in with material of a different colour; the inner pair was of much thinner stuff, but much longer, and very wide. The really peculiar feature of these breeches was the great

266

amount of material used to produce the bagginess. While from 4 to 6 yards of cloth sufficed for the hose proper, the puffing required 20 or even sometimes from 40 to 60 yards of very thin silk, called *Kartek*, or *Rasch*.

These figures are not an exaggeration. If the cloth was very narrow

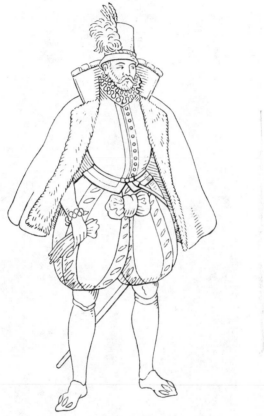

Fig. 331. GERMAN MEN'S DRESS, END OF THE SIXTEENTH CENTURY
German form of the *tonneaux*.

from 80 to 100 yards could easily be used to make this garment, because it was cut much longer than the length of the leg required, and arranged in thick pleats round the body, or gathered round the hips so as to produce the great bagginess desired. The lower edge of this baggy mass was sewn to the lower edge of the outer hose and to the lining. The hose were divided into strips, and reached to the middle of the calf. The lining was much tighter than the hose, and

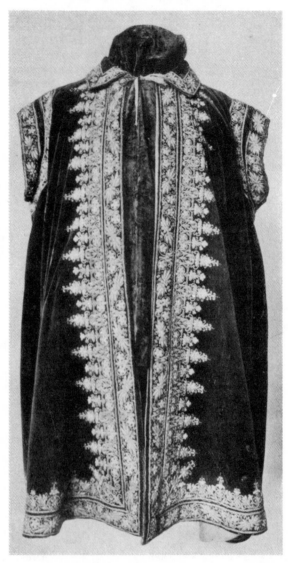

Fig. 332. WEDDING CLOAK OF DUKE WILLIAM V OF BAVARIA, 1568

came only to the knee, so that the bagginess fell from the thigh to the knee. (See Fig. 325.)

Directly connected with the evolution of trousers was the invention of stockings to clothe the feet and the legs to above the knees. When in the middle of the century the short outer hose were lengthened to

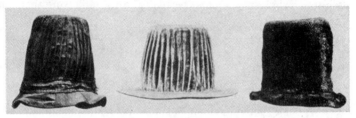

Fig. 333. Men's Hats, Sixteenth Century

or below the knee, the close-fitting leggings coming up to the hips were seen to be superfluous, and the lower part of the leg was thereafter clad in stockings. Like the garment whose place they were taking, they were made of cloth, leather, or silk, with one seam up the back. The foot was either made separately and sewn on or cut

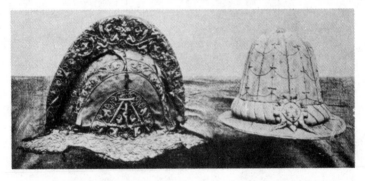

Fig. 334. Stiff Helmet-shaped Hat, End of the Sixteenth Century

in one piece with the leg. In the latter case a gusset was inserted at the ankle to provide the width necessary for the sole of the foot.[1] Stockings, however, would not have been so universally adopted, nor would they have been retained so long, had not the process of knitting been invented at almost the same date, for the knitted stocking did away with many of the disadvantages of the cloth stocking. The costliness of knitted stockings was, however, such a serious handicap

[1] This gusset was retained even with knitted stockings, and also later when they were woven. It was often decorative.

to their adoption that cloth stockings continued to be worn by many people till nearly the close of the century.

In Germany knitted stockings were for a long time made only of wool or cotton. Silk stockings were considered such a luxury that in many places—*e.g.*, Magdeburg in the year 1583—their use was absolutely forbidden, and even persons of royal rank wore them only

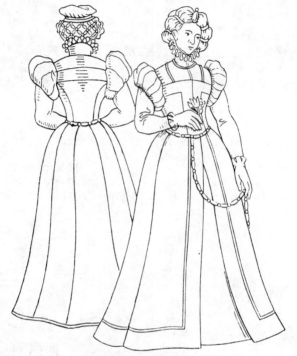

Fig. 335. GERMAN WOMEN'S DRESS, SECOND HALF OF THE SIXTEENTH CENTURY

on Sundays. Men wore stockings of the same colour as their breeches ; only black stockings could be worn with black breeches. Ere long in Spain and in the Netherlands black stockings were universally worn, but in Germany they were largely restricted to officials, especially the clergy. Soldiers liked to wear leather leggings over their knitted stockings.

About the middle of the century boots and shoes also underwent various changes. They were now less broad, and their shape was more in accordance with the contour of the foot. Shoes were again so high that they enclosed the foot up to the ankles. They continued to be slashed and ornamented, quilted and embroidered. They were

made mostly of dark material, as expensive as people could afford
—velvet, silk, or very fine leather.

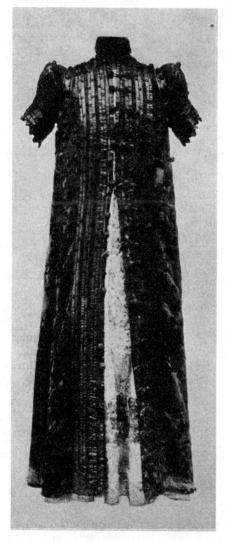

Fig. 336. Over-dress—So-called "Wide Dress"

Women's Dress. The character of women's clothes changed much
more rapidly than that of men's. The transition to the Spanish

styles was so rapid and complete that hardly any intermediate fashions appeared. What variety there was did not outlast the second half of the century. After that the transformation was complete.

The introduction of Spanish fashions into Germany gave increased importance again to under-dresses, and it was the proper thing to wear two dresses, one over the other. (See Fig. 336.) The under-dress had a long, close-fitting bodice, while the over-dress fitted only at the shoulders, gradually increasing in width downward. Such over-dresses were called " wide dresses." They were closed only at the top. They were either sleeveless or had short sleeves, although pendent sleeves were also worn. These wide dresses continued in general use till 1570; after that time only ladies of the upper classes wore them.

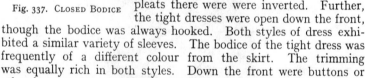

Fig. 337. Closed Bodice

" Tight dresses," or dresses with bodices sewn on, were merely a development of previous styles. The slashes and puffs were given up, and the bodice was longer and tighter. The chief change, however, was that the bodice came much higher up, and was closed all down the front. These tight dresses maintained their place together with the wide dresses, and even continued to be worn when the latter had gone out of fashion. Both styles were without a train, and had no pleats, or only very few. What pleats there were were inverted. Further, the tight dresses were open down the front, though the bodice was always hooked. Both styles of dress exhibited a similar variety of sleeves. The bodice of the tight dress was frequently of a different colour from the skirt. The trimming was equally rich in both styles. Down the front were buttons or other fasteners.

The skirt had formerly been cut as a complete circle, or made of two or—according to the width of the material—four oblong pieces, with an equal number of gussets at the seams. Now, however, skirts were without pleats, and tighter than they had been ; the waist of the skirt, therefore, was made tight-fitting, and the skirt was no longer cut as a complete circle, but as two-thirds or three-fourths of one.

The bodice was always closed in front. It ended in a long point, and was in two styles according as it was meant to reach to the neck or to cover only the breast. The high-necked bodice (Fig. 337) was in two parts, joined by a seam at the shoulders and by another running down the middle of the back. Two tucks running over the shoulder-blades and down the back made it fit smoothly at the back, while tucks and intakes caused it to follow exactly the lines of the figure.

On the other hand, the low-necked bodice (Fig. 338) was so cut that each front piece made, with the corresponding back piece (to which it was connected by a piece at the shoulder), one whole. The bodice had thus one back seam and one front seam and two side-seams fairly far back. This low-necked bodice, like the other, was made to fit closely by tucks where it was unduly wide.

Tight sleeves were cut as shown in Fig. 310, and baggy sleeves were made like those of the *Harzkappe*. Wide sleeves were cut as shown in Fig. 338, *b*. The thick, baggy shoulder-rolls and the sleeves with erect, padded shoulders were sewn to the top of the shoulder-strips so that these were completely concealed.

As a rule the bodices were stiffly lined, and those with a high neck were slightly padded to make them perfectly smooth. The fastening was done with laces or hooks and eyes, or occasionally with buttons.

The neck-frill passed through the same changes as that worn by men, and soon attained large proportions. Osiander, who expressed great disapproval of the frills, tells us what they were like and how they were made. *Inter alia*, he says : " From foreign countries we have introduced and learned how to make large, long, wide, thick neck-frills of fine, delicate, expensive linen. They have to be starched and dressed with a hot iron." And again : " These frills have to be supported by fine silver or other

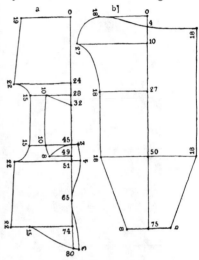

Fig. 338. Low-necked Bodice
(*a*) Front and back piece ; (*b*) sleeve.

wire, specially made for the purpose." (See Fig. 398.) These supports were broad, elastic collars made of fairly strong wire, sloping outward so as to resist better the pressure of the frill.

Frills similar, but narrower, were worn at this period round the wrists by women of every age and station.

During the second half of the sixteenth century the stocking made its appearance as a new, or, at least, entirely different, item of dress. We have already seen how it came to be invented because of an important alteration in men's nether garments. Previous to that time most women wore short socks made of cloth, whose only purpose was to protect the foot against any pinching of the shoe. Women, with their long skirts, had no need of a garment to conceal their legs or keep them warm. If they felt such need, they used separate hose such as men wore. Nor was there any real necessity for women to clothe the leg below the knee at the time when knitted stockings had become universal wear for men. So it is safe to say that it was because women saw how much a shapely leg gains in attractiveness from a close-fitting stocking that their vanity led them to add this further item to their wardrobe. They soon began to devote great attention to this new article of wear, and ere long extended their interest to their garters, which were of silk and richly embroidered. At that time white stockings were regarded as the most elegant, black being the colour coming next in favour.

Women's shoes were exactly like men's, and, like them, were slashed. Additional decorations were silver cord and dainty frills. The usual

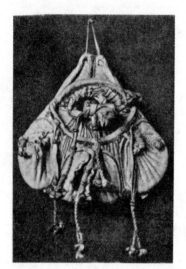
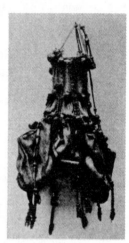

Figs. 339, 340. LEATHER BAGS, SIXTEENTH CENTURY

material was *cordouan*, or Spanish leather—very soft goatskin tanned in a special way and dyed in all colours. Silk and velvet in all shades were also used. Like the men, women also wore inner shoes, or *Trippen*, but theirs were, of course, much daintier. To make a pattering sound with the over-shoes while walking was a practice greatly favoured by women.

At that period heralds occupied an important position. Their duties included the bringing of important news and the conduct of negotiations. (See Fig. 271.) Their costume was both handsome and striking. Their most imposing garment was a wide cape open at the sides—the *Wappenrock*, or coat with armorial bearings. It reached nearly to the knees. Breast and back were embroidered with the arms of the master in whose service they were. The cape was made of two approximately oblong pieces of cloth joined by shoulder-pieces.

ITALY

Men's Dress. The tightness and stiffness of Spanish costume did not commend itself to Italian taste. The transition to new styles therefore proceeded very slowly, and took the form of a gradual change rather than an unquestioning acceptance of the new fashions. Points and puffs gradually disappeared. The doublet was lengthened.

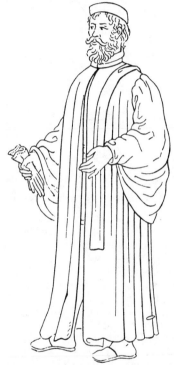

Fig. 341. ITALIAN (VENETIAN) MEN'S DRESS, MIDDLE OF THE SIXTEENTH CENTURY

The shirt was made high at the neck, with a ruff. The short jacket was retained, but a small skirt was added to it. The long, open over-coats were gradually given up, especially by young men, and were now worn only by older people of the better class, by scholars, by the Venetian nobility and high officials ; and even these no longer wore them in the old close-fitting style. (See Fig. 341.) The over-coat was now much wider than before, and reached to the ankles ; it had sleeves, tight at the top and at the wrists, but wide in the middle, which were called *maniche a comeo*, or elbow-sleeves. (See Fig. 342.)

These overcoats went by the name *zimarra*. They were rarely worn with a girdle. If one was used, it was fastened quite loosely. The coats were made of heavy patterned silk or of velvet, and lined in summer with silk, in winter with light fur.

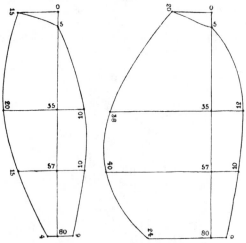

Fig. 342. ELBOW-SLEEVES

Young men went about in short closed coats with a high neck and a very long slit at the breast. These, sometimes lined with fur, and always worn with a waist-belt, widened just a little from the bust to the waist, and were much wider from the waist downward. Back and front were of the same shape, and were sewn together by shoulder- and side-seams. The sleeves were elbow-sleeves like those of the wide coats.

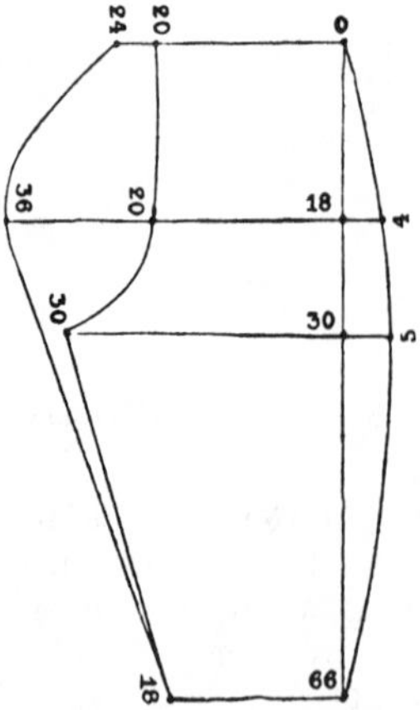

When the sixteenth century opened men's hose were still of the two usual forms—viz., either footed hose of elastic material, close-fitting, covering the entire leg and the lower part of the body, or a garment consisting of two parts, the upper one, the over-stock, reaching from the hips to the knee or lower, while the other, the under-stock, supplementing the upper part, consisted of long, close-fitting footed hose which extended to the ankle and covered the foot. These were put on beneath the breeches, and fastened at the waist by the girdle and at the knees by garters.

Fig. 343. ITALIAN BREECHES

The breeches that were supported by the girdle and by being

fastened to the under-vest were close-fitting at the leg. They were longer than was necessary, and so wide round the body that they formed folds under the waist-belt. (See Fig. 343.) The frontal opening was still covered by a pouch-shaped flap. The breeches were slashed, and the slashes were lined with material of another colour. If they were long, the knees and legs were also slashed. The underhose were never slashed. Breeches of this kind continued to be worn in Italy during the whole century. Only in the northern and southern

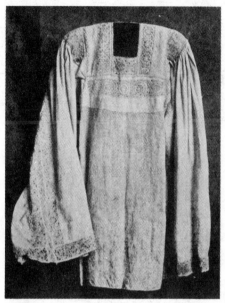

Fig. 344. MAN'S SHIRT OF THE RENAISSANCE
Sixteenth century.

districts were they ousted by the Spanish breeches, which were there so popular that they were worn even by the lowest classes. At the beginning of the sixteenth century the long, slashed breeches that had been so fashionable toward the end of the fifteenth century went entirely out of fashion.

The Italian doublet worn in the middle of the sixteenth century was cut like the Spanish type, but it was not padded to the same degree. It was moderately high at the neck, or had a stand-up collar. It was either quite short or came down to the thigh. The sleeves were slightly padded, and mostly very tight. Sometimes there were no sleeves, and in that case a second, sleeved doublet was worn beneath it. The breeches too were of the Spanish type, but less padded (Fig. 345), and the slashes were always trimmed.

277

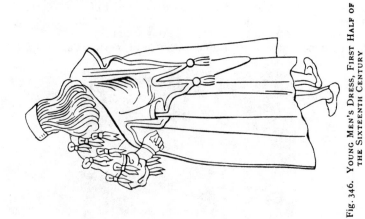

Fig. 346. Young Men's Dress, First Half of the Sixteenth Century

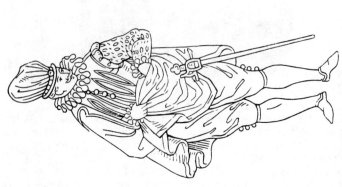

Fig. 345. Costume of Young Venetian, Second Half of the Sixteenth Century

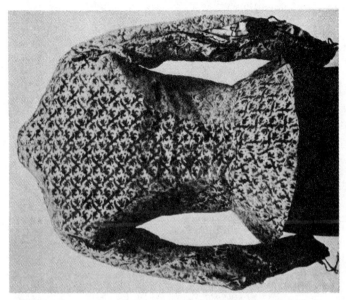

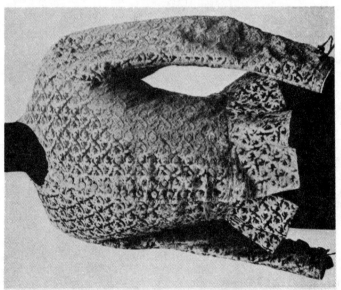

Figs. 347, 348. Greenish-yellow Velvet Jacket Sixteenth Century—Front and Back Views

Women's Dress. At the beginning of the sixteenth century women's dress in Italy showed a similar striving after simplicity. The tight bodices and dresses that were tight down to the hips, as well as the wide, trailing dresses, went more and more out of fashion, and were replaced by garments that were tight only across the bust. Dresses

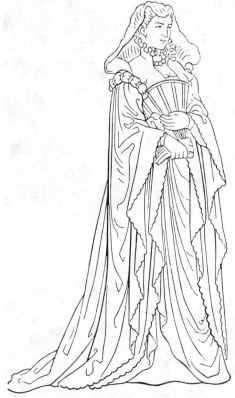

Fig. 349. Costume of High-born Lady of Siena

with separate short bodices were still worn, but the bodice was now wider, and the fastening was no longer in front, but at the side. The low neck was retained, but it was now trimmed with some fine white material. Long trains were abandoned except for Court dresses.

Under-dresses, all the cloak-like over-dresses, and also the shoes continued as before. But hats and hairdressing exhibited a return to simpler styles. Of the numerous forms of headdress, the net caps, small toques, and in particular the round rolls called *balzo* were retained ; the last named were worn both by women and men. They were made of gilded copper foil or gilded leather.   The disappearance of many of the various forms of headdress was due to the fact that women and girls now began to pay great attention to their hair, and to use pearls, flowers, and jewels in their *coiffure*.   Veils again came into fashion, and soon became an indispensable item of headdress.

The foreign influence that came in about the middle of the century met with even greater resistance among women than among men,

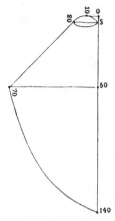

and although in those districts that fell under the dominion of Spain dress became more and more dominated by Spanish fashions, its whole character was different.   The absence of drapery and the stiffness of Spanish costume did not please the taste of Italian women. These did not lace themselves more than was necessary to raise the breast.   They retained not only the voluminous skirt, but also the train.   The skirt was so long that the wearer had to lift it from the ground while walking. The farthingale found no acceptance—stiffened petticoats were worn instead.   For the Italian women shoulder-puffs were merely decoration, and were never allowed to become too high (see Fig. 349).   It was only in the Spanish districts that the covered breast and high neck and large ruffs made any headway.   In

Fig. 350. Cut of Sleeves
in Fig. 349

Venice, Rome, Florence, Pisa, and Ferrara women of all classes covered only the shoulders, leaving the breast bare.   The collar varied, of course, with the style of the dress at the neck.   It either had a narrow goffered ruff or surrounded the neck and shoulders in a high circle trimmed with lace.

The first change was in the sleeves. These were only moderately wide, and the bagginess was confined to the top of the arm, which was slashed and lined with coloured stuffs or ornamented with puffs.   Sometimes the back of the sleeve was left open, revealing a white under-sleeve of small puffs.   Both back and front of the bodice were low, and the bodice was thinly padded to fit the outlines of the body.   It was much longer in front than at the back ; the

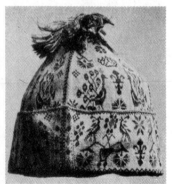

Fig. 351. Italian Child's Bonnet,
Sixteenth Century

hooking was at the side.   The other style of bodice, however, which was closed in front, still continued to be worn ; the front of this bodice was more or less pointed. The seams joining the sleeves to the bodice were trimmed not with shoulder-rolls, but with close rows

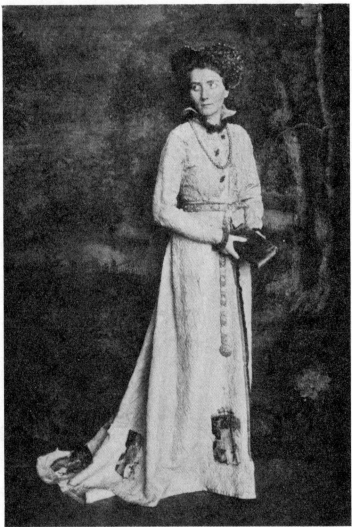

Fig. 352. Renaissance Gown with Bavarian Coats of Arms, Middle of the Sixteenth Century

of white frills with plain or scalloped edges. In Venice the back of the bodice was also shaped to a point at the waist, though it was much shorter than the front, but in other parts—for example, in

Bologna—the front of the bodice was very long and the back as short as possible. The lower edge of the bodice formed an elegant waist-belt, trimmed with pearls, jewels, or silk, the end of which

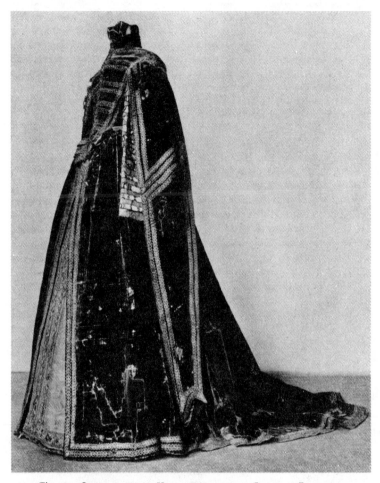

Fig. 353. Over-dress and Under-dress of the Countess Palatine Dorothea Sabine of Neuburg (d. 1598)

hung down in front from the point of the bodice. (See Fig. 352.) The neck was very low in the districts which were not under the dominion of Spain, and the straight top edge of the bodice did not come higher than the armpits. It was frilled or trimmed with lace. Even when it was V-shaped it was very low.

283

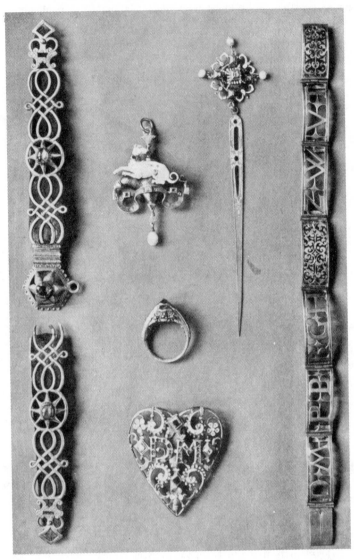

Fig. 354. Jewellery from the Royal Mausoleum at St Martin-in-Lauingen

In the districts round Milan and Naples the low-necked bodice and the open-fronted bodice gave way to the high Spanish style (Fig. 353). But in Naples itself an opener style was worn by ladies of high station. The Italian bodice was partly Spanish and partly German in cut. Toward the end of the century the front of the bodice was padded—frequently to such an extent that it bulged outward at the stomach. In some cases it resembled the *Gansbauch*. As the front was now much longer than the back, and ended in a sharp point, the bodice was not now closed at the side, but either at the back or front; the fastening was done not with hooks and eyes, but with a draw-string. The draw-string was invisible, however, as it was in the lining, and hidden by the material over it, which was fastened with buttons or hooks.

The skirt varied in length, for although moderately long dresses with a short train were generally worn, the over-skirt was long or short according as the wearer desired or not to display the petticoat worn underneath. In Pisa the skirt came only to the knee, so that the under-skirt was fully displayed.

The sleeves underwent little change. They were of medium width, tight at the wrist and shoulder, widest at the elbow. In rare cases they were widest at the top, tapering toward the hand. In most instances they were slightly padded or lined with some coarse stuff, such as fustian. Occasionally under-sleeves were worn, the shape of which was dictated by local fashion. In some places, such as Siena, sleeves were immoderately long; in others they were actually pendent (see Fig. 349). In Bologna they were so very long that they had to be tied together behind in order to allow freedom of movement. But the greatest variety in sleeves was seen in the open-fronted over-dresses. All the shapes that had been current were retained during the second half of the century. The commonest styles of these dresses were those which gradually widened from the shoulders down and those which fitted closely at the waist (Fig. 353).

THE SEVENTEENTH CENTURY

WITH the opening of the seventeenth century a set was made in almost all European countries against Spanish fashions. Stiffness in dress was abandoned, and a return was made to more natural styles of clothing. During the period of the Thirty Years War Germany passed through an independent evolution which had its effect even on French fashions. The long war touched every class and every calling, and gave the entire manhood of Germany a warlike appearance. Not only young men, noble and middle-class, but even scholars and clergy appeared in leather doublets and with swords, " booted and spurred." Ere long the French gave to the new fashions a definite form, and the year 1650 forms a fairly sharp dividing line. From that time France became the leader of European fashion. This period covers the transition from Spanish to French costume. Although toward the end of the sixteenth century Spanish dress had already undergone great modifications, its original form had continued till then to be the prevalent fashion for Court dress.

SPAIN

Till well into the middle of the century Spanish dress retained the character it had assumed during the time of Philip II (reigned 1556–98).

Men's Dress. In men's dress thickly padded knee-breeches gradually became the leading fashion. The starched ruff was exchanged for the broad, smooth collar worn by the soldiers. About the year 1630 boots with wide tops took the place of those with reversed tops reaching to the knees. The soft felt hat replaced the stiff variety (see Fig. 369). All the same, Spanish dress still retained its neat, compact character. Even the short doublet still continued to be worn, although the padding and the slashes and puffs were no longer fashionable. The long sleeves opened longitudinally and pendent sleeves were worn into the middle of the eighteenth century. Toward the end of the seventeenth century the characteristic slashed breeches were replaced by much shorter knee-breeches. Silk stockings and low leather shoes enclosing the entire foot and decorated with rosettes of ribbon completed the attire (see Fig. 363). Wigs made their way very slowly into Spain, and it was not till the year 1700 that they were universally worn. On the other hand, the opening of the seventeenth century saw gentlemen beginning to wear eyeglasses, the size increasing with the rank of the wearer.

Women's Dress.   About the year 1621 women began to abandon
the closed bodice.   The low neck came in, exposing shoulders and

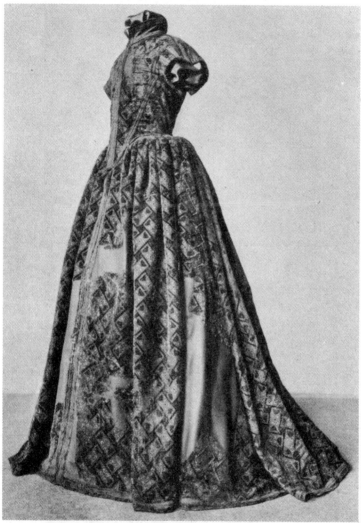

Fig. 355.   Over-dress of the Duchess Dorothea Sabine Maria of
Sulzbach (*d.* 1639), Wife of Otto Heinrich

back, but covering the bust.   As a matter of fact, Spanish women
disliked any fullness at the breast, and sheets of lead were fastened
over the breasts of young girls to retard their development.   Apart

from the introduction of the low neck, the shape of the over-dresses was unchanged. The over-dress fitted closely down to the hips, and

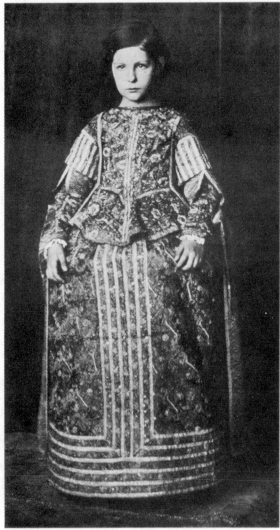

Fig. 356. Gown of the Infanta Isabella of Spain,
Seventeenth Century

was open all down the front. Farthingales were smaller, and began about the year 1665 to be ousted by numerous petticoats, often eight to ten in number, made of good material. Farthingales were now worn only at Court and on outstanding occasions. The sleeves of the over-dress, hidden by shoulder-rolls and flaps, were open all down the front, and buttoned only at the wrist. When going out of doors ladies wore the mantilla, a short cloak of black silk.

The hair was now dressed lower, but it was still combed back from the face. The front and side hair was rolled back, while the rest was plaited and massed at the nape of the neck and fastened with ribbons,

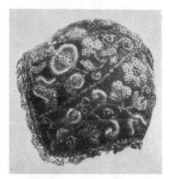

Fig. 357. SPANISH BONNET FOR AN INFANT
SEVENTEENTH CENTURY

hairpins, and ornamental buttons. Pearl chains and hanging ostrich feathers were much used as hair ornaments.

By the end of the seventeenth century French fashions had become fairly established, and in the course of the eighteenth century they completely supplanted Spanish costume.

FRANCE

The fashions that prevailed at the end of the sixteenth century continued in France practically without change till about the year 1620. But from the death of Henry IV onward the lavish use of expensive materials, ornaments, and jewellery had again become so general that in 1633 a law passed in 1629 was renewed forbidding all except princes and nobles to wear clothing decked with precious stones and gold embroidery, or caps, shirts, collars, cuffs, and other linen embroidered with gold, silver, cord, or lace, either real or imitation. These edicts, however, were as ineffectual as all other similar ones had been.

This increasing love of finery reawakened the preference for loud, glaring colours, which had died out at the end of the sixteenth century. By the year 1630 only the Huguenots wore dark colours.

Men's Dress. It was the marriage of Louis XIII with Anne of

Austria in 1615 that gave the signal for a revolution in dress. Although Spanish fashions were reintroduced at Court, only courtiers and their families wore them. But even in this Court dress the influence of

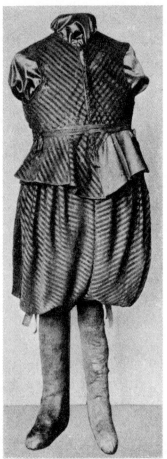

Fig. 358. DOUBLET AND BREECHES OF DUKE PHILIP LUDWIG OF PFALZ-NEUBURG (*d.* 1614)

new ideas was recognizable. The old stiffness was gradually eliminated. In men's dress the change was first seen in hats. Instead of being stiff and narrow-brimmed they were now soft and broad-brimmed, like those worn by Henry IV. About 1650 the crown was high and conical, but it gradually became lower and cylindrical in

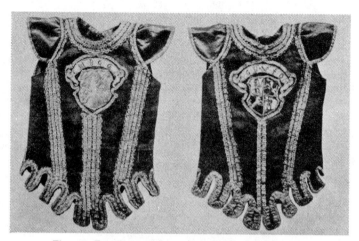

Fig. 359. Two Pea-jackets worn by Pages, about 1607

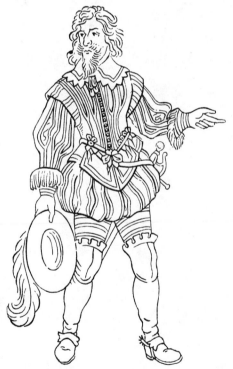

Fig. 360. French Men's Dress, Beginning of the
Seventeenth Century

shape. The brim was tilted up at one side, and held in that position by a clasp. Behind the clasp came the plume of feathers.

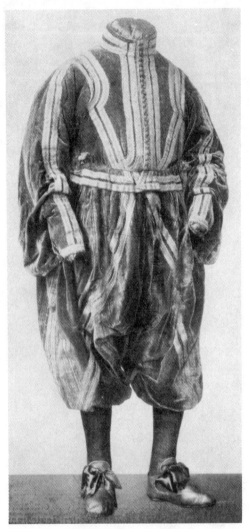

Fig. 361. GREEN VELVET SUIT AND SHOES OF DUKE MAURICE OF SAXE-LAUENBURG

The large ruff at the neck was the next item of dress to change. Now it either fell loosely on to the shoulders in the form of two or three strips one over another, or was replaced by a smooth, embroidered collar (Fig. 360), either stiffened with wire and standing out from the neck all round or unstiffened and lying flat. These three styles of collar were all worn till about 1630 From that time onward the last-mentioned style became universal.

There were also changes in the other items of attire. The short breeches (*trousses*) reaching only to the middle of the thigh were

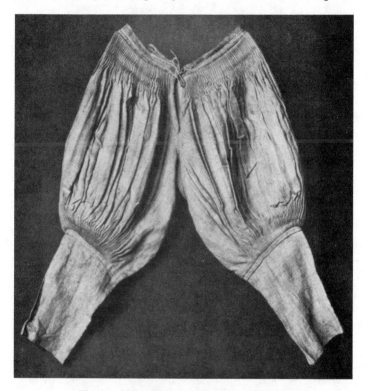

Fig. 362. BAGGY BREECHES (PLUDERHOSE), 1620

now almost without padding (Fig. 362), and the baggy appearance was only the result of a very stiff lining. The projecting flap (*braguette*) was done away with, and was replaced by a simple slit that could be buttoned. The long silk riding breeches were protected by a pair of tight *Streufflinge* (*bas attachez*) fastened at the top to the breeches and tucked inside the riding boots. For the winter these were of the same material as the breeches and doublet ; for summer wear they were made of stout white linen. They were daintily trimmed or quilted. The doublet (*pourpoint*) was still slightly padded throughout, but not stiffened nearly as much as before. It was also now much longer in front than at the back, and the tails were cut in

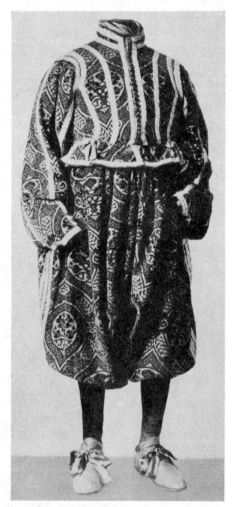

Fig. 363. RED VELVET SUIT AND SHOES OF DUKE MAURICE OF SAXE-LAUENBURG

one piece with the body of it. Both front and back had long slashes richly trimmed, and side-pieces were now not infrequent. Instead of the shoulder rolls or shoulder-hoops men wore shoulder-pieces surrounding the top of the sleeves and sewn into the sleeve-holes with the sleeves. (See Fig. 365.) These shoulder-pieces were also worn with pendent sleeves. The rounder they were cut, the flatter they lay. When they were being sewn in they were folded longitudinally, the edges being sewn in. The sleeves were either slightly padded throughout and close-fitting, or were slashed at the top and given a baggy lining of differently coloured stuff. In this case the upper part was very long, and frequently, also, somewhat wider than usual.

The breeches were fastened to the doublet as before, but no longer to the inside of it. Tapes or ribbons with metal tags (*aiguillettes*)

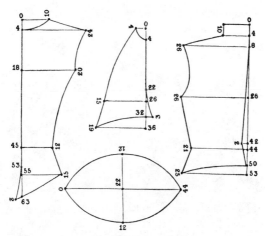

Fig. 364. FRENCH-SPANISH DOUBLET, BEGINNING OF THE SEVENTEENTH CENTURY

about 8 cm. in length were drawn through holes made for the purpose in the doublet and tied on the outside in neat bows.

Sometimes the doublet, with the exception of the sleeves, was left quite plain, and an ornate ' cape ' (*Goller, collet*) of exactly the same shape, with pendent sleeves, was put on over it. The doublet was visible through the slashes in the cape.

The alterations in the cloak included the addition of a broad, oblong collar, which lay flat at the back. The trimming and embroidery were also more extensive. Fur lining was frequent, as were also fringes of gold or silver round the lower edge. As a rule the cloak came half-way down the thigh. It was slung either over one shoulder or over both. The lower part of it was usually drawn across the body to the opposite side, and fastened in that position.

Popular and universally worn as the Spanish doublet then was, it was chiefly a summer garment. In winter men wore instead of it a coat made like it, but with a skirt reaching nearly to the knees. This coat, called *casaque*, and often beautifully trimmed, was worn even in summer by menservants, pages, and grooms. It was frequently sleeveless, like the *collet*, or had hanging sleeves. The actual covering

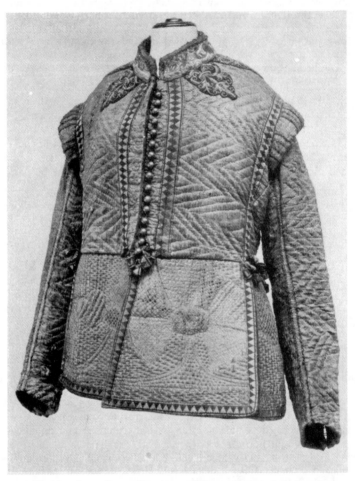

Fig. 365. Olive Green Doublet of Quilted Silk, about 1630–40

of the arms in that case consisted of the sleeves of the doublet worn beneath it.

The dress of men of the middle classes was the same as that of the nobles, only less expensive and ornate. Most of them, however, preferred the *culotte béarnaise* introduced by Henry IV to the slashed Spanish knee-breeches. But it too was modified. By 1613 it was much tighter than at the end of the sixteenth century. Within the next ten years it became tighter still, was lengthened to the calves, and was fastened below the knees with broad ribbons tied in a bow. In this form the *culotte* of Henry IV was soon adopted by the nobility ;

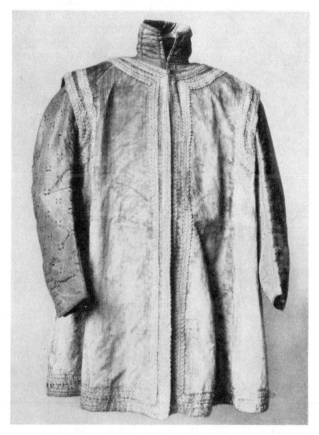

Fig. 366. Cloak of Pale Yellow Velvet, about 1630

it was trimmed down the outside seam with rows of close-set buttons, and occasionally with an additional broad trimming. A few buttons at the foot were left unbuttoned so as to allow a baggy puff of fine material to be seen underneath. The breeches were still fastened to the doublet by ribbons, which were allowed to hang down below the doublet unless they were tied on the outside of it. The front flap (*la braye* or *bavaroise*) was now mostly fastened with very large buttons. They were in full view—ornamental as well as useful.

About 1629 the doublet was still cut in the former way, but was shorter in the waist, and altogether less close-fitting than before. In order to show the fine white under-linen the doublet was slit at the back (Fig. 367). The slit was made to button, but a portion of it was left wide open. As a rule, also, the doublet was buttoned only at the top, in order not to hide the shirt. The sleeves were much wider than they had been ; they had a moderately deep cuff, and were open in front from the top to the wrist so as to show a light-coloured or white loose under-sleeve. (See Fig. 368.) The sleeve-

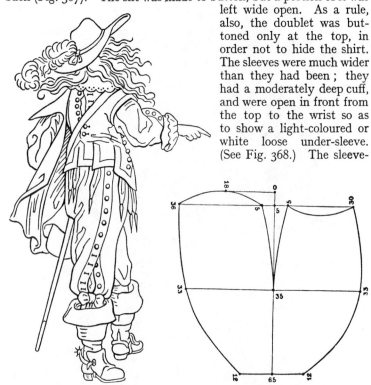

Fig. 367. French Men's Dress of the Year 1629

Fig. 368. Open Sleeve of French Doublet, 1630

edges were provided with close-set buttons so that they could be closed if desired. These sleeves were rarely cut straight, but were usually widest at the elbows. Hanging sleeves were now going more and more out of fashion, and were never worn with these open-fronted sleeves.

The cloak was now longer and closer-fitting. It had frequently short, wide sleeves, and was sometimes collarless. Not rarely it was slit from the foot up to the small of the back. These cloaks began at this time to be called *casaques*, the name that had been applied about twenty years before to the short, close-fitting coats. Sleeveless cloaks were still worn.

The soft felt hat began soon after 1620 to be made with a much broader brim (Fig. 369). It was lower in the crown, and the top was rounded. It was usually dyed white or light brown. Dark colours were rare. Black hats were almost never worn. It was a common

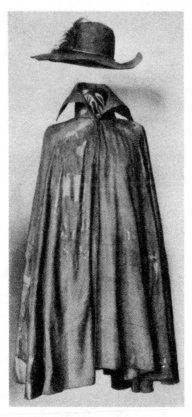

Fig. 369. HAT AND CLOAK, FIRST HALF OF THE SEVENTEENTH CENTURY

practice to adorn the hat with two or three long ostrich feathers of different colours—usually red, white, or blue.

About 1630 fashion produced as an alternative to the usual short doublet another style, with fairly long tails. The sides were sewn together only down to the waist—at that time very short—so that the skirt was open at the sides. This gave the garment four tails. (See Figs. 370 and 371.) The two front tails were always cut in one piece with the doublet, but the two at the back were frequently sewn on. As the tails were broader at the foot than at the top the edges

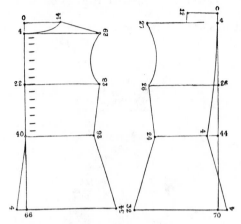

Fig. 370. Long-tailed Doublet of the Year 1636

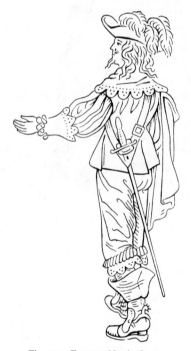

Fig. 371. French Men's Costume, about 1636

overlapped. The breast and back of this doublet were usually adorned with long slashes (Fig. 372), through which material of another colour showed, and bows of ribbon were attached in front and also close together round the waist. Similarly, the sleeves were either open all down the front or slashed so as to expose the baggy

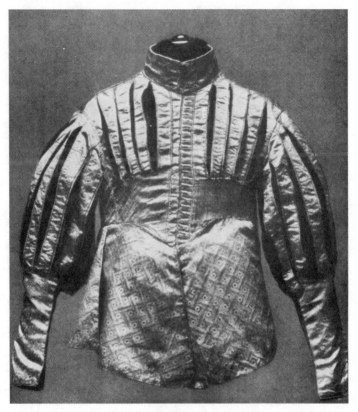

Fig. 372. DOUBLET OF WHITE PATTERNED SATIN, 1630–35

mass underneath. In a few years' time this style of doublet lost all semblance of a waist and the only trimming was a double or triple row of lace following the lines of the edges.

From 1634 onward the breeches ceased to be fastened at the foot. They were left open. The foot hem was trimmed with hanging strings or bows of ribbon or with lace (Figs. 374 and 403), hiding the garters. The rows of small buttons and the trimming on the outside of the breeches had long gone out of fashion. One single button was sewn on at the knee to hold a bow of ribbon about 20 cm. long. Since the waist of the doublet had been shortened, the breeches were no longer attached to it, but were kept up by means of a cord through the top seam, fastened above the hips.

About 1640 the cylindrical hat was very high in the crown ; the

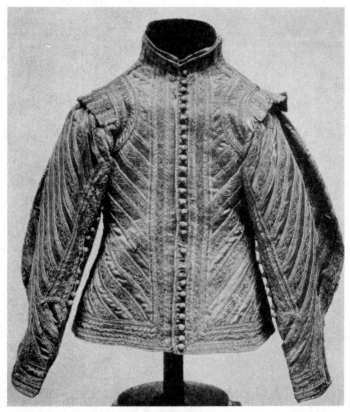

Fig. 373. POURPOINT OF RUST-RED SILK WITH YELLOW AND BLUE EMBROIDERY, ABOUT 1650

width of the brim was about 10 cm. This fashion never became popular, and lasted only a few years. Most hats had a broad brim and a high conical crown.

After the lapse of ten years—up to 1650—dress had again entirely changed. The *pourpoint* had become very short and very tight, but on the other hand the breeches had greatly increased in width (see Fig. 374), so that separate under-pants, tied below the knees, had to be worn. The breeches had the same width at the top and at the

foot. The ends of the legs were open, and trimmed with close-set
tags. At the top were bows of ribbon arranged to form a triangle

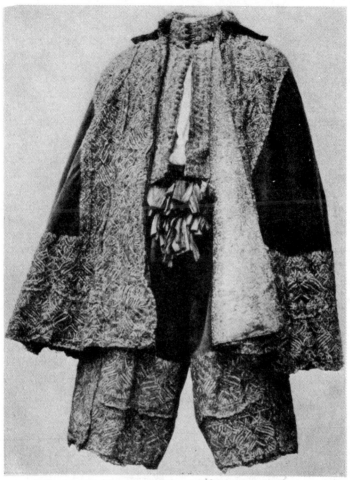

Fig. 374. SUIT OF CHARLES X OF SWEDEN (REIGNED 1654–60)

which hung down and hid the front opening. Similarly at the foot
was a bunch of ribbons sewn down with a button.[1]

The fashion of trimming the nether garments and doublet with
lace not only continued, but was carried even further. All seams were

[1] Instead of these breeches male servants such as pages wore the short,
slashed Spanish hose with thick, firm padding. In other respects their dress
was exactly the same as that here described.

303

thus trimmed, except in the case of everyday dress. If shoes were worn instead of boots, the tops of the stockings were turned outward and deeply trimmed with lace.

Sometimes—especially on festive occasions—a cloak was worn above this costume. During the whole of the first half of the seventeenth century the cloak was an essential item of men's full dress ; it had still the same form as it had had all along, reaching half-way down the thigh. It was slung over one shoulder and wound round the body.

The costume just described indicated a turning-point in the development of men's dress. It was the basis of all the new types of male

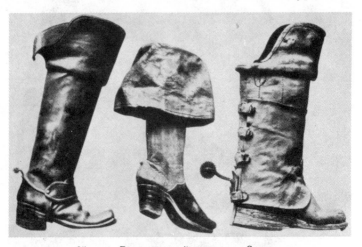

Fig. 375. BOOTS OF THE SEVENTEENTH CENTURY

clothing that appeared right up to the time of the French Revolution. The changes affected not only the coat and the breeches, but also collars and cuffs, shoes and hats. Even the styles of hairdressing underwent a complete transformation.

Of the various collars worn at the beginning of the century the only one that survived the year 1630 was the lace collar fastened in front and falling loosely on the shoulders. This had gradually increased in breadth, and ere ten years had passed had attained such a size that it hung down over the shoulders. As, however, only very rich people could afford these large collars of lace they soon came to be made of fine linen, only the trimming being of lace. This lace trimming became narrower and narrower, till about 1650 it went out of fashion altogether. For ten years previously the collar itself had been losing greatly in breadth. These collars rarely deviated from the ordinary shape and make. A straight piece of material was pleated on the edge next the neck ; these pleats were then fastened down and

304

starched. A style of collar favoured by soldiers was the *welsche* or
' foreign ' collar. It was worn right on till about the middle of the
seventeenth century. The cord used for tying the collar ended in
tassels whose shape varied from time to time. They were small to
begin with, but gradually became larger and larger. The cuffs
changed along with the collars, and their shape was always exactly
the same as that of the latter. Throughout the whole of the first
half of the seventeenth century the cuffs were turned back over the
sleeves (Fig. 371).

During the first half of the seventeenth century the nobles wore
boots with spurs attached, and wore them even on festive occasions
and in drawing-rooms. The fashions in footgear changed several
times, with the rest of the attire. At the
beginning of the century boots were narrow,
and came up only a little beyond the knee.
From 1610 onward they were longer. The
tops were lined with coloured material and
reversed to show this. (See Fig. 375.)

During the second half of the seventeenth century men's dress underwent more
numerous changes than ever. These were
due to the caprice of the French king, but
they exhibited a continuous evolution of the
various items of attire, with the result that
men's dress had altered so much by the
year 1700 that the dress of that day was
altogether different from what it had been in
1650.

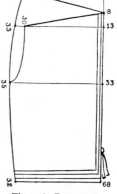

Fig. 376. BREECHES,
MIDDLE OF THE SEVEN-
TEENTH CENTURY

About the year 1650 men were still wearing
the very wide breeches of ten years earlier.
Owing to their great width these were called
larges canons. Their width was now so excessive that they had to be
pleated at the waist, and resembled a short skirt (Fig. 376).

This excessive width of the breeches led to a complete revolution
in the character of this garment. It came to be a very wide one-piece
skirt reaching from the hips to just below the knee, and bore the
name *la jupe* (petticoat-breeches). The waist was trimmed all round
with bows of coloured ribbon, and similar bows were tied low down
at the sides. This garment hid almost entirely the knee-breeches
worn underneath it. These latter were now slightly tighter than
before, and were fastened at the knees with a draw-string.

Stockings had not greatly changed. They were ornamented with
a broad, stiff edging of lace, rucked where it joined the stocking and
turned down so that it covered half the calf. The shoes' had also
remained as before, but the ornamentation consisted now of broad,
stiff ribbons instead of rosettes (Fig. 377). Boots, now used only for
riding, were as they had been about 1650.

While the ordinary middle-class man was still wearing wide breeches tied below the knee and a doublet with tails of varying length, gentlemen of the upper class wore, along with the breeches just described, a short-sleeved, tight jacket (also called doublet, or *pourpoint*). It was fastened only at the top ; the corners were either rounded or left square. The front did not meet across the breast or

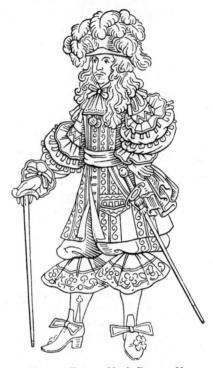

Fig. 377. FRENCH MEN'S DRESS, 1665

abdomen, and there, as at the arms, the sole clothing was the richly embroidered shirt of fine linen, the sleeves of which were baggy and gathered into puffs with the help of coloured ribbons.

Men still wore the lace collar. As the long hair or large wigs which were fashionable at the time hid the collar at the back and shoulders, this was very narrow at these parts.[1] Only the front of it was broad.

Shortly after the year 1660 the short jacket-doublet and the full breeches (which were also worn as riding breeches) came to be con-

[1] A survival of this lace collar is still seen in the ' bands ' worn by the clergy to this day.

sidered very unsuitable for daily use. The closed skirt was therefore abandoned, and instead of the short doublet, or over it, was worn the *casaque*, which for years had replaced the cloak even for full dress.

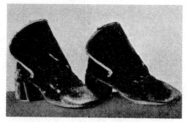

Fig. 378. VELVET SHOES, SEVENTEENTH CENTURY

It was made of the best materials available, and was liberally trimmed with lace or galloon.

As, however, this wide garment in its old form was not quite suitable for its new purpose it was made closer-fitting and arranged for

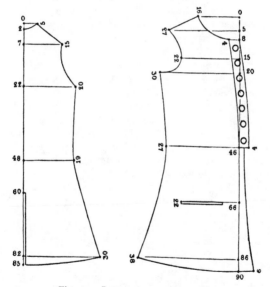

Fig. 379. JUSTAUCORPS, ABOUT 1665

buttoning. (See Fig. 379.) The short sleeves were retained, but they were lengthened by the addition of a piece which could be worn as a turned-back cuff.

This new garment, which was called *le justaucorps*, and which soon came to be richly decorated with galloon, immediately became a chief item of male costume, and continued—although with repeated modi-

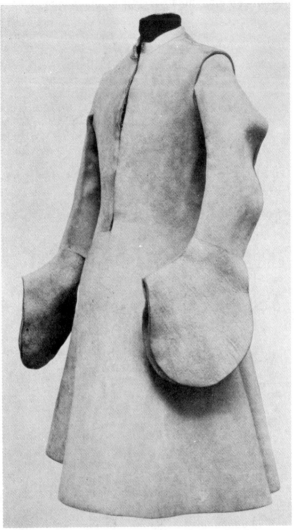

Fig. 380. LONG LEATHER COAT (KOLLER) OF ELK SKIN,
ABOUT 1700

fications—to be worn till about the end of the eighteenth century. (See Figs. 377 and 381.)

For ten years this *justaucorps* retained its original cut. It was patently a development of the *casaque*. It was, of course, far more

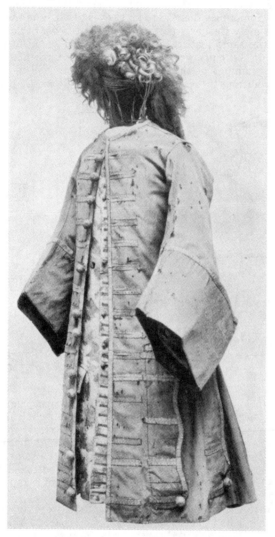

Fig. 381. JUSTAUCORPS OF RUST-BROWN SILK, ABOUT 1690

ornamental, with the front, back, and sides embroidered with perpendicular lines of gold galloon. Even the sleeve-holes were occasionally embellished in the same way.

Subsequent changes affected only the elbow-length sleeves. The cuffs turned back were sometimes broad and sometimes narrow. Some were wide, others close-fitting. They were open or closed at the back. Sometimes there were no sleeves at all. As the reversed cuffs were simply the lower part of the sleeve thrown back they were always of the same material and colour as the lining of the coat. The edges of the cuffs were trimmed with the same material that made the trimmings of the coat. The cuff was kept in its proper position by buttons ; these were retained long after they had ceased

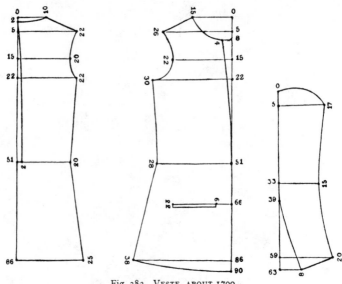

Fig. 382. VESTE, ABOUT 1700

to serve their original purpose. The lower arm showed fine white shirt sleeves which protruded beyond the tight coat sleeves and ended in a broad lace cuff fastened at the wrist with coloured ribbon. The whole front of the coat was arranged for buttoning (Fig. 379), and there were buttons and buttonholes also at the short slit at the back. The coat was not always worn buttoned, but was sometimes left open. In both cases a sash was worn round the waist (see Fig. 377).

About 1670 the doublet, the *pourpoint*, underwent an important change. It lost its jacket-like character, and became a kind of coat. In this new form it received a new name, *la veste*. (See Fig. 382.) It now reached almost to the knees, was somewhat tight round the chest, and open at the sides down to the hips. It also had a slit at the back, and buttoned all down the front. This *veste* formed men's indoor dress. For the street the *justaucorps* was put on over it.

About the year 1670 the *justaucorps* also underwent some alterations. The skirt, especially in front, was much wider, and this

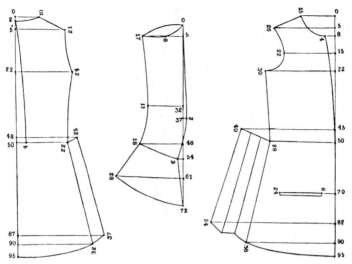

Fig. 383. JUSTAUCORPS, ABOUT 1680

additional material was gathered at the waist on both sides in two
or three large pleats. (See Fig. 383.) These pleats were secured by
a button sewn on each. The
front and back of the skirt
were not entirely sewn together, but merely joined by
a few stitches, so that there
was a long slit at each side.
The sword passed through that
on the left side. The sleeves
were made longer and longer,
till finally they came to the
wrists (Fig. 381). The reversed cuffs were very large ;
their lining was the same as
that of the coat. The pocket
flaps were made larger and
larger, and had buttonholes,
but the buttons were merely
trimming. About the year
1700 the foot of the skirt of

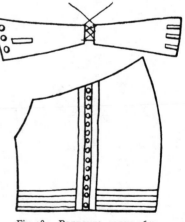

Fig. 384. BREECHES, ABOUT 1650

the *justaucorps* was greatly widened. To make it stand out stiffly
all round it was padded with horsehair.

311

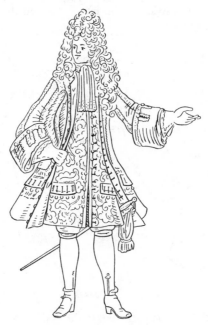

Fig. 385. FRENCH MEN'S DRESS, 1690

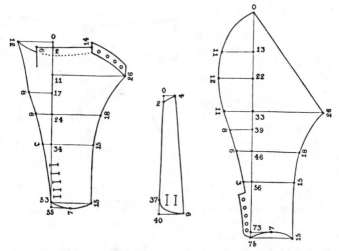

Fig. 386. BREECHES, ABOUT 1700

The nether garment known as *la culotte*, which was worn with the *justaucorps*, still had the shape that had been customary about the year 1650 (Figs. 376 and 384), but it was now tied below the knees

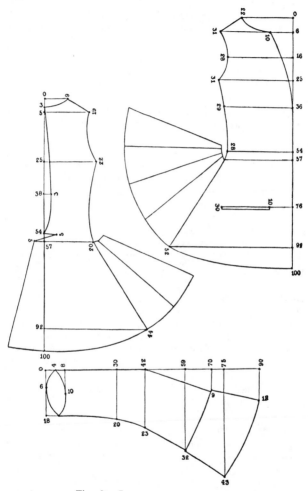

Fig. 387. JUSTAUCORPS, ABOUT 1700

and adorned at the sides with galloon. On festive occasions the short doublet was worn below the coat (which in that case was not buttoned) and the top of the breeches was decorated with hanging ribbon bows.

Soon after the appearance of the *justaucorps* the lace collar made way for the neckcloth (*cravate*), which had been worn by German

313

soldiers about the year 1640. It was a strip of white material, 30 cm. in breadth and 1 m. in length, placed round the neck and knotted in front. Between 1665 and 1680 it was tied with large loops of ribbon, the ends of which came down to the breast and were there spread out in fan-shape. Some men, instead of knotting the neckcloth, fastened it with strings which ended in tassels (Fig. 377). Later these strings were replaced by coloured ribbons, which were at first narrow and afterward broad.

The most striking changes were in the style of hairdressing. Wigs came in, and the natural hair was neglected. Wigs were worn at Court as early as the time of Louis XIII, but fell into disuse again as long as Louis XIV retained his own beautiful long hair. When he began to grow bald, not only he, but also his whole *entourage*, took to wigs.

At first wigs were a faithful imitation of natural curled hair. By the year 1670 they were a mass of small curls hanging down in great confusion. They then began to increase in size, and, instead of reaching to the shoulders, fell down the back. The large *allonge* wig was the most popular style from 1680 till the beginning of the eighteenth century. Large wigs of natural human hair, fair or light brown, were the most expensive. Black wigs were the cheapest. Horsehair and goat-hair were also used. Already under Louis XIII beards were decreasing in size. The chin beard went entirely out of fashion. Only a small moustache was left, and even this disappeared after the year 1700.

From 1660 onward the hat was broad-brimmed and high-crowned. Short feathers were stuck all round the crown so as to encircle the brim. Long feathers were used only at the back. About 1670 one side of the brim was turned up. Ere long another portion of it was turned up, and about the end of the century a third side was similarly treated, thus making the three-cornered hat. The turned-up parts were kept in place by means of a cord passed through them. The brim was trimmed with broad gold braid, and the feather was laid so high round the crown that only part of it reached beyond the brim.

Women's Dress. In the first half of the seventeenth century women's dress closely resembled that worn by men, but it too underwent extensive alterations about the year 1620. Farthingale and hip-pads disappeared. Two dresses were still worn one above the other. About 1630 half the length of the over-dress was caught up and gathered in order to show the under-dress and the lining of the over-dress. A woman in her best attire always left the front of her over-dress unfastened. Only the exposed parts of the under-dress were trimmed with costly materials. This style of dress became universal. The over-dress, *la robe*, was longer than the under one, *la jupe*, and had a short train, whereas the latter just reached to the feet.

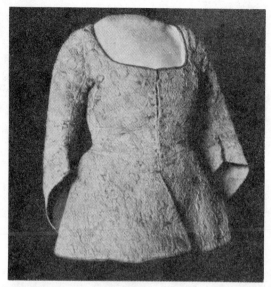

Fig. 388. LADY'S JACKET, SEVENTEENTH CENTURY—FRONT

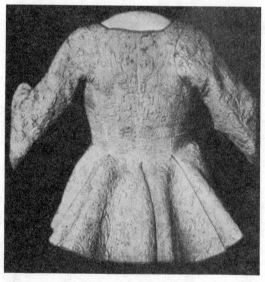

Fig. 389. LADY'S JACKET, SEVENTEENTH CENTURY—BACK

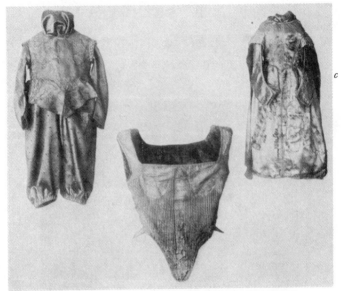

Fig. 390. (*a*) Young Boy's Suit—belonged to Count Ludwig Philip
of Hilpoltstein (*d.* 1632)
(*b*) Corslet (Mieder) worn with Over-dress of the Countess
Palatine Dorothea Sabine of Neuburg (*d.* 1598)
(*c*) Child's Frock of Countess Maria Magdalena of Hilpoltstein
(*d.* 1629), Daughter of Duke John Frederick

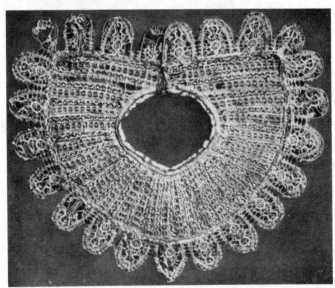

Fig. 391. Lace Collar, First Half of the Seventeenth Century

The bodice, called *corset*, or *pourpoint*, retained for a time its sixteenth-century form, with a square neck-opening in front and a stiffening of whalebone. While in other respects the bodice was unchanged, the back was cut 10 cm. higher and the cut in front was square. Owing to the whalebone stiffening all curvature at the waist disappeared. If open-fronted, the bodice was fastened with hooks and eyes ; otherwise it was laced at the back. About 1650 the bodice exactly resembled the men's doublet. The stiffening was omitted, the lower edge was cut quite straight all round, and the fastening was with buttons. For a time tails were added, as with the doublet, but the fashion soon disappeared. The desired girth round the hips was attained by wearing numerous petticoats. When the tails were discontinued the bodice changed its character and became again part of the over-dress.

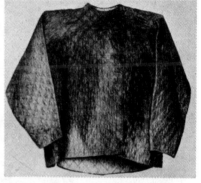

Fig. 392. QUILTED GREEN SILK JACKET, BEGINNING OF THE SEVENTEENTH CENTURY

The under-dresses worn with these over-dresses were short-waisted, like the bodices ; the short waists had a broad peak that came low down over the abdomen. The rolls at the top of the sleeves were replaced by shoulder-pieces. At the beginning of the century these were quite narrow and wadded, but after a few years they were wide and open in front. Although buttons were present, these were not used ; thus the baggy, light-coloured under-sleeves were shown (Fig. 394). Ladies of the upper classes, however, still imitated the gathered and slashed sleeves of the men, and the style just described was confined to the middle classes.

The low neck still continued, and was so low that the upper half of the breasts was exposed. A collar of finest linen trimmed with lace was worn, which gradually came lower and lower on the shoulders, till much of the back was exposed (see Fig. 393). This was the fashion about the middle of the century ; about the same time sleeves were greatly shortened.

About this time, too, light, pliant materials were preferred to heavy, costly fabrics, and even ladies of high rank wore brocade and damask only on great occasions. Velvet, satin, and woollen stuffs were also much worn. As a rule the under-dress was of stronger material than the upper one. Less heavy material was used for the over-dress in order to obtain a more graceful draping ; the draped material was lined with still lighter stuffs. There was a decided preference for strong, brilliant colours rather than for those that were faint and mat.

The upper dress was dark in colour ; the under-dress was lighter, while the lining of the former was as showy as possible.

In the first half of the seventeenth century women's clothing had hardly any trimming at all—only the under-dress showed any ornamentation. The upper dress was decked out with bows of coloured ribbon at the breast, at the point of the bodice, and at the sleeves. These had to be of the same ribbon as that of which the

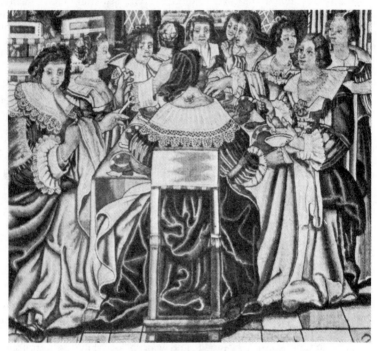

Fig. 393. LADIES' PARTY
From a Gobelin of the seventeenth century.

waist-belt was made. About the middle of the century women took to lace. Previously it had been used only to trim the collar and the turned-back cuffs. Now it was used at the neck and sleeves. (See Fig. 393.)

Women's shoes were like men's. The heels, which had been moderately high and broad about 1630, became higher, but less broad. On the instep was a rosette of ribbon.

Soon after 1600 an entirely different style of hairdressing was adopted. High *coiffures* were given up. The hair was combed back and arranged in curls that fell to the shoulders. For a time women wore fine, lace-edged kerchiefs or small, close-fitting caps coming to a point over the forehead. About 1630 the hair was parted over the brow, one portion being combed smooth or curled and combed forward to the forehead, the rest being gathered at the back of the head and adorned with strings of pearls or an ostrich feather. By the middle of the century the hair was combed smoothly back from the forehead and parted so as to fall at the sides in long curls, while the back hair was plaited into a pigtail and wound into a coil at the back. Even with this *coiffure* small caps were worn. Large hats were rare. They were worn only by ladies when on horseback; they resembled those worn by men.

Pearls were the favourite form of jewellery. Strings of large pearls were worn round the neck and wrist and in the hair. Other precious stones were rare.

About 1640 these fashions ousted even in Germany the last traces of Spanish costume, and became the established styles not only in Germany, but everywhere else.

From the middle of the seventeenth century women's dress developed on its own lines, in complete independence of that of men. Ladies wore an under-dress (*jupe*) of rich material embroidered with silver or gold, and over it an open-fronted *robe* with a very short train. It had

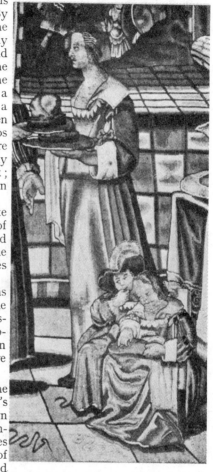

Fig. 394. NURSE AND CHILDREN
More of the Gobelin shown in Fig. 393.
Seventeenth century.

short, baggy sleeves; from under these emerged wide lace sleeves or sleeves trimmed with lace falling over the elbows.

About 1660 the *robe*, or gown, was made of velvet (not too dark in colour) or of heavy silk. It was quite closed at the waist, and only the skirt of the smooth, light-coloured silk under-dress could be seen.

The low neck was surrounded by a lace collar of the same breadth all round. Out of the short, baggy sleeves protruded other sleeves of finest linen, trimmed with lace and gathered by coloured ribbons into several large puffs.

The neck became lower and lower, while the waist was even longer than it had been, and more pointed in front. About the year 1670 the corset reappeared, and brought about a great tightening of the waist. The corset, which was of Spanish origin, and had been invented as far back as the first half of the sixteenth century, compressed the waist to the utmost. It consisted of a large number of

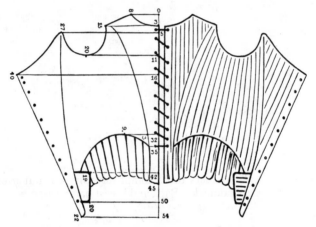

Fig. 395. CORSET, SECOND HALF OF THE SEVENTEENTH
CENTURY

whalebone rods placed close together, covered on both sides by material, and sewn in. The first corsets had a double set of strings. The one in front was always fastened ; the one at the back could be opened at will. (See Fig. 395.) Girls had to wear this corset from a very early age. It not only constricted the waist, making it thinner and longer, but, by being laced from the foot upward, it pressed the breasts up, while the long, pointed front kept the figure straight below the waist.[1]

The corset now replaced the bodice of the under-dress. This was therefore fastened only round the hips. It was forced down in front and at the back by the stiff flaps of the corset, and firmly fastened in

[1] The slimness at the waist attained by wearing the corset was rendered still more striking by the reappearance at the same time of hip-cushions (*postiches*), even though these were not at first large.

About the same time face-masks began to be worn, and continued into the first decades of the eighteenth century. Ladies considered it improper to appear in the street without such a mask. See Fig. 417.

that position. The side-flaps of the corset were underneath the skirt, those at back and in front over it.

The bodice of the over-dress was cut to fit exactly over the corset. Its sleeves became shorter and shorter, till they disappeared almost altogether about the year 1680, leaving as sole cover for the arms the wide, slightly puffed lace sleeves of the under-dress. The broad lace collar was given up and replaced by a narrow, slightly crimped frill that appeared above the corslet. At the same time a fashion of some decades earlier reappeared—the open wings of the *robe* were turned back to display the lining. These wings were, however, not taken quite round to the back as formerly. Only the edges were turned widely outward and gathered into puffs by clasps. These were called *bouillons*, or puffs. The train of the over-dress was considerably lengthened, but the under-dress remained in this respect as it was.

A few years later the front wings of the over-dress were turned back completely, and gathered at the back into a large bunch, exposing the lining. The train had again been lengthened, and ladies of high rank had it borne behind them by a page, usually a Moorish boy.

Just as the *robe* had been lengthened at the foot, so the bodice was now made higher at the neck. The leader of fashion at the time was the canting Marquise de Maintenon, the last mistress of Louis XIV, and she declared war on all exposure of the person. To please her not only had the shoulders to be completely covered, but even low necks had to be abandoned. Back and breast had both to be covered as far as permitted by French Court etiquette, which demanded a certain amount of *décolletage*. Mme de Maintenon did not even approve of bare arms, and so sleeves were lengthened almost to the elbows, and broad lace cuffs were sewn on to cover half of the lower arm.

As the stiff corset could not be brought higher than the breasts, a broad, stiff frill of lace was attached to the top of it. The *robe* was once more gathered only at the waist, and came up to the shoulders, leaving the chest uncovered. This arrangement would have shown the corset had not a richly embroidered bib hidden the corset and filled the gap. The embroidery on these bibs was very beautiful, and was frequently done with gold and jewels.

The edges of the *robe* close to the sides of the bib were trimmed with ribbon, braid, or lace. Fashionable ladies were in the habit of accentuating their waist by a narrow belt fastened with a large buckle close to the point of the corset.

On the head was worn the *fontange* (or topknot), a staged framework of wire covered with white lace and trimmed with coloured ribbons. It was in some cases a head and a half in height. The hair was brushed back from the face and piled high. Curled fringes were worn by few, but the long curls coming to the shoulders, which had been fashionable since 1670, were still common. The practice of powdering the hair—which almost necessarily involved the painting of the face—began about this time ; beauty patches also made their appearance. On the other hand, less jewellery was worn. A single row of large pearls sufficed, and pearl earrings were used.

THE NETHERLANDS

After undergoing numerous alterations the costume of the Dutch had come by the year 1630 to be very like that worn in France.

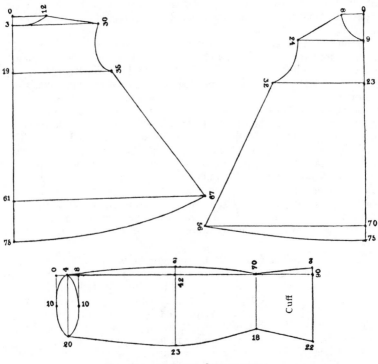

Fig. 396. Dutch Over-jacket

French fashions were unquestioningly adopted. These included the *casaque*, worn over the doublet in the form of a loose jacket. Something like this (but not so wide, and with sleeves diminishing in width toward the wrists) had long been known in Holland (Fig. 396), and continued to be worn by the lower classes for a considerable time afterward.

A fashion peculiar to the Dutch was the wearing of long, wide-topped gaiters of deerskin or coloured cloth. These had feet, and were pulled on over the stockings. Two or even three pairs of different colours were worn at the same time, with top-boots over them all. With shoes shorter stockings of different colours were worn. The inner stockings overlapped the outer to some extent, so the outer ones were therefore made shorter or were not pulled up so high.

Toward the middle of the century Dutch costume was exactly like

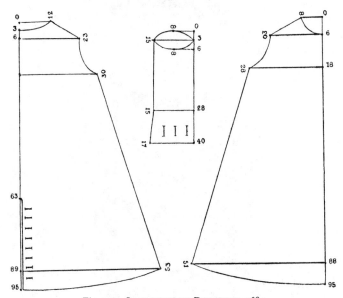

Fig. 397. COAT WORN BY DUTCHMEN, 1680

that of the French, except that closed sleeves were preferred to open ones and conical hats to cylindrical ones.

Shortly after 1650 hats gradually became lower in the crown, and narrow brims came into fashion. They continued to decrease in size for nearly twenty years, until it was impossible to make them any smaller. *Pari passu* with this change in headgear the nether garments became wider, and were trimmed with lace and bows of ribbon, as in France. This fashion was ere long followed by the adoption of ' slops,' or pantaloons, which suited the Dutch taste for roomy, baggy clothes, and afforded plenty of opportunity to indulge their love for trimming. These pantaloons were lengthened and widened till they entirely lost their original character ; the top, foot, and sides were trimmed with lace and bows of ribbon until no room was left for more. In contrast to this, the small jacket worn with the ' slops ' was very

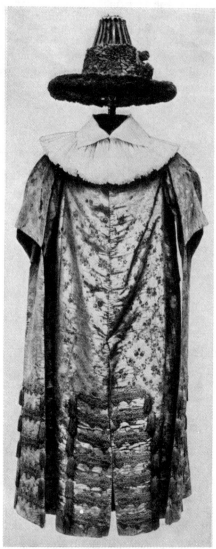

Fig. 398. Councillor's Cloak, Hat, and Ruffle as worn
in the Sixteenth Century

plain. It was not so tight and short as the French jacket, but trimming was entirely absent. It was buttoned at back and front, and a long sash was worn. The hat had a crown of medium height. This whole style lasted for twenty years, but finally gave place to coat and wide breeches. As in France, the Dutch coat was at first quite

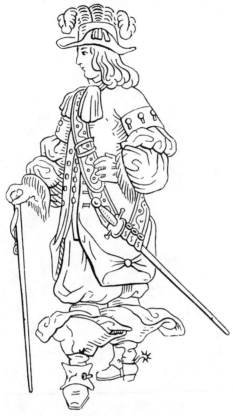

Fig. 399. Dutch Men's Dress, Second Half of the
Seventeenth Century

plain. It had no waist. This style suited the Dutch taste, and continued to be worn for a long time without any change except a lengthening of the sleeves, although neighbouring countries introduced many improvements. The Dutch coat was remarkable both for its width and for its length—it often came to below the knees. (See Fig. 399.) This made it so inconvenient for walking or riding that the back and front corners of each coat-tail were buttoned or hooked together. This practice was immediately imitated by the

325

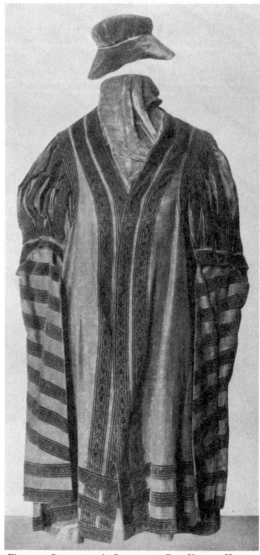

Fig. 400. Councillor's Cloak and Red Velvet Hat,
Seventeenth Century

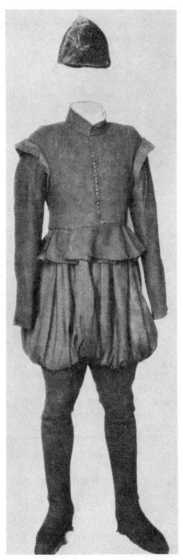

Fig. 401. Costume of the Junker or Squire of Bodegg,
Beginning of the Seventeenth Century

French. By the beginning of the eighteenth century the latter had greatly improved it, and it was soon adopted by soldiers. The endeavour to get rid of all inconvenient hindrances to freedom of movement led to the abandonment of the pantaloons, which were

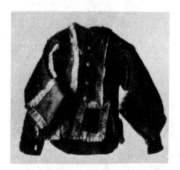

Fig. 402. BOY'S JACKET OF YELLOW CLOTH
ABOUT 1700

replaced by very wide breeches tied at the knees. The great width of the breeches made top-boots necessary; these were very wide at the tops. They in turn necessitated a great increase in the size of the gaiters. The Dutch preferred a small hat to a large one, and showed little inclination to adopt the wigs which began to appear about the year 1670.

GERMANY

Soon after the opening of the seventeenth century French costume made its way into Germany. At first it was confined to the upper classes, the middle classes continuing to wear the traditional forms of dress. French influence was first seen in the doublet and the ruff; other changes followed more slowly. The Thirty Years War led to the use of the Swedish leather cape by soldiers. It was sleeveless, and was worn over the doublet. Low shoes of necessity gave place to heavy riding boots with spurs.

This simple, unadorned style of dress did not last very long. First came the lace collar (Fig. 391)—which by the year 1630 had quite driven out the ruff—and the cuffs, which were of the same pattern as the collar. Then the breeches were trimmed at the side with a close-set row of medium-sized, semi-conical metal buttons, and the cape was ornamented with rosettes of cord or ribbon with long metal tags.

The most important item of the costume was the leather jerkin of tanned elk or buffalo hide. In general appearance it resembled the French tailed doublet of the year 1630. The fact that it was made

328

of leather, however, and that it had frequently to serve as armour, necessitated various alterations in cut and make. The leather was tanned after the chamois-dressing process, and this made it very elastic, so that it conformed to the shape of the body. The back could therefore be cut in one piece. Owing to the thickness and stiffness of the leather the tails could not be cut very wide, but as such

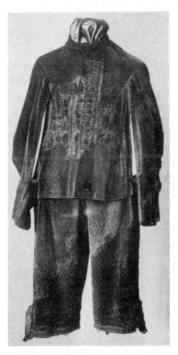

Fig. 403. Doublet and Breeches of Duke John Frederick
of Hilpoltstein (d. 1644)

width was necessary to protect the thighs of the wearer against the enemy's blows and thrusts, the tails in front and at the back were cut so as to overlap ; the edges of the front tails thus lay over those at the back. (See Figs. 404 and 406.)

If the leather of the tails was defective, or was thin in places, a special flap was inserted and sewn on at the waist (Fig. 404). In this way the garment came to have six instead of four tails. Those in front lay over those at side and back, and the back part of the inserted flaps covered the front edge of the back flaps. Sometimes these flaps were carried up under the arm, and in that case the upper part of the jerkin was cut in the Franco-Spanish fashion. In some cases the tails at the back (or even any of them) could not be cut in one

329

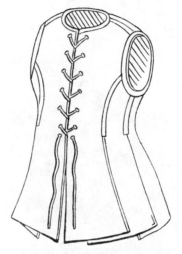

Fig. 404. LEATHER JERKIN WITH SIX 'TAILS'

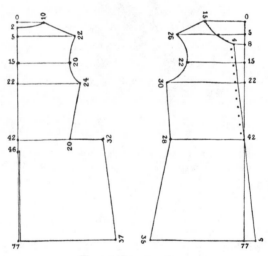

Fig. 405. LEATHER JERKIN

piece with the body of the garment, and had to be separately sewn on (see Fig. 406). As a rule the jerkin was fastened by lacing, rarely with clasps, and still more rarely with buttons. Its length and the

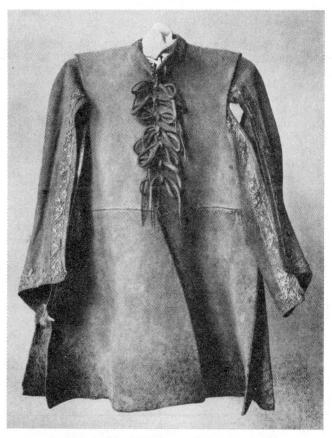

Fig. 406. Leather Jerkin, with Sleeves lined with Yellow Silk, Seventeenth Century

length of the bodice varied with fashion and personal taste, as did the sleeves. Sometimes it had sleeves, and at other times it had none. It was rarely dyed, and was usually of the natural light yellow colour. If it had to be dyed the colour was always a dark tan.

THE EIGHTEENTH CENTURY

BY the end of the seventeenth century the development of European costume, in the true sense of the term, had attained its highest point. From that period onward the dimensions were smaller for a time. Wigs were not so high, the trimming on the various garments was less liberal, the coat became the dress coat. Under Louis XVI fashion struck out in what seemed new directions, but the changes were more in ornamentation than in general cut. The development in the sphere of attire also seemed to be hastening toward revolution. But this was preceded by one more period which, from a purely artistic point of view, produced fashions of great charm, and of a variety previously unknown (1700–90). In the realm of fashion the leadership of France was as unassailable as it was in the political sphere. Any novelty, it is true, made its way but slowly, and not always simultaneously in different places. Distance from Paris was decisive in this matter. Towns in the Rhine district were frequently years in advance of large cities like Vienna or Berlin. It was the coming of fashion plates that helped to bring about a more rapid diffusion. These began to appear from the year 1770 onward in Paris. Then at regular intervals from about 1786 came papers like the *Journal des Luxus und der Moden*, sent out by Bertuch in Weimar.

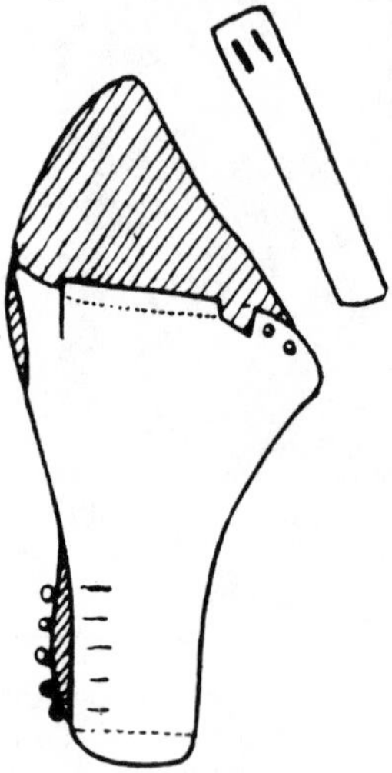

FRANCE

Men's Dress. The first important change affected the wig as worn by men. From the beginning of the eighteenth century wigs had become much smaller. The prime movers in this change were the army. Large wigs proved uncomfortable for riding and fighting and other active exercises, and cavalry officers endeavoured to overcome the inconvenience by tying back the long side-curls with ribbon.

Fig. 407. BREECHES

German officers found this sufficient, and thus introduced the fashion of pigtails (see Plate V), but French officers tied the ends of the wig and tucked them into a small silk bag that could be fastened at the top, and thus invented the hair-bag, *le crapaud.*

Plate V

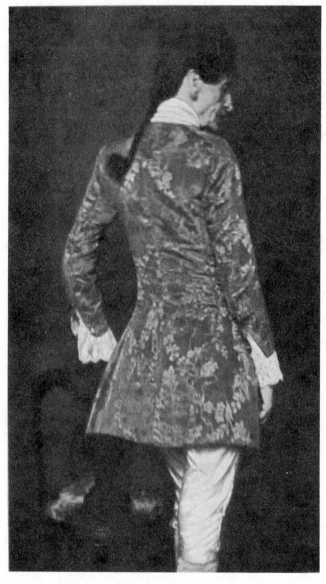

SLEEVED WAISTCOAT OF GREEN DAMASK
FOR INDOOR DRESS
About 1720

In the year 1700 wigs were already no longer worn, as they had been a few years before, in two large masses of curls in front, with a third mass falling over the back. The curls were now of equal length, and distributed all round, over breast, shoulders, and back (see Plate VIII). The back portion was divided into two parts, each with a knot at the end. Later these took the form of two long pendent

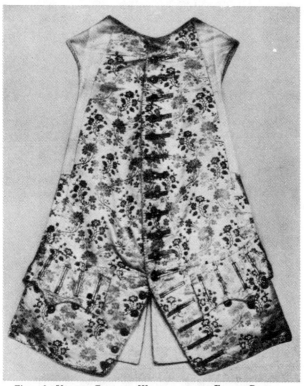

Fig. 408. YELLOW BROCADE WAISTCOAT WITH FLORAL DESIGN, ABOUT 1700

queues. This fashion became universally popular, and was retained by aged courtiers till the time of Louis XVI. It fell out of fashion again, however, by the year 1720, when wigs were beginning to be much smaller.

Breeches also underwent important alterations. When men had got tired of the wide ' slops,' or pantaloons (about 1660), the *culotte* worn underneath came into its own again. This was still very wide, and was fastened below the knees with a draw-string. But as the top of the stocking was now being pulled up over the breeches—a

333

practice which the shape of the legs of the breeches made difficult
—the breeches were much tighter at the knees. Some years later
the whole leg was made much tighter. This change in the breeches

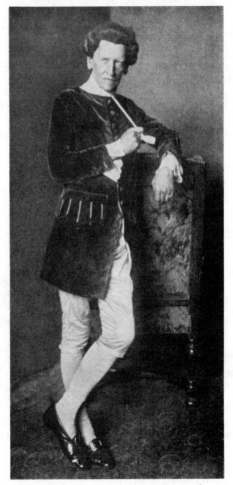

Fig. 409. SLEEVED WAISTCOAT (SMOKING JACKET) OF COPPER-RED VELVET,
FIRST HALF OF THE EIGHTEENTH CENTURY

was facilitated by the great improvement which had been made in
their cut about the year 1700 (see Fig. 407). The necessary width at
the seat was obtained by extending the back upward. Since the
end of the sixteenth century the front opening—*la bavaroise*—had

Plate VI

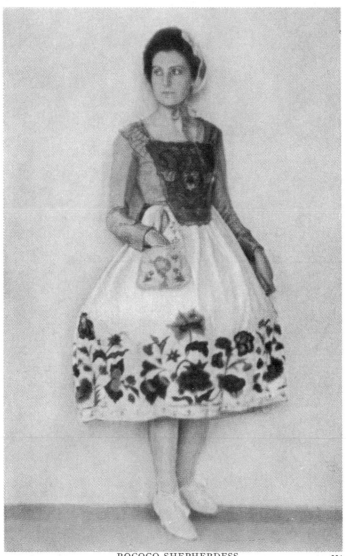

ROCOCO SHEPHERDESS

About 1730

been made to button, and this arrangement was now applied to the fastenings at the knees, which were also now buttoned.

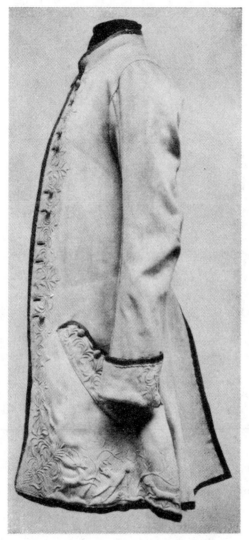

Fig. 410. Hunting Coat of Yellow Buckskin with Stamped Ornamentation, First Half of the Eighteenth Century

The *pourpoint* was again made tighter, and was buttoned either altogether or from the waist upward. The general cut was unchanged,

335

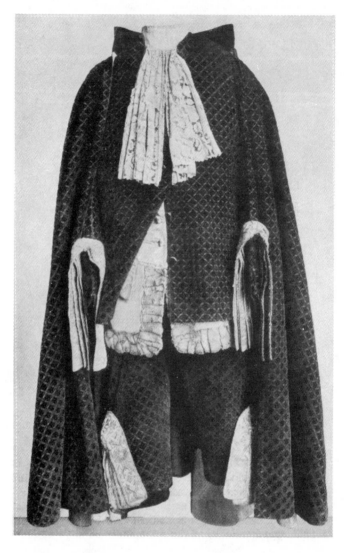

Fig. 411. Suit of the Grand Master of the Order of St Hubertus, about 1720

but the next years saw changes in other ways. The waist varied in length ; the cuffs were either broad and open at the back or narrow (either open or closed) or very broad and closed.[1] The buttons of the

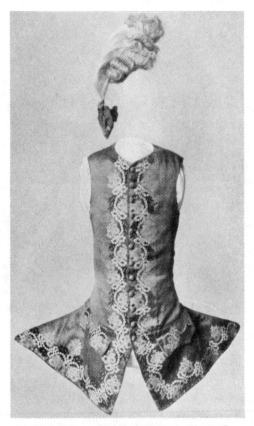

Fig. 412. Waistcoat of Red Brocade with Woven Pattern,
Middle of the Eighteenth Century

coat and of the waistcoat (which was like the coat, and came down to the knees—see Fig. 408) were somewhat large, and became an important article of commerce in France and England. Toward the middle of the century they were made of goat's hair or of silk, and later of metal. Gold or silver trimming and embroidery were not now so liberally used as they had been under Louis XIV, but they appeared at the same places as in his time—at the coat-edges in front,

[1] Cuffs closed at the back were usually called *parements en pagode*, a name that showed a preference for Chinese models.

the slit at the back, on and all round the pocket-flaps, and at the cuff-edges. The material and colour of the cuffs were the same as the lining of the coat, and in most cases now the same as the waistcoat. From 1730 the lining no longer extended beyond the large turned-back cuffs, but was confined to the cuffs alone. Hunting and riding coats were mostly without reversed cuffs. (See Fig. 410.) The ribbon bows at the right shoulder of the coat—called *aiguillettes*, and originally meant to hold up the sword-belt—were left as an ornament,

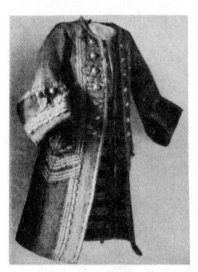 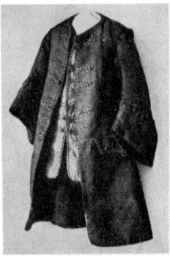

Fig. 413. Boys' Suits, Beginning of the Eighteenth
Century

though they were now of no use ; they came down in four long ends to the elbows. After 1725 they went gradually out of fashion.

The costume just described was called *l'habit à la française*. Louis XIV added to it as Court dress a richly trimmed shoulder-cloak similar to the Spanish one reaching to the knees. About 1730 this costume underwent important changes. In imitation of the women's farthingales rods of whalebone were sewn into the skirts of men's coats to extend them. At the same time the waistcoats from the waist up were fastened merely with a few buttons, so that *le jabot*, or frill of lace that surrounded the neck of the shirt, was displayed. This was of the same width and pattern as the cuffs. The appearance of the *jabot* drove out of fashion the long, hanging, richly embroidered ends of the muslin *cravate*. The *cravate* with shorter ends was also soon ousted by the neckcloth knotted at the back and adorned in front with a diamond pin. These neckcloths were also usually of white muslin. Only military men wore over them still another neck-

Plate VII

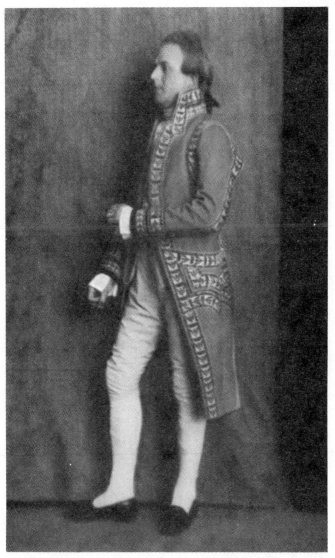

FOOTMAN'S LIVERY OF YELLOWISH CLOTH   338
About 1780

cloth, of coloured silk (red or black), which allowed a narrow strip of the white one underneath to peep out above it.

In the second half of the seventeenth century the French adopted one of the Dutch fashions. For riding purposes the corners of the coat-tails were turned outward and buttoned or hooked together. Other nations borrowed this practice from France, and it became universal about 1700. The cut of the coat was not changed, and the skirts were in no way stiffened. This style of coat was adopted

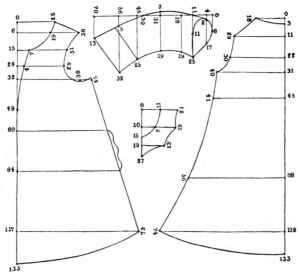

Fig. 414. ROCKELAURE—TOP-COAT, ABOUT THE MIDDLE OF THE EIGHTEENTH CENTURY

everywhere by military men, and it led to the creation in England of the riding coat—the 'frock.' In the new style the coat was made closer-fitting and the front skirts were removed.

In rough weather an overcoat with pockets and a small cape was worn. It was buttoned, and was called after its inventor, the Duke of Rockelaure. (See Fig. 414.) The garment for travelling was a long, wheel-shaped cloak. For morning dress gentlemen wore a sort of loose dressing-gown. It was made of velvet or silk, lined with silk, and fastened by ribbons round the waist. A waistcoat of the same material was worn beneath it (see Plate X). The headdress was a tall 'night-cap' of silk. The hair-bag, *le crapaud*, was at first only for ordinary wear. For ceremonial or Court occasions gentlemen had to appear with their hair combed back and held together by a ribbon that dangled round the shoulders. Military men, especially in Prussia, wore the stiff pigtail. The front hair was combed back, and that at the sides was crimped into curls. At first three or four curls at each side constituted the fashion. Later there were only two, and about 1790 these were transformed into small, slightly convex *toupets*, or tufts, called *ailes de pigeon* (pigeon's wings). When this fashion came in the hair above the forehead was gathered into a roll, but afterward it too took the form of a pointed *toupet*, called *vergette à la chinoise* (Chinese dusting-brush).

Because of this artistic *coiffure* the three-cornered hat could not be worn ; it was carried in the hand or under the arm. It was low in the crown, and the brim was no longer bolt upright (Fig. 440). This *chapeau-bas* had no plume, only a trimming of gold or silver braid.

Stockings were no longer worn over the breeches, but under them. They were pro-

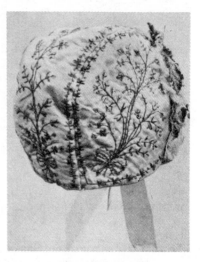

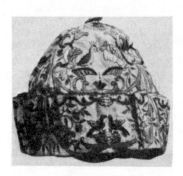

Fig. 415. CHILD'S BONNET (FRENCH) OF THE EIGHTEENTH CENTURY

Fig. 416. CHILD'S BONNET (FRENCH) OF THE EIGHTEENTH CENTURY

tected by close-fitting linen gaiters—*housseaux*. Full attire included walking-stick and sword. The latter was so popular that its use was subject to fixed regulations. Lackeys, servants in livery, commercial apprentices, musicians, and cooks were forbidden to wear one.

Women's Dress. Toward the middle of the eighteenth century women's dress underwent even greater changes than that of the men. The way had been prepared for them in the reign of Louis XIV. Dresses were again supported by the farthingale, which had gone out of fashion a century before. This stood out around the wearer in bell-shape (Fig. 418). The *fontange*, or topknot, soon disappeared entirely, and its place was taken by a simple but high *coiffure* of curls. The new farthingale, which was not very wide at first, was a framework of hoops made of cane, whalebone, or steel fastened together with strings. Owing to their resemblance to the baskets under which poultry was kept in France they were called *paniers*, or hen-baskets.

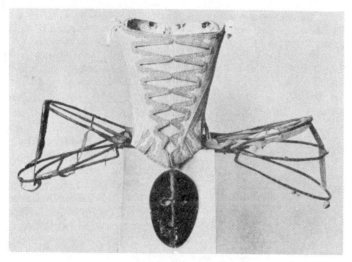

Fig. 417. FARTHINGALE FRAME, CORSLET, AND MASK, MIDDLE OF THE EIGHTEENTH CENTURY

Already in the time of Louis XIV the farthingale had begun to grow wider. It was at its widest about 1725, when the lowest hoops were

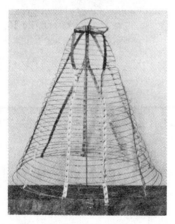

Fig. 418. FARTHINGALE FRAME

often 5 or 6 metres in circumference and the topmost 3 metres. At each side of the top hoop two semicircular pieces of steel were fixed

341

to prevent the skirt from widening suddenly and to keep it in a semi-circular shape. Though this was the usual style of farthingale, there were various minor modifications of it. The circumference varied ; the farthingale was sometimes slightly compressed toward the back. These modifications had different names, such as *la culbute, le bout-en-train, le tatez-y*, etc. All kinds were extremely inconvenient, and frequently brought their wearers into difficulties not only in the streets, but in carriages and when they were passing through doors.

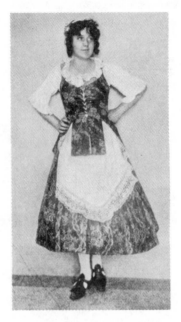

Fig. 419. Dress of a Girl of the Middle Classes, about 1720

They took up the space of three or four people, and women had to twist and turn to avoid obstacles. In spite of this the fashion became popular so quickly that at the beginning of the reign of Louis XIV women in all countries, from princesses to working-women, wore this peculiar attire, and a woman without a farthingale was looked down upon. The coming of the farthingale did not at first cause any change in the dresses worn over it, but when it began to increase in circumference the long, trailing gown, open in front and gathered at the back, was no longer a suitable dress. So the gathering at the back was omitted, the train was left off, and the dress was in various ways tucked up with draw-strings.

The only changes in the under-dress were a greater width and more liberal trimming. About the year 1700 a new style of adornment

342

Plate VIII

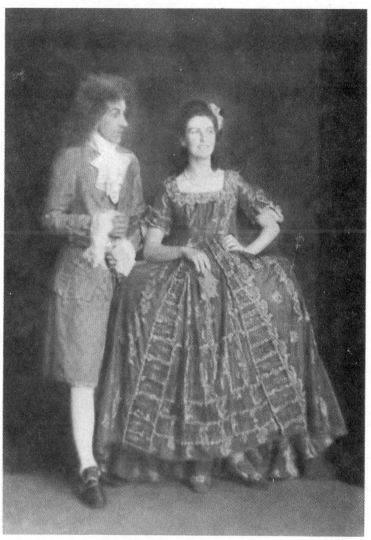

DRESS COAT AND SILK GOWN
About 1730-40

had been devised—viz., *les falbalas*—flounces or furbelows. These were strips of material, crimped or pleated, sewn horizontally round the skirt. They were not always of the same material as the dress, whereas the wide ruffles that came in about the same time—the *volants*—were always of the same material as the garment they were used to adorn.

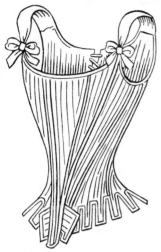

The bodice, *le corsage*, while it remained on the whole as it had been, was now laced at the back instead of in front ; the sewn-on skirt had a slit at the back. The change was due to the adoption of the English corset, which was laced at the back. It came into fashion soon after the year 1700, and was very quickly adopted. Like the French type (which was laced in front), this corset was covered with beautiful material and worn instead of a bodice. The English corset, unlike the French, was an arrangement of whalebone

Fig. 420. CORSET OF THE FIRST HALF OF THE EIGHTEENTH CENTURY

rods, from 4–6 cm. broad and 1 cm. thick, which went all round the body, even across the breast. A stout wire at the top kept it in the

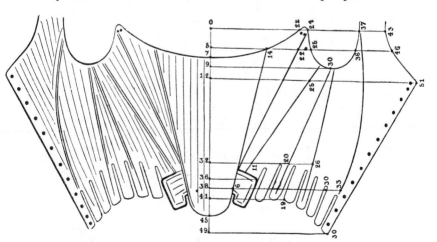

Fig. 421. MEASUREMENTS AND CUT OF CORSET SHOWN IN FIG. 420

proper convex shape. The rigidity of the corset was increased by having the foot of the central front section doubly strengthened

343

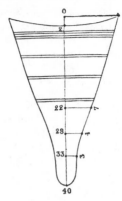

Fig. 422. CORSET, FIRST HALF OF THE
EIGHTEENTH CENTURY

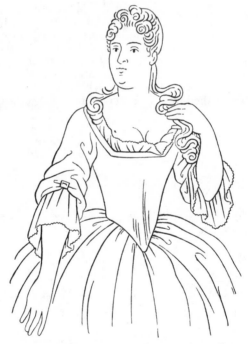

Fig. 423. LADY, FIRST HALF OF THE EIGHTEENTH CENTURY

with whalebone laid longitudinally and across. It was made so
that an edge projected. To produce this edge the coarse linen
lining was cut several centimetres narrower at the foot than the

material covering the corset. When it was sewn to the edges of the material the latter was bent upward. At the back and in front the English corset had broad laces which were passed over the top of the skirt to keep it down, while the narrow laces at the side were hidden under the skirt. In the front of this corset, in the top of the lining

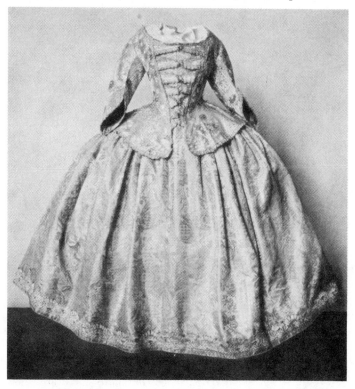

Fig. 424. DRESS OF YELLOW DAMASK, MIDDLE OF THE EIGHTEENTH CENTURY

—as in the front bib (*la pièce*) of the French corset—a small pocket was made to hold fragrant herbs. Both the French and the English styles were laced from the foot upward.

Shortly before the death of Louis XIV ladies began to wear wide over-dresses. These resembled long cloaks with sleeves, without any shaping at the waist ; they hung from the shoulders to the feet, gradually widening downward. These were called *contouches* (Fig. 425). They were open all down the front, and were worn both in the house and out of doors. They were made of silk or of wool, and were fastened—sometimes only at the breast, and in other cases right down to the foot—with bows of broad ribbon. These *contouches* were so universally worn about 1730 that hardly any other style of dress was

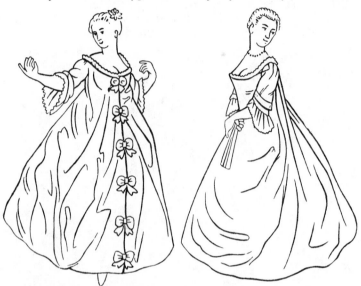

Fig. 425. LADY WEARING A CONTOUCHE (MORNING GOWN), FIRST HALF OF THE EIGHTEENTH CENTURY

Fig. 426. WOMEN'S DRESS, FIRST HALF OF THE EIGHTEENTH CENTURY

to be seen. Another popular material for them was white or pink taffeta. Young girls wore gauze or embroidered muslin over a dress of taffeta of a strongly contrasted colour.

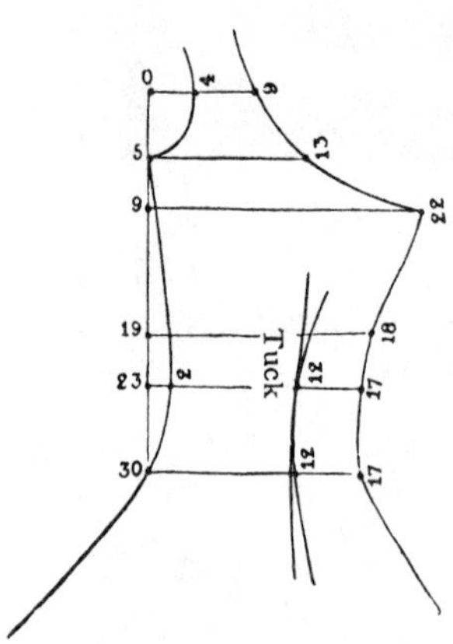

Short *contouches*, reaching to the knees and worn only indoors, were popular in Germany, and were known as *Cossäcklein*. Like the longer *contouches*, these were low-necked, and were trimmed with narrow lace. In that respect, as well as in the style of the sleeves, they resembled the other dresses worn at the time.

About the year 1740 the *contouche* was made with a lining in the form of a close-fitting bodice. It was sewn to the dress only in front; the back was joined to it only at the neck. The rest of the dress fell loosely down as before (Fig. 426). The back of the lining, which was

Fig. 427. HALF OF FRONT PIECE OF THE SCHLENDER

Plate IX

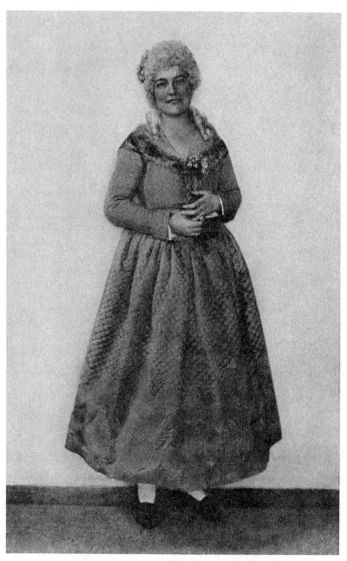

GOWN OF LIGHT BLUE QUILTED SILK   346
About 1740

made of coarse linen, was cut in one piece, and only slightly stiffened with whalebone. The front was like that of a corset that laced at the

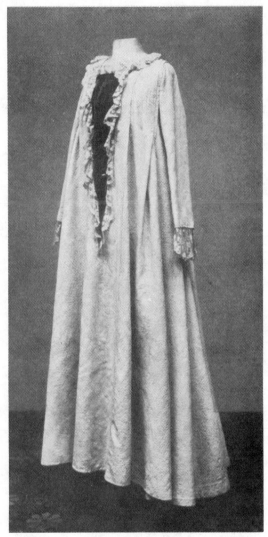

Fig. 428. Contouche of White Linen covered with Designs in Quilt Stitching, Middle of the Eighteenth Century

back. The cut of it was the same, and it too had a stiffening of whale-bone. The front piece was divided in the middle and arranged for

347

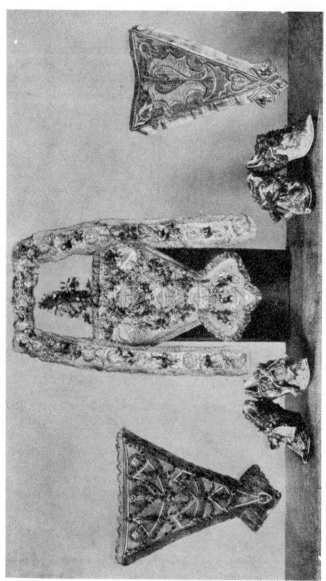

Fig. 429. Stecker (Bibs) and Set of Trimmings with Gold and Silver Lace. Shoes of Pink Velvet. Middle of the Eighteenth Century

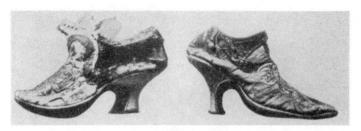

Fig. 430. Two Shoes, First Half of the Eighteenth
Century

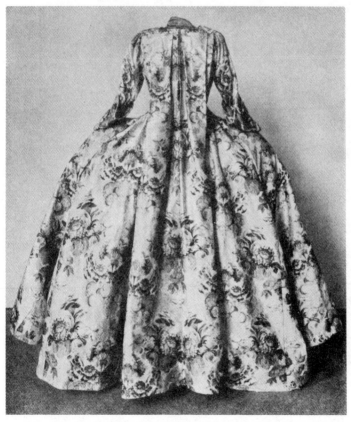

Fig. 431. Back View of a Gown of Damask, Middle of the
Eighteenth Century

349

lacing. This fastening, however, was not visible, for the corresponding part of the dress was stretched across the front of the lining and sewn

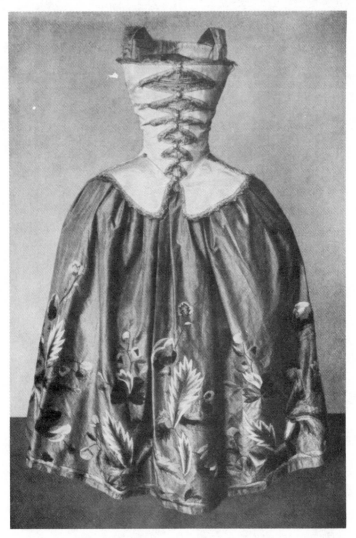

Fig. 432. Embroidered Skirt of Blue Silk with Corslet of White Silk, Middle of the Eighteenth Century

close to the lace-holes, leaving as much of the edge as was necessary to conceal the laced part. This garment, which in other respects was

Plate X

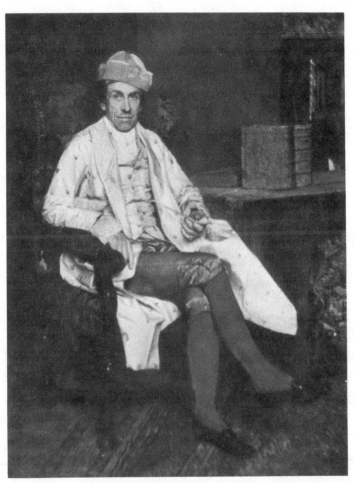

LOUNGE COAT FOR INDOOR WEAR AND SLEEVED
WAISTCOAT 350
About 1750

exactly like the *contouche*, was called in Germany the *Schlender*. Sometimes the front of the bodice was entirely separate from the skirt, and was cut like the under-bodice. The skirt was then sewn to the lower edge of the back and pleated. This gave the *Schlender* exactly the same appearance as an ordinary *robe*.

About the year 1750 farthingales greatly diminished in size. At the same time the *contouche* gradually went out of fashion. Its place was taken by the *robe*, or gown, called *robe ronde*, open from the waist

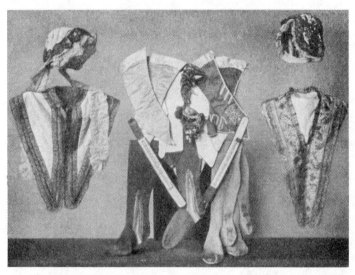

Fig. 433. BONNETS AND TIPPETS (PALATINES) WITH GOLD LACE. GREEN AND PINK SILK STOCKINGS WITH GUSSETS. GREEN AND PINK LEATHER GLOVES WITH WHITE STITCHING

down. This dress was something essentially novel. A separate corset was now rarely worn underneath the bodice, because the lining of the *robe* was practically a corset. The fastening of the bodice of this *robe ronde* was always in front, and was either like that of the *Schlender* or was a *Stecker*, or *pièce* (Fig. 429). In the latter case the cut of the material and the arrangement of the whalebone in the lining were copied from the French corset. The material and trimming of the under-dress worn with the *robe ronde* were always exactly the same as those of the *robe*.

Toward the middle of the century women began to wear as morning attire garments resembling the *contouche*, made of fine white material and trimmed with flounces. About the same time it became the fashion to wear at the morning toilet various kinds of powder-mantles and dressing-jackets.

As the *contouche* was as low-necked as all the other dresses, various kinds of neckerchiefs were worn with it. A favourite style was a small triangular *follette* of black or coloured silk (Plate IX). Similar to this were the tippets (*palatines*), large neckerchiefs made of gauze, *crêpe*, or lace, trimmed with lace, and fastened in front with silver braid or small buttons (Fig. 433). For winter wear the tippet retained its former cape form, and was either of velvet or fur or of short black or white feathers. Up till about 1750 some women still wore the mantilla, a short cloak of velvet, taffeta, or lace, with frills of the same material or small ruches of gauze.

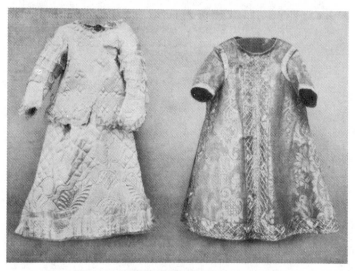

Fig. 434. CHILDREN'S FROCKS, EIGHTEENTH CENTURY

The long-continued use of topknots (*fontanges*), the back part of which was a cap covering the head, had accustomed women of the middle class to having a portion of their hair concealed, and they were now loath to renounce the practice. With the appearance, therefore, of low *coiffures*, with which fashionable women wore no headdress, women of the middle classes invented various caps and coifs, which they wore both in the house and out of doors. (Plate VI.) These were of white gauze or other fine material, and were trimmed with lace and ribbons. Some of them were made over a framework of wire, while others had no such foundation. The most popular were the *dormeuses*, or *négligés*. Some of them came down to the eyes ; others left uncovered not only the forehead, but also a portion of the hair. The style depended on the purpose which they were meant to serve.

Till about the year 1750 changes had been confined to the dress, *coiffure*, and headdress. Shoes remained as they had been, and slippers were worn indoors as before (Figs. 429 and 430). In bad weather galoshes were put on over the shoes. The customary green

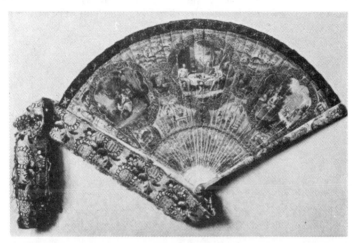

Fig. 435. FAN WITH MINIATURES, FIRST HALF OF THE EIGHTEENTH CENTURY

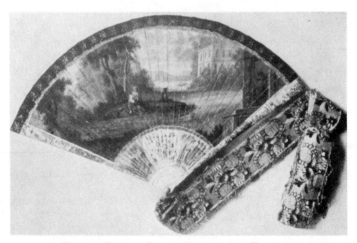

Fig. 436. REVERSE SIDE OF FAN SHOWN IN FIG. 435

silk stockings with pink gussets (Fig. 433), however, gave place to white ones. Women continued to use cosmetics and beauty patches, but masks (Fig. 417) were no longer worn. Gloves were now not only of leather or silk, but also, from 1740 onward, of silk net. Fans were indispensable (Figs. 435 and 436). Strings of pearls were not now so frequently worn, but diamonds were very fashionable.

During the second half of the eighteenth century fashions underwent a complete change. The feeling prevailed that the old styles had become impossible, and efforts to improve them were being made

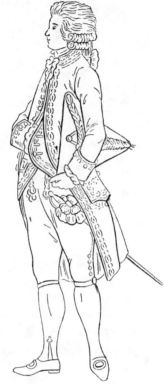

Fig. 437. MEN'S DRESS, ABOUT 1780

when the French Revolution broke out and brought about profound alterations.

Men's Dress. The first results of the attempt to attain a simpler, more practical, and more comfortable style of dress were a great diminution of ornamentation and a great lessening of the width of men's clothes. (See Plate XIV.) In place of broad trimmings and rich embroidery on coat and waistcoat came narrow braid and simple *girlandes*. The turned-back cuffs now came hardly half-way up the forearm, and lay close to the sleeves. The most remarkable change in the coat, however, was one that came in about 1770. In imitation of the English riding coat the lower ends of the coat front were cut

Plate XI

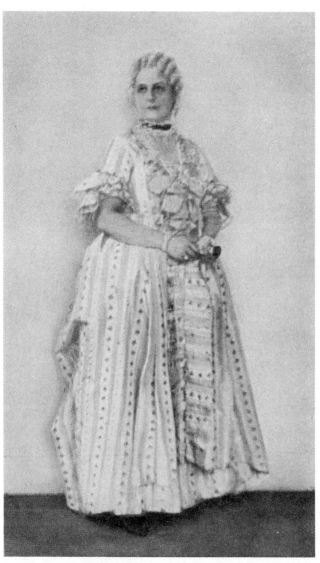

LIGHT BLUE STRIPED ROCOCO COSTUME
About 1750   354

away, thus producing a new style, *le frac,* or the swallow-tail coat. In other respects this resembled the *justaucorps,* known as *habit à la française,* but while the latter was collarless, the former had always a small stand-up collar, *le collet* (Fig. 438). As Louis XVI wore this

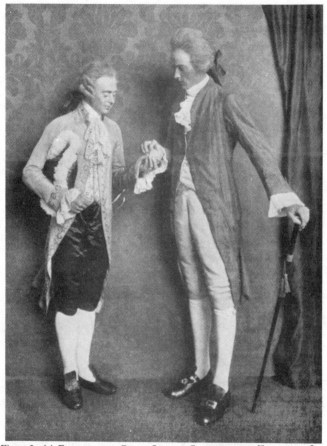

Fig. 438. (*a*) Embroidered Dress Coat of Greenish-pink Taffeta, 1780
(*b*) Dress Coat of Striped Green Taffeta (Middle-class Costume)

new style, it soon became universal, and was in 1780 the recognized Court dress in place of the *habit à la française.* The waistcoat was also shortened and cut away like the coat, so that the lavish embroideries were perforce restricted to a narrow edging.

From about 1780 onward the waistcoat was gradually ousted by *le gilet.* This was copied from the English sleeveless waistcoat. It reached to the abdomen, and was quite straight at the foot, with no tails or skirt. Unlike the waistcoat, the back of the *gilet* was of the same material (though of inferior quality) as the front ; it was arranged

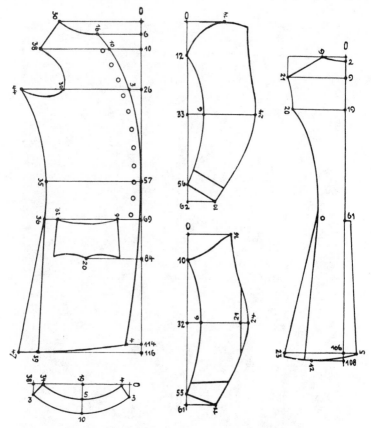

Fig. 439. Cut of Dress Coat shown in Fig. 438, *b*

for lacing up to the shoulder-blades. Owing to this false back and the absence of sleeves there was a great saving of material; this was also effected in the short-fronted waistcoat. This intermediate garment —half waistcoat and half *gilet*—was called *gilet-veste*, or *veston*. Ere long the *gilet-veste* and the *gilet* completely drove out the waistcoat proper, and the name *veston* was applied to both.

The embroidered dress coat (Plate XIV) and the skirted waistcoat were the Court dress in France till the downfall of the monarchy, but from 1788 onward the lavish ornamentation disappeared. This simplification gave the dress coat the appearance of the *frac habillé*, which till now had been merely the garment worn for balls or when making morning calls on distin-

guished persons. With the dress coat the *gilet* was never worn, but always the waistcoat or *veston*, together with the sword. On the whole, however, swords had ceased to be worn since the adoption of the English swallow-tail and the round hat. Gentlemen now carried instead a stick of Spanish cane with a large knob when wearing a round hat.

Nether garments still consisted of long silk stockings and breeches reaching below the knee, where they were not only buttoned, but also fastened with a buckle and strap. Along with the dress coat and *gilet* France had also adopted a different (an English) style of breeches, which too came into general use. Instead of the buttoned front opening they had a fairly broad flap, *le pont*, or *la patte*; they were supported by shoulder braces—*les bretelles*. Shoe-buckles were now much larger than those previously worn.

Women's Dress. There had been little change in women's dress during the last years of the reign of Louis XV. In 1750 the farthingale began to decrease in size, and about 1760 it was replaced by numerous stiff petticoats. About this time the excavations in Greece had led to the introduction of Greek fashions—*à la Grècque*—but it was hairdressing that was chiefly affected. The only

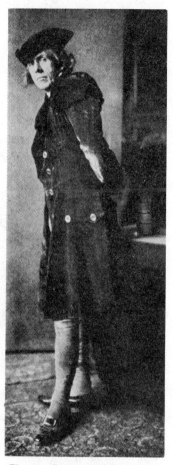

Fig. 440. Reddish-brown Velvet Coat, Second Half of the Eighteenth Century

other novelty was a garment that was half cloak, half jacket. The neck in front was lower than before, but at the back it became higher and higher. Greek fashions soon ceased to affect dress, but Greek *coiffures* continued and developed. *Chiffons* were wound round the head—*i.e.*, broad strips of gauze, attached to the hair in various ways. About 1772 the hair began to be dressed higher

357

and higher, till the distance from the chin to the top of the hair frequently measured 70 cm. or more. On the top of this mass of

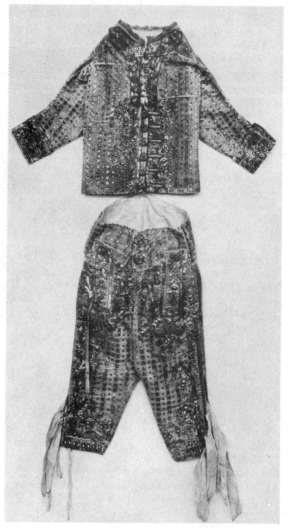

Fig. 441. Suit (1785) of the Young Prince of Asturias, later King Ferdinand VII of Spain

hair were stuck three ostrich feathers and a bow which was fastened by some kind of ornament. Pearls, flowers, and aigrettes were also

358

Plate XI

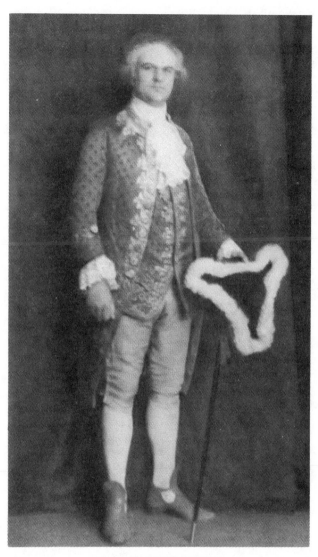

COAT OF RED BROCADE
About 1760

358

used. The disproportion between a lady's height, increased by the enormous *coiffure*, and the lessened girth due to the disappearance of the farthingale was so great that it displeased Marie-Antoinette, and after the accession of her husband in 1774 her first step was to reintroduce the farthingale at Court. She gave it a form, however, that it had never yet had. It extended only at the sides, and was as straight as possible in front and at the back. The framework was made of iron ribs, 1 cm. in breadth and 1 mm. in thickness, encased in fine leather. It consisted of several parts. Chief of these were two fairly long rods, slightly bent outward, fastened together at the ends on both sides with three hoops, whose diameter was in proportion to the girth of the wearer. These three hoops at each side were so hinged to each other and to the two long rods that they could be raised and lowered at will. When lowered, the lowest two hoops were in the same horizontal plane as the rods. Linen tapes affixed to the hoops kept these at the proper distance from each other, and when the lowest hoop was let down the two others practically trisected the space between the lowest hoop and the waist. Other tapes, some running to the hoops and some to the rods, connected the framework with the waist-belt. This farthingale was put on so that the rods came to about the middle of the body or a little lower, and from that height the skirt fell perpendicularly at both sides (Fig. 443). In spite of the width of this framework ladies were able to reduce it at will to almost their natural

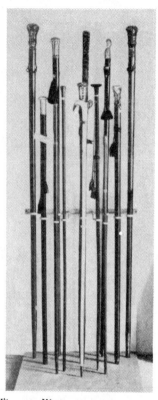

Fig. 442. WALKING-STICKS OF THE EIGHTEENTH CENTURY

size, because the hinges allowed the projecting hoops and the dress to be raised till they could if necessary be held up by the upper arms. Narrow lanes and doorways had now no terrors for ladies dressed thus. As these farthingales looked as if their sole purpose was to support the elbows they were called *à coudes*. A beautiful example is shown in Fig. 443.

This farthingale gradually came into general use, and continued to be the accepted form of Court dress up to the time of the French Revolution. For ordinary wear it began to diminish in size about the

359

year 1780, and went almost completely out of fashion about 1785. At Court too about the same time excessive dimensions were less often seen. Finally it was worn only on ceremonial occasions.

Over the framework of hoops was worn a petticoat (a skirt without a bodice), *le jupon*. Its length varied according to the fashion of the moment. It was longer at the sides than in front and at the back, the extra length being equivalent to the distance from the waist to the extreme end of the hoops. It had no folds in front and very few at the back, where the slit was situated, but at the sides it was so full

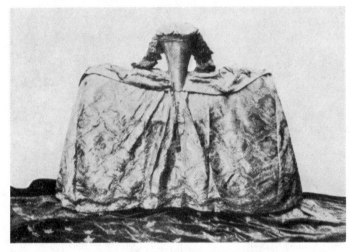

Fig. 443. WEDDING DRESS OF QUEEN SOPHIA MAGDALENA OF SWEDEN, 1766

that it could pass over the hoops without being at all stretched. Over this was worn a dress, *le manteau* (Fig. 444). This consisted of a close-fitting, low-necked bodice, *le corsage*, with tight, elbow-length sleeves, and an open-fronted skirt with a train.

The back of the bodice of the *manteau* was made of six strips, in each of which at both sides, close to the joining seams, a piece of whalebone was inserted. Several rods of whalebone were also sewn into the front piece. The arrangement for lacing the bodice was in the lining, and was hidden by a strip of material falling over it. The sleeves were arranged in two small pleats running up and backward. The length of the skirt, or *la queue*, of this *manteau* was 110 cm. in front, 125 cm. at the back, 122 cm. at each side. (See Fig. 445.) The width was that of seven panels each 47 cm. wide. The skirt was sewn directly to the bodice at the back, but from the back of the hip forward it was attached to a strong band, which was hooked in front. The sewing was done so as to distribute the folds and place one at

360

each seam of the bodice. Inside the skirt were four equidistant rows of small brass rings, running from top to bottom at distances of 25 cm. apart. Through these were passed the strings which enabled the wearer to raise and drape the skirt at will.

Sometimes the skirt of the *manteau* was cut much fuller. In that

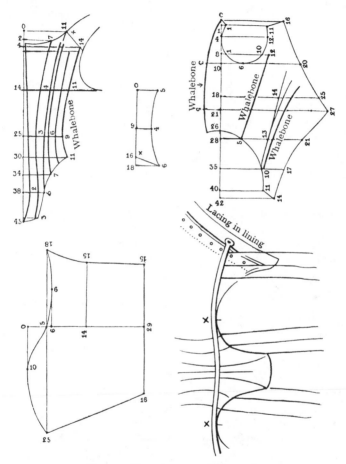

Fig. 444. MANTEAU OF THE YEAR 1776

case the back panel was cut in one piece with the middle panel of the back of the bodice, which was then slightly taken in at the waist. (See Fig. 446.) The whalebones in the back were distributed as in the previous case, but the skirt was not sewn directly to the bodice.

In some cases the back panel of the skirt was carried up at its full

361

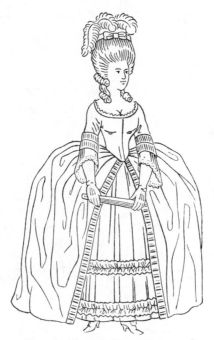

Fig. 445. WOMEN'S DRESS, ABOUT 1778

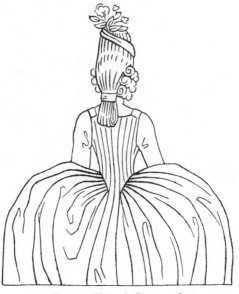

Fig. 446. WOMEN'S DRESS, 1787

width to the neck of the bodice and arranged there in a few deep
pleats. The edges were sewn to the lining. This garment closely

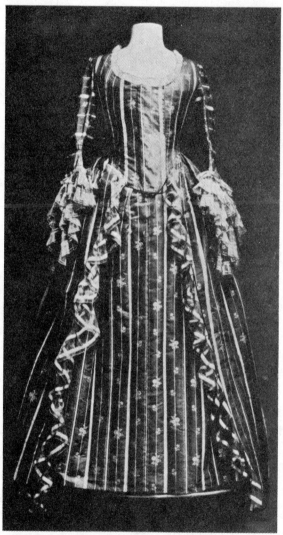

Fig. 447. RED AND WHITE STRIPED SILK DRESS, END OF THE
EIGHTEENTH CENTURY

resembled the *Schlender* worn in the first half of the century. It had
been a favourite with Watteau the painter at the beginning of the

century, and remained steadily in favour for nearly seventy years. The front edges of the skirt of the *manteau* did not come quite as far as the fastening of the bodice, so that they were 20 cm. or more apart, exposing the under-dress all down the front.

The neck of the bodice of the *manteau* was as a rule closed to the top, so that the front—*Stecker, la pièce*—was rarely necessary. The upper edge of the bodice was trimmed with lace of moderate width (Fig. 447), and right in front was a large bow of coloured ribbon or a diamond clasp. The tight sleeves, out of which long lace *engageantes* fell to the forearms, reached at least half-way down the upper arm, and were variously adorned at the ends. The front edges of the skirt—which was occasionally lined—had a trimming like that of the sleeves. The skirt itself either fell quite plain to the feet or was gathered as far as the knees into very large folds, which were loosely filled with paper to retain their baggy shape. The under-skirt—which might be either like or unlike the *manteau* in material and colour—was liberally ornamented with its own material or with lace, silk ribbon, or even strips of fur. Similar variety was shown in the styles of ornamentation, the commonest being *volants*, flounces, and especially the smooth pleatings, called *en platitude*, attached to the skirt either in straight lines or in larger or smaller curves. Frequent use was also made of the so-called "plastic ornaments." These were pieces of the dress material lined with wadding and sewn on in curves and wreaths. The need of warmer clothing was met by wadding and quilting (see Plate IX). A thin layer of wadding was laid on a lining of strong linen. Over the wadding was placed the silk material, which was then sewn with fine stitches through the wadding to the lining. The stitching was so done that beautiful patterns were produced, covering the entire dress with tendril-like lines—a design which can be seen on the wadded bodices of the seventeenth century and on doublets of the sixteenth century. It was called *matelassé*.

The *manteau* enjoyed a longer vogue than the broad farthingale, for even after the latter had gone out of fashion the *manteau*, in almost unchanged form, continued to be worn with the *culs*. As a matter of fact, even in later days it changed only its name, for all the new forms of dress that came in about 1790 were cut on the lines of this garment.

When, soon after the year 1780, the farthingale gradually disappeared its place was taken by small pads or cushions, called *poches*, fastened at the hips. (See Fig. 449.) These did not last long. In their stead came a fairly large cushion, *le cul*, so named after the material (*cul de crin*) of which it was made. The Germans called it *cul de Paris*, after the city where it was first introduced.

The skirt worn with the hip-pads and with the *cul* was usually pleated all round, and reached to the feet. On the other hand, the dress, *le manteau*, had again a train, whereas when worn with the farthingale it had been gathered or tucked. Occasionally, also, the

Plate XIII

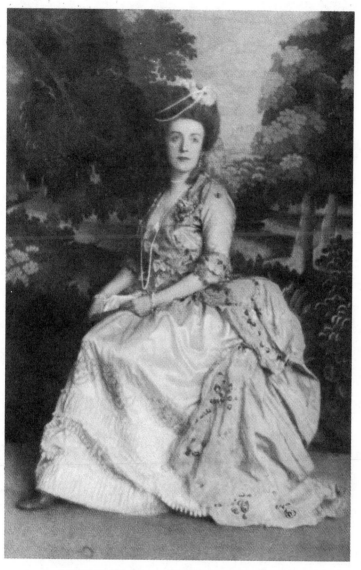

LIGHT BLUE GOWN WITH ROSE DESIGN, 1770

bodice was made of a material other than that of the skirt. In such a case the skirt was called *un tablier*.

In spite of a few not unimportant changes in the cut the bodice when finished retained the form it had hitherto had. The back was

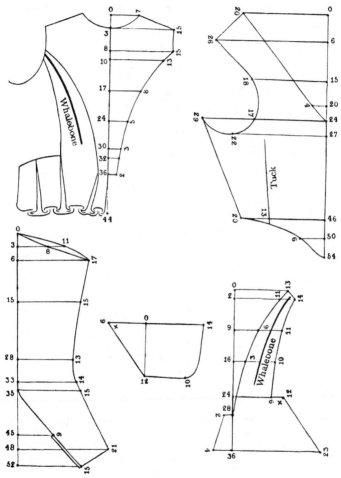

Fig. 448. PATTERN OF JACKET, 1790

now cut in one piece, but was considerably narrower at the foot than before. It was also less wide in front. A side-piece was inserted between front and back. As had previously been the case, the fastening of the bodice was in the lining, and was concealed by the edge of the dress material. There were fewer whalebones than before—two close together in the back, one in the middle of each side-piece, one at each seam connecting back and sides, and one on each edge of the lacing in front. The neck of these bodices was still very low in front, and so, in imitation of the general practice of Englishwomen, it became the fashion about 1790 to cover the bust. This was done

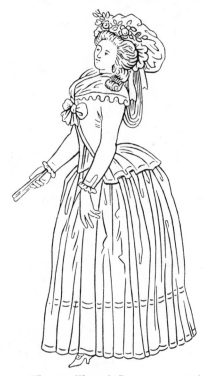

Fig. 449. WOMEN'S DRESS, ABOUT 1776

by means of a large triangular piece of fine white cloth, called a *fichu*, which was put on either under or over the bodice. In the latter case it was crossed over the bust and tied at the back in a large bow. As a rule the *fichu* was arranged to lie as loosely as possible in front, and for this purpose bent frames were sometimes used. They were called *carcasses*, but the French gave them the nickname *trompeurs*, or *menteurs*. The English called them " liars." The German name was *Lügner*. Their use, however, was not confined to women with defective busts; they were worn also by women with faultless outlines.

About the year 1790 separate jacket-like garments became very

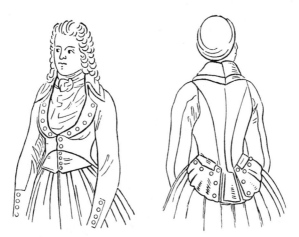

Fig. 450. Caraco, Women's Garment, End of the
Eighteenth Century

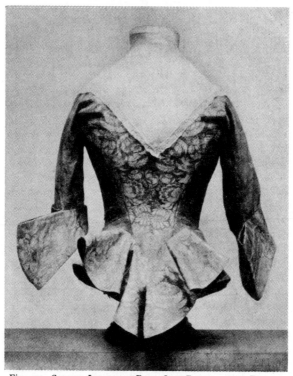

Fig. 451. Caraco Jacket of Blue Silk Damask with Floral
Design, toward the End of the Eighteenth Century

fashionable. They were called *caracos*, and were as a rule close-fitting (Fig. 451). Most of the various styles (which soon went out of fashion

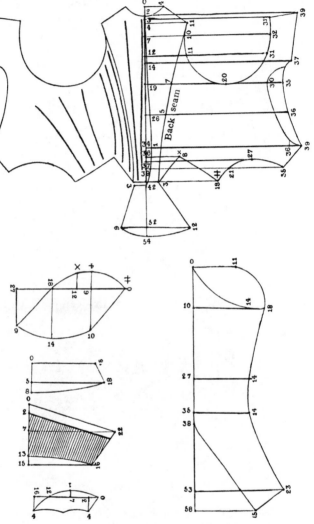

Fig. 452. Cut of the Caraco in Fig. 451

again) were called *jaquettes*, and the name *caraco* came to be applied only to the style that resembled the male dress coat (Figs. 453 and 454). This enjoyed great favour among German women, who had borrowed it from the riding habit of Englishwomen. Frenchwomen preferred a simpler form of the *caraco*.

The bodice of the under-dress, over which a *caraco* or a gown closed only at the top was worn, was always of the same material as the skirt to which it belonged. It was as close-fitting as possible. It was laced at the back, and the front and sides were stiffened with whalebone. Mostly, however, the under-dress was without a bodice. A light corset was worn instead ; it was concealed by a broad front, *la pièce d'estomac*, of the same material as the dress. This front was either laced or otherwise attached at both sides to the *robe* or the *caraco*, so that the *robe* also fitted close to the body. In one style of the *caraco* the bib was sewn to the over-dress and buttoned down the front, so that it looked like a waistcoat.

Following a fashion that was current in England about the year 1786, women began to wear instead of an over-dress a light corslet, called *Mieder* by the Germans. This was usually of black taffeta with a white lining ; it had a long peak in front and at the back, like the bodice of a dress. It was stiffened with whalebones a hand's-breadth apart, and quilted with white silk. These corslets were either laced behind or buckled in front. In the latter case the edges were about four fingers' breadth apart, and were fastened with broad cloth tapes and steel buckles.

About 1780 it became the fashion to put on over the elegant costume worn indoors and outdoors—this including the short over-dress known as *fourreau*—a *tablier* (pinafore or apron). This was of some fine white material, and was

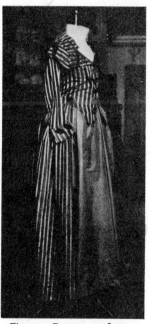

Fig. 453. Dress with Long Caraco Jacket of Brown Striped Silk, about 1795

trimmed all round with a broad frill called *falbala* (flounce, or furbelow). These *tabliers* were as a rule very wide, and almost as long as the dress. They had two large pockets sewn on. The fashion lasted only a few years.

During the cold weather of spring and autumn ladies wore *mantelets* —short capes of silk material, trimmed all round the edges with flounces of the same material or with lace. These were so broad in the middle that they completely covered the wearer's back ; they grew narrower toward the front. The ends were long enough to reach to below the knee. Made of velvet and trimmed with swan's-down or with fur, they were worn even in winter, but a more usual winter wear was actual furs, called *pelisses*. These varied in style, but were usually short and very wide ; they were fitted with wide half-length sleeves.

The *coiffure*, which at the time of the accession of Louis XVI was already very high and included much ornamentation, continued to

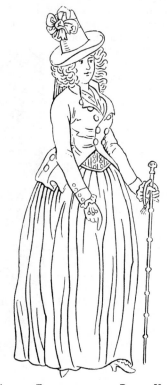

Fig. 454. ENGLISHWOMAN IN RIDING HABIT

increase in height, and had to be supported by wire frames and pads of various kinds. In 1778 it was often more than 50 cm. in height, and the ornamentation included gauze, pearls, ribbons, tinsel, plumes, and flowers. The side-curls of former days were still continued (see Plate XIII)—sometimes long and sometimes gathered below the ears —while either the whole of the long back hair fell down loosely with curled ends or half of it was combed upward and arranged in *chignon* shape. These two concurrent styles went under the name of *cheveux à la conseillère*, for they were the fundamental styles on which the hairdressers rung all their changes. All historical events, phenomena of nature, motifs from mythology, even the happenings of the day, supplied suggestions for ladies' *coiffures* and for descriptive names. One style bore the name *coiffure à la flore*—in this a small basket of flowers was perched on a steeply rising mass of hair. *Coiffure à la victoire* meant a wreath of laurel or oak leaves. Ladies even wore *parterres galants* or *chiens couchants* made of hair. This inventiveness was not confined to Parisiennes. They had worthy rivals in the women of London, Berlin, Vienna, Leipzig, Dresden, Göttingen, and Frankfort-on-the-Main. An event of great significance for the women of Paris took place in the year 1785. The Queen, who had just given birth to a child, lost her magnificent fair hair, which had made that colour fashionable and caused it to be called *cheveux de la reine*. Her hairdresser cut the remaining hair quite short, in order to introduce a new style, *la chevelure à l'enfant*. This had no effect, however, on the hairdressing of German and English women. Even in Paris variations in *coiffure* continued to be worn, and ere long the *cheveux à la conseillère*, or the *coiffure à l'urgence*, as it was also called, was once more the basis for numerous other styles.

Although these styles of hairdressing exceeded both in size and variety those that had preceded them, signs of a change of taste were already perceptible. The piled-up masses of hair began to lose their popularity, and women now crimped their hair and arranged it in a new fashion called *hérisson,* or the ' hedgehog ' style. The back hair was still disposed in the *chignon* fashion, or was allowed to fall down behind with curled ends. Ornamentation, however, had entirely changed, because fashion now ordained that some kind of headdress must be worn. The use of white powder, which had come in with the new century, was continued, but about the year 1790 light yellow or red powder replaced the white, though only for a short time.

It was about the year 1780 that it became fashionable to wear hats and bonnets even with the high *coiffures*. When once this practice had become general fashion strictly prescribed whether and when a hat or a bonnet must be worn. The hat was declared to be informal —*en négligé*. The bonnet was indispensable for *la grande parure*, or full dress. About 1786 a headdress called *chapeau-bonnette* was permissible for both purposes. It consisted of a piece of material so arranged that it made a large puff at the top, held together by a ribbon, the rest of the material falling down at the back of the head. The ribbon was tied at the back in a knot, which was surmounted by a plume of coloured feathers. A veil completed this headdress. All kinds of ornamentation were added to please individual taste.

Le bonnet, a piece of material (satin, taffeta, or linen) of any desired shape, was fixed to the hair in any fashion that suited the wearer and worn with strings of beads, ribbons, laces, feathers, or flowers. There were no definite rules—the skill and taste of the hairdresser, who was ever inventing new modes, were the only law on the subject. Like the styles of hairdressing, the *bonnets* had all kinds of curious names—there were *bonnets à la turque, à l'espagnole, à la béarnaise,* or even *à gueule de loup.* The happenings of the day brought in new styles with new names. For example, the calling up of the Notables in 1787 gave rise to a style called *bonnet à la notables.*

Although the bonnet was part of full dress, it could also be worn with informal attire. Indeed, it was an essential part of it, if the expression *en négligé* is used in the meaning it then had, as the opposite of *grande parure*—Court, official, or ball dress—and not in its present-day meaning of 'undress,' for the bonnet was worn *en négligé* both by middle-class women and elderly ladies merely for comfort's sake. Fashionable women and young ladies wore it especially when going to church or as part of walking costume.

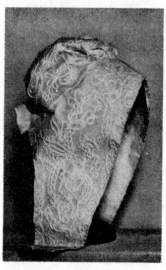

Fig. 455. Bonnet of White Embroidered Linen, about 1800

From the year 1785 onward bonnets assumed larger dimensions, while *coiffures* became smaller and, in particular, lower. From this date the shape of the bonnet differed more and more from that of the hat, for up till this time the two sometimes differed from each other only in name.

The hat, *le chapeau,* became fashionable soon after 1780. The sole difference between it and the bonnet lay in the almost horizontal brim. The hat, however, soon began to take various shapes. It was in most cases fairly large, so that it was not hidden by the high *coiffure.* Usually it was of light material—straw or silk. It could be either high or low in the crown, broad- or narrow-brimmed. Similarly variety was shown in the way it was worn. It was perched on the top of the hair, or placed sideways, or tilted forward. Sometimes it was low down, at other times high up on the head, but in all positions it had to be secured by ribbons or pins; otherwise it fell off.

Still greater variety was shown in hat-trimming. Feathers, flowers, and ribbons were used. From 1786 women began to wear hats of beaver fur, *castors,* imitating the shape of men's hats, but with the addition of rich, gay trimmings. In Paris in the year 1790 ladies, willingly or unwillingly, decked their hats with large tricolour cockades or ribbons.

There had been little change in footwear since the middle of the century. From 1780 onward heels were lower. The long upper also disappeared, so that the shoe now covered little more than the toes.

EIGHTEENTH CENTURY—FRANCE

About 1790 buckles began to be fashionable. Soon after 1785 shoes became so comfortable that slippers (*mules*) ceased to be worn.

The fan still retained its popularity, although a formidable rival

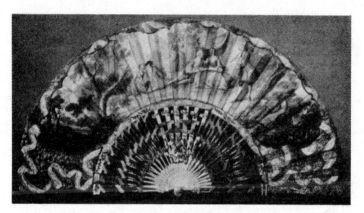

Fig. 456. Fan with Carved Frame and Miniatures, Middle of the Eighteenth Century

appeared in 1789 in the sunshade or parasol. As the sunshade was carried chiefly out of doors, the fan was restricted to the drawing-room. About the same time the long walking-sticks known as *badines* came into use.

THE PERIOD 1790–1820

DURING the years 1791–92—years so fateful for the French monarchy—all ornamentation disappeared from clothing, and although earlier fashionable styles continued for a time, even these last relics of former days vanished when the Reign of Terror opened. Rich and poor alike were careful to dress as negligently as possible, for anyone whose outward appearance brought him under

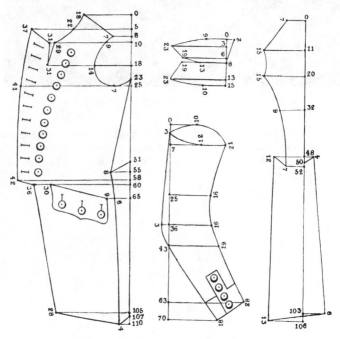

Fig. 457. ENGLISH RIDING COAT, 1786

suspicion of being an aristocrat went in danger of his life. During that time even wealthy men went about wearing the blue linen pantaloons and short jacket (*carmagnole*) of the working man and the red cap of the galley-slave—the symbol of the Jacobins. The French even went to the length of introducing a Revolutionary costume, and in imitation of Greek models they exchanged dress coat and breeches for chiton and chlamys, and wore sandals in place of shoes. Such extremes of Revolutionary sentiment appealed to women with far

374

more success than to men. The Greek chiton, or tunic (a garment after the style of the chemise then worn by Englishwomen), was selected as the type of the new dress movement, which reached its climax.in the year 1800 with its *costume à la sauvage*. All underclothing was discarded; breast and arms were bare. Only the thinnest possible materials were used to make these garments, below which were worn close-fitting, flesh-coloured tights, with brightly coloured insertions and garters. Shoes—mostly made of red leather—had no heels. The hair was bobbed *à la Titus* and curled, and covered with a turban.

Coloured, patterned materials disappeared entirely. The favourite shades were white and grey. A thin shawl or a tinted ribbon at the waist was all the colour allowed. Men's dress too exhibited the same absence of colour and design. Ostentation in dress was not in accord with Republican sentiment.

Men's Dress. Dress coat and breeches were the first to be affected by the new ideals. The coat was constantly being remodelled, and different styles were worn concurrently. Finally two of these drove all others from the field—one worn exclusively by men of the middle classes, the other a military officer's dress coat.

The model for both of these was the English dress coat. The back was cut narrower, thus both diminishing the size and lessening the number of coat-tails. About the

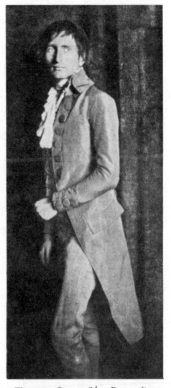

Fig. 458. GREEN SILK DRESS COAT, ABOUT 1786

year 1786 a third style was added —the English riding coat, which was used at first in France solely as riding dress. (See Fig. 457.) The chief difference between it and the other coats of the day was that it had two rows of buttons—*i.e.*, it was double-breasted—and could therefore be buttoned to the right or the left. If one desired to wear it open the two fronts could be buttoned back. This soon became the usual coat worn by the middle classes, but as fashions were continually changing it was altered again and again. (See Figs. 458 and 459.) For example, the front was shortened, while the tails were made narrower and longer. The shoulder-seams were put farther back, and the sleeve-holes greatly enlarged. Other changes, due merely to the caprice of fashion, affected the length of the sleeves, the length and width of the tails, the kind of buttons, the colour of the material. The Revolution, which overthrew everything, really left men's coats pretty much as they were. The French word *habit* now exclusively denoted this garment. It was, as has

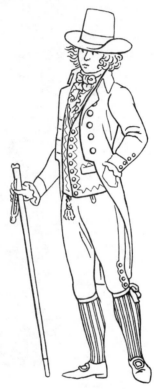

Fig. 459. MEN'S DRESS, 1790

been said, altered again and again. The waist was shortened, the breast-flaps were at times extremely large, but the coat continued to be double-breasted, and retained its square cut. (See Figs. 460 and 461.) The other style of coat, with rounded edges and one row of buttons, was now only a riding coat, although it was often worn by others than horsemen. The collar was high (see Fig. 462) and was either doubled down or lay quite flat. Within a short time numerous other changes were made, and several styles, differing considerably from each other, were being worn at the same time. All of them,

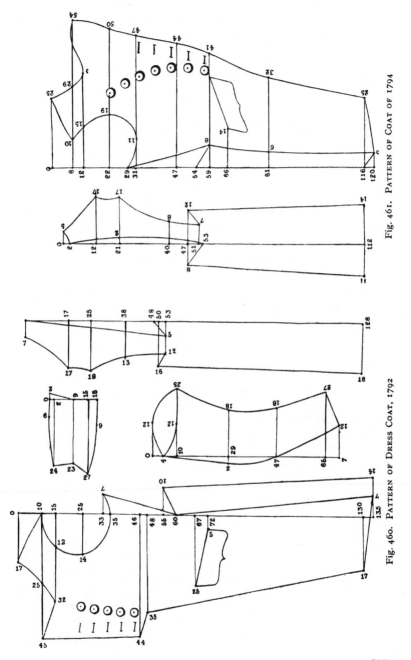

Fig. 461. Pattern of Coat of 1794

Fig. 460. Pattern of Dress Coat, 1792

377

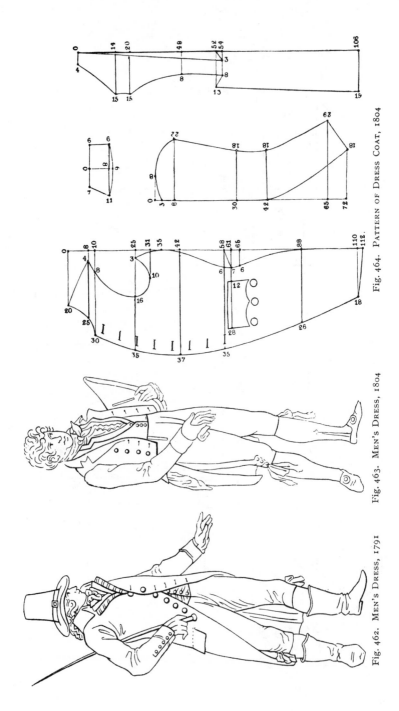

Fig. 464. Pattern of Dress Coat, 1804

Fig. 463. Men's Dress, 1804

Fig. 462. Men's Dress, 1791

however, were short-waisted. About 1804 the upper part was considerably lengthened and the collar took an entirely different shape (Fig. 463). For quite a number of years the coat retained this cut, although numerous small changes were made, and many modifications, which chiefly affected the collar and the tails.

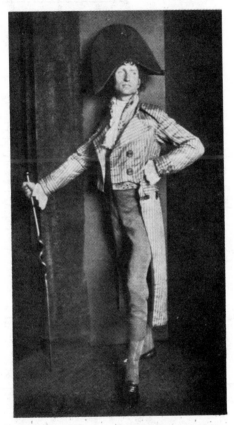

Fig. 465. DRESS COAT OF STRIPED SILK, ABOUT 1792
The so-called " *incroyable* ".

While the coat worn by the middle classes was thus altering and varying the dress coat proper had been out of fashion in France since about 1792, and in other countries too except as Court dress. It was Napoleon who reintroduced it at his Court after his coronation as emperor. (See Plate XIV.) But this garment also bore traces of the Revolution era, and the cut of it was greatly changed. Embroidery was fashionable again, but it was no longer a matter of individual

379

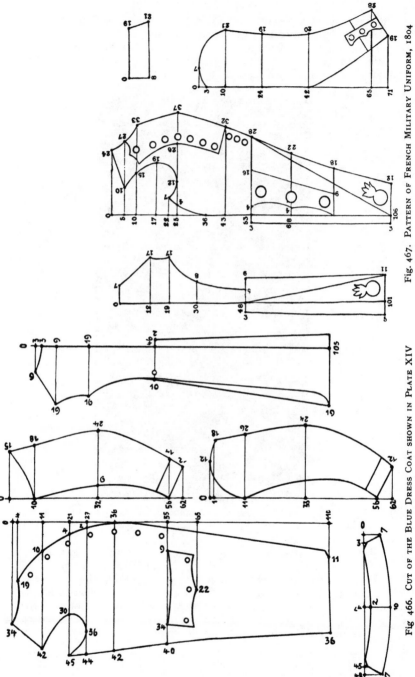

Fig. 467. Pattern of French Military Uniform, 1804

Fig. 466. Cut of the Blue Dress Coat shown in Plate XIV

taste. It was governed by precise regulations in accordance with
the rank and standing of the wearer. Buttons and buttonholes were

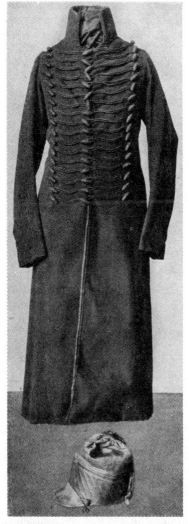

Fig. 468. So-called "Polish" Coat belonging to King Ludwig I
of Bavaria, Beginning of the Nineteenth Century

merely ornamental, because this coat was never buttoned. Two
hooks and eyes were fixed inside, however, half-way down the breast,
so that it could be fastened.

381

The military officer's dress coat (Fig. 467) resembled that just described, as did also the coat worn by most of the regiments of the French Imperial army.

After the coming of the dress coat in 1780 the *justaucorps* had

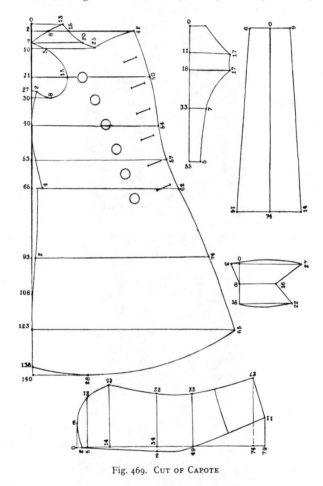

Fig. 469. CUT OF CAPOTE

gradually gone out of fashion. By 1790 it was worn only by men of low rank. The cut of it had in the meantime changed so much that it differed from the dress coat only in the greater breadth and length of the tails. From its resemblance to the English riding coat it was called *redingote*. Men of standing wore it only as an overcoat or *surtout*. When they desired a coat other than a dress coat they chose

Plate XIV

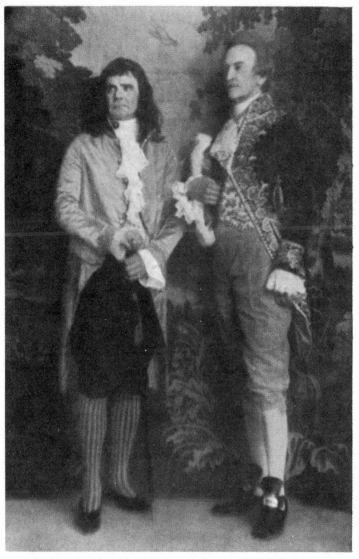

DRESS COAT OF LIGHT BLUE SILK   DRESS COAT
OF LILAC VELVET

About 1790   382

some foreign style, mostly a Polish coat, lavishly trimmed with cord and tassels. When the Revolution had banished all differences of

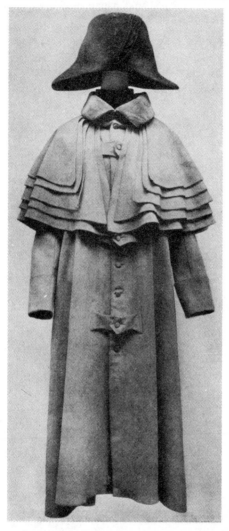

Fig. 470. Gentleman's Overcoat, about 1800, the So-called "Garrick"

rank and made men attach greater importance to comfort in dress even gentlemen of high rank frequently wore the *redingote* in preference to the dress coat, giving it the nickname of *pauvre diable*. It was not till 1810, however, that the *redingote* was generally worn, and by that time it had been so frequently altered and shortened that it retained very little to suggest that it had been originally an overcoat. From 1815 onward it was again much longer.

From 1807 onward the " Polish " coat also became fashionable again (Fig. 468). The *redingote* was still a popular overcoat, and was lengthened and widened to make it more suitable for that purpose. Less attention was paid to fashionable style than to comfort, and the

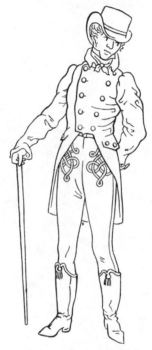

Fig. 471. MEN'S DRESS, 1810

new *redingote* was therefore made to button all down the front. It is clear from all this that the cut of the *surtout* when used as *redingote* had not been greatly altered, and so to distinguish the two the *redingote* was called *la capote* (Fig. 469). About 1800 another style of overcoat came in ; it proved a formidable rival to the *capote*, for it retained its place beside it for many years. This was the English " Garrick," with its numerous capes (Fig. 470). It was half coat half cloak. By draw-strings and straps that could be buttoned it could be widened at will, and thus served many purposes. As a matter of fact, it ousted the ordinary cloak for a considerable time, and reduced it to the rank of a mere travelling dress.

About the year 1805 another English coat, of very novel design, the
" spencer," was introduced. It was intended to protect only the
upper part of the body against cold, and had therefore no tails and

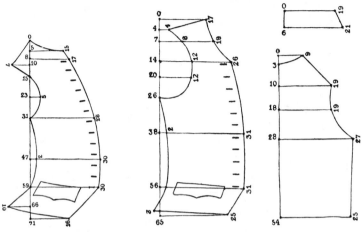

Fig. 472. SCHOSZWESTE
(VESTON) OF 1786

Fig. 473. VESTON OF 1804

very short sleeves. It was usually made of light-coloured cloth, and
was meant to contrast strongly with the darker coat worn beneath it.

The *veston* (tailed waistcoat, lounge coat, or jacket) (Fig. 472), which

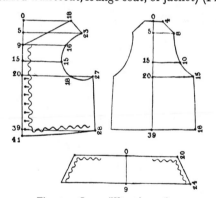

Fig. 474. GILET (WESTE) OF 1802

was worn with the dress coat, was in front very like the waistcoat
that had recently been in ordinary use. But the tails were a few
centimetres shorter, and those in front were farther apart from each
other. It differed also from the ordinary waistcoat in that the back

385

was not exactly the same length as the front. It reached only to where the tails began, and was usually made of strong linen. The

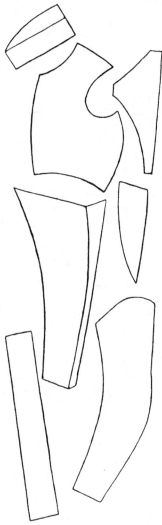

Fig. 475. Dress Coat of 1820

Revolution banished the *veston* (Fig. 473) from France in favour of the *gilet*, and it was not till the time of the Empire that it came in again with the dress coat. Like the latter, it returned in a slightly

different form.   To distinguish it from the tail-less waistcoat (*gilet*)
the Germans called it the *Schoszweste*, or tailed waistcoat.   The *gilet*
they called simply *Weste*.

The *gilet* was at first very long and had only one row of buttons
(Fig. 474).   During the Revolution it had two rows, and was repeatedly
shortened.   At that time it was usually made of fine, light-coloured
material such as cashmere, and was lavishly embroidered, but striped
or patterned materials were also frequently used.   The broad collar
was kept upright by thin whalebones sewn into the front edges.

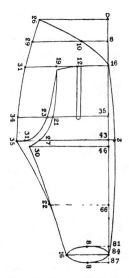

Fig. 476.   Breeches of 1790

About 1804 the waistcoat became longer again, and was worn open
low down in front ; by and by it had a turn-down collar.   Changes
were very frequent.   For example, actually or apparently several
waistcoats were worn together.   The collar was now broad, now
narrow.   The foot of the waistcoat was cut straight or into small
tails, which were long one day and short the next.

About the year 1780 breeches had been greatly improved in England.
The front opening had taken the form of a flap (*le pont* or *la patte*)
(Fig. 476).   This change continued till about 1840, when the perpendicular slit returned.   But the flap was not the only improvement.
From 1790 onward the breeches were becoming more practical and
convenient.   The slight excision in the hollow of the knee was
retained.

When it became the custom to wear boots instead of shoes out of
doors the knee-buckles of the breeches were replaced by ribbons,

either tied in bows or hanging down. These bows were worn even after 1790, when the breeches were lengthened to the calves (Fig. 462). Breeches were made longer and longer, till in 1800 they were full length, although the lower part was hidden by the high boots (Fig. 471).

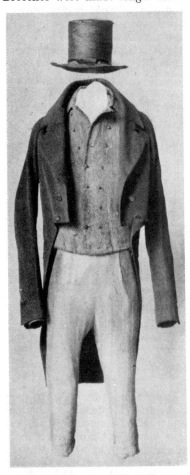

Fig. 477. Dress Coat and Silk Stockinette Trousers of King Ludwig I of Bavaria, Beginning of the Nineteenth Century

At that period breeches were made as tight as possible (Fig. 465). They were therefore not made of cloth, but were knitted like stockings (Fig. 477), and were called in Germany *Strumpfhosen* (stocking breeches). Like the cloth breeches, these stocking breeches were light in colour. The front opening was embroidered with cord, in the case of cloth breeches with quilted designs.

About 1810 men began to wear trousers (*pantalons*) long enough to cover the legs of the boots. They were now somewhat wider than formerly (Fig. 478). In the years 1815–20 they were noticeably short. Even riding breeches were very tight from 1810 onward. They were prevented from slipping up by straps passing under the soles of the boots.

In spite of all these new fashions knee-breeches continued to be worn. They retained the form they had had in the year 1790. They were the only style worn with the dress coat or at Court or on ceremonious occasions, and did not go out of fashion till 1830.

Boots, especially top-boots, were for a considerable time worn by the middle classes along with the English dress coat. The French Revolution brought this costume into prominence, and Fashion adopted it.

The hat was a subject of contention for a much longer period than any other article of attire. The style called *à l'Androsmane* lasted for decades as a rival with others. The round hat gradually gained most favour. It had been since 1790 the popular wear with the middle classes, but on ceremonial occasions, and with any kind of uniform, the hat with a turned-up brim was the only style worn. Although habit and the prejudice of rulers who suspected a revolu-

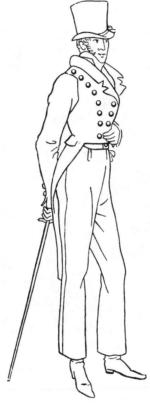

Fig. 478. MEN'S DRESS, 1818

tionary in anyone who wore a round hat stood in the way of the new style, this neat and useful headgear was widely adopted. By the year 1812 it was being worn throughout almost the whole of Europe by the educated, unofficial classes, and it has maintained its ground ever since.

The hat with turned-up brim continued to be worn with any kind of uniform and on ceremonial occasions. (See Figs. 465 and 470.) About the year 1800 the front brim was pulled well forward, while at both sides it was bent up. This shape has been retained to this day.

389

The Revolution affected the styles of hairdressing as profoundly as those of dress in general. It put an end to the use of powder, and brought about a complete, though gradual, change. The changes came slowly, because many people were unwilling to adopt the new fashions, and there were many styles competing for the public favour. For example, the 'dogs' ear' and the 'hedgehog' styles were entirely different from each other—they had nothing whatever in common.

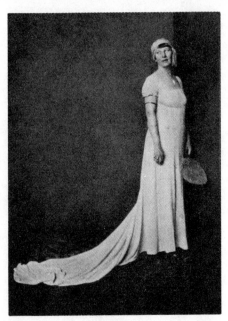

Fig. 479. WHITE EMPIRE DRESS, ABOUT 1807

In the former the hair was long, especially in front, and fell down to the shoulders ; in the latter it was cut short all over and brushed straight up. When the hair was not quite so short it was called *à la Titus*.

Women's Dress. The cut of the dresses to which the name 'Grecian' is given is sufficiently indicated by the mention of the garment which furnished the earliest model—viz., the English chemise. Although this resembled the usual female garment that still bears that name, it was both longer and wider, and, further, in addition to the draw-string at the neck, had another below the breast, by means of which it could be pulled in and draped at will. This was the style worn throughout the whole time of the Republic (see Fig. 485). The only changes made in it were that the neck became lower and lower, and the waist, as indicated by the draw-string, came closer and closer

390

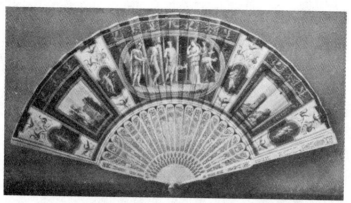

Fig. 480. Fan, Hand-painted, of the Eighteenth Century

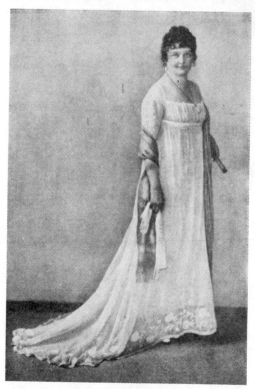

Fig. 481. Chemise Dress of White Embroidered Lawn,
about 1800

up to the breast. The sleeves were shortened—occasionally, indeed, there were none—but the train grew longer and longer.

This dress, which in its way was nearly perfect, changed its appearance entirely when, about the year 1800, a bodice (*le corsage*) was added, to which the dress was sewn. The dress was still wide at the top, and had therefore to be arranged in large pleats. This bodice

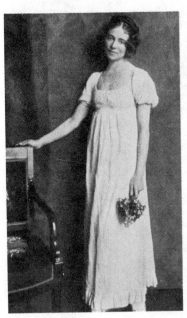

Fig. 482. HOUSE GOWN, 1810

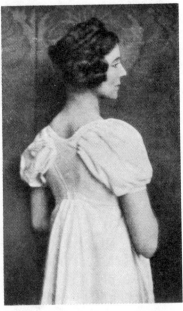

Fig. 483. HOUSE DRESS OF WHITE WASHING MATERIAL, ABOUT 1810

was as short as it could possibly be, and very low in front. It was laced sometimes in front and sometimes at the back ; the lacing was hidden under a piece of the material. The bodice was very simple in cut. It consisted either of two similar pieces, a back and a front, sewn together at the sides, or of a front piece cut very wide so as to go far back and a very small, almost square, back piece. It made no difference to the cut whether the bodice was laced in front or at the back.

With the reintroduction of the separate bodice sewn on to the dress the latter was soon made so as to have fewer folds. These were put as far as possible at the back, and this gave the whole dress an entirely different appearance. Fashion soon dictated a dress without any folds, and by the year 1807 dresses were so tight that it was almost impossible for the wearer to walk in them. They had to be so close-fitting that the outlines of the figure were clearly seen. For this reason only one very thin petticoat was worn, and even this was sometimes left off.   These dresses went by the name of *robes en caleçon*.

The width of the skirt at the foot rarely exceeded 250 cm. The skirt was in two pieces, a front and a back ; a third piece was sewn

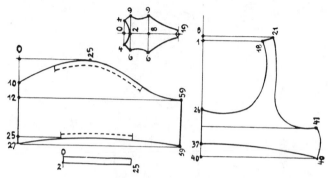

Fig. 484. PATTERN FOR FIG. 483

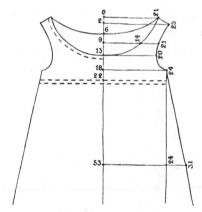

Fig. 485. WOMEN'S DRESS, 1793

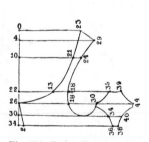

Fig. 486. DRESS BODICE, 1802

in diagonally as a lateral gusset.   If even this did not give the required width two smaller gussets taken from the top of the sides of the front piece were inserted.   The front was sewn to the bodice quite smoothly, while the back piece was disposed in pleats on each side of the slit. The width thus lost at the top of the skirt was regained by the insertion of a gusset rounded at the top.   From the year 1809 onward the back piece had only from four to six close-set pleats, about 2 cm. in depth, and the upper breadth of the back piece had to be correspondingly diminished (see Fig. 490).   This was done by cutting

393

gussets out of the top and inserting them upside-down at the foot (see Fig. 490). For dresses with trains the cut was the same, as the train was merely a prolongation of the back piece.

In the case of dresses whose back piece was pleated the back of the bodice was about 10 cm. broader than was necessary ; to it the pleated portion of the back piece was sewn. This part was provided

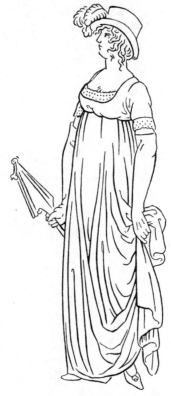

Fig. 487. Women's Dress, 1802

with a draw-string by which the waist of the bodice could be con-tracted, independently of the lacing arrangement inside. There were two similar draw-strings at the neck of the bodice, one passing from the shoulder to the back and the other to the front. The sleeves of these dresses were pleated at the top in front ; the seam was under the arm. The short sleeves were cut in exactly the same way as the long ones. For dresses with few pleats at the back the bodice was like the one already described.

These tight dresses without folds remained unchanged and were fashionable till after the year 1820. The bodice was short, but it underwent considerable modifications. In particular after 1812 it was made higher, so that after six years high-necked bodices were again worn. The wide, low-necked style was worn only at dances and on other festive occasions.

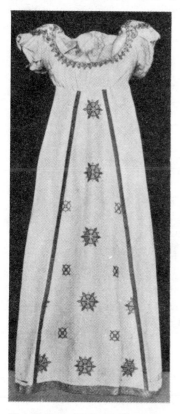

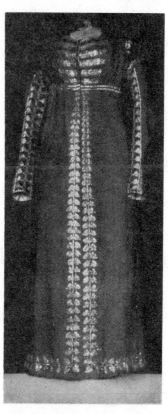

Fig. 488. Evening Gown, White Silk with Gold Ornamentation, about 1800

Fig. 489. Dress of Red Woollen Material with Silver Embroidery

Short sleeves disappeared about the same time as the low necks, and the long sleeves that succeeded them varied from time to time, the general form being that shown in Fig. 493, *a*. The favourite style was that of open sleeves caught up in several places by buttons or gathered, and this fashion lasted for several years.

Since the introduction into France of English fashion about the year 1790 there were many varieties of trimming, but all of them were simple. Only the foot of the dress and the wrists of the sleeves were trimmed. Later the front of the dress was also ornamented (see Fig. 489).

The commonest trimming was thin cord or narrow braid. On ball dresses artificial flowers were frequently used. About 1805 lace began to be employed, and not long afterward embroidery. From 1810 onward the material of the dress itself was used for the trimming in

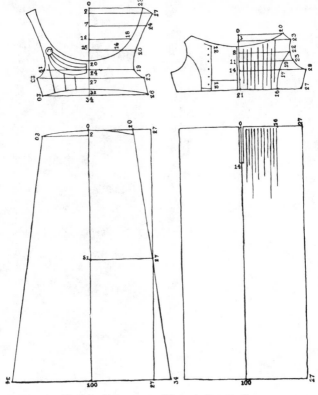

Fig. 490. PATTERN OF WOMEN'S DRESS, 1805

the form of frills, thin rolls, and diagonal strips. In most cases the trimming was of the same colour as the dress. Exceptions to this rule were rare until about 1812.

The reappearance of the bodice was accompanied by that of over-dresses made in the Grecian style. They bore the name of 'tunic.' The close-fronted dress worn with them was now called the 'dress.' Speaking generally, the tunic had the same cut as the dress, the chief difference being that it was open in front. A touch of the antique was highly prized. (See Figs. 495 and 496.)

396

The Emperor Napoleon made the open tunic, which had been known as the *manteau de cour*, an obligatory part of Court dress. The former name was now dropped, and from this time the open tunic was known as a *robe*, with an additional epithet to denote its style, such as *robe turque* or *robe à la prêtresse*. These *robes* continued in fashion till about 1810, but they then disappeared altogether from a lady's wardrobe.

These *robes* gradually developed into entirely new articles of attire,

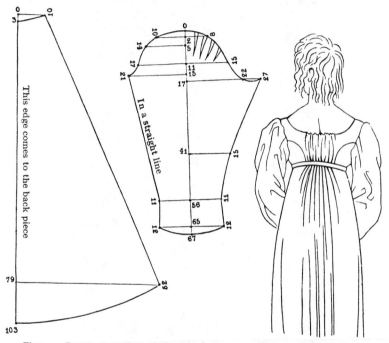

Fig. 491. PATTERN OF WOMEN'S DRESS, 1805   Fig. 492. WOMEN'S DRESS, 1805

worn, under the name of *redingotes*, either as comfortable morning dresses or as cloaks to give extra warmth in cold weather. The morning dress was called *douillette*, and was almost like the *robe*. The front edges met. These dresses were always high at the neck, with long, close-fitting sleeves. The cloaks, called *pardessus*, were comfortable and roomy, but in other respects of varied design. In the year 1812 they were much worn with a broad collar of coloured material and gathered sleeves.

A peculiar kind of over-dress was worn throughout the whole of the first decade of the nineteenth century—a sleeved over-apron, or

397

robe en tablier. These *robes* had the cut and appearance of an ordinary dress made to fasten at the back, but they were merely fastened with a few buttons or bows of ribbon. Some of them were as long as the dress worn beneath them, others came to a little above the knees. A very popular style was the spencer, which was worn

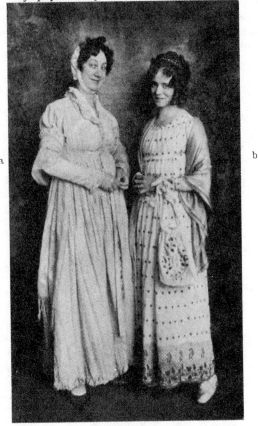

a   b

Fig. 493. (*a*) MIDDLE-CLASS DRESS, EMPIRE STYLE, 1809
(*b*) WHITE DRESS WITH GREEN AND PINK PATTERN AND TRIMMING, 1815

almost continuously from 1800 till about 1830. The spencer was a short, long-sleeved jacket worn over the dress. It was mostly closed, but some women wore it open. There were numerous styles. It closely resembled the bodice of a high-necked dress closed in front, but it was not so close-fitting. The colour and material were different from those of the dress worn with it. In winter it was often lined with fur.

In cold weather many women wore furs. Little can be said about these, as every one followed her own taste. Foreign styles were preferred—Hungarian, Polish, Russian. Some fur coats were made after the fashion of the *douillette*. The fur was usually covered with some kind of dark-coloured velvet or heavy silk.

All sorts of wraps and shawls were worn, partly for warmth and partly for show. About 1800 large rectangular shawls or plaids, like the Greek chlamys, were fashionable, and were worn in the Greek style. They were made of taffeta, muslin, or *crêpe*, mostly white, but often of some delicate shade. Their great size—they were from 4 to 5 metres wide and from 7 to 8 long—allowed them to be worn

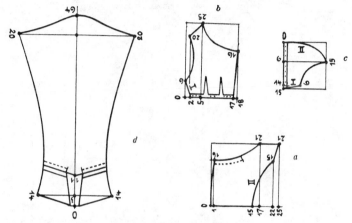

Fig. 494. PATTERN OF FIG. 493, *b*
(*a*) Front ; (*b*) back ; (*c*) side ; (*d*) sleeve.

in many ways and to be draped in graceful lines. Wealthy women wore shawls of delicate Oriental cashmere. These were smaller than the others, which were soon reduced in size, and imitation cashmere shawls were quite frequent. Owing to the high price of the ordinary square shawls, however, others came into fashion. These were 5 or 6 metres long and 1 metre broad—the "long shawls." About 1812 these also were ousted by the *redingotes*.

At this period cloaks, although not strictly speaking fashionable, were much worn in rough weather. Fashion in cloaks, as in furs, was left to the wearer's own taste, and cloaks consequently varied greatly in shape and material and trimming. They had only one feature in common—they were all more or less cape-shaped.

The disappearance of the large kerchiefs called *trompeurs* was followed in 1794 by the appearance of various methods of covering the neck and bust, but none of them enjoyed a long vogue. The gradual heightening of the bodice from 1814 onward rendered all such devices superfluous. In 1797 women imitated men's fashion and wore cravats, but these were so voluminous that women looked as if they had goitre. This fashion did not last long, and women were soon again exposing not only the neck, but the bust. In 1803 both neck and bust were again hidden under linen or lace chemises which came up to the neck and ended in a tiny stand-up collar. This fashion was even more short-

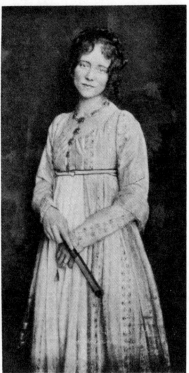

Figs. 495, 496. GREEN AND WHITE EMPIRE OVER-DRESS, 1810

lived. Other collars which came in about 1808 likewise succumbed almost immediately to the popularity of the low neck, but the downfall of the Napoleonic Empire put an end to the latter for a long time except at balls and on similar festive occasions.

Footwear underwent great changes after the Revolution. High heels were abolished, and flat soles were worn (see Fig. 495). Shoes were so much wider that they had to be kept on by ribbons tied cross-wise. From about the year 1808 low boots, ankle-high, were also frequently worn.

The stormy times of the Revolution did not greatly affect the styles of dressing the hair. The use of powder was abandoned, but the high *coiffures*, large side-curls, and elongated *chignons* all remained. Only women with strong Republican sympathies sought to imitate the 'dogs' ears' style worn by men. Most women continued to dress their hair as they had been accustomed to do, until they were tempted

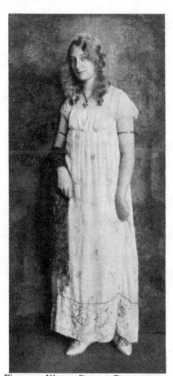

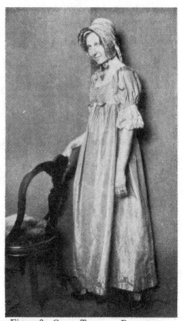

Fig. 497. White Empire Dress with Gold Embroidery, about 1806

Fig. 498. Grey Taffeta Dress and Taffeta Bonnet, about 1820

to adopt the Grecian style of long, hanging curls. This fashion led to various extravagances. The natural hair was sacrificed in favour of curled wigs, and women vied with each other in the display of lavish ornamentation. They were not content with perukes which were expensive and elaborately curled. Each had to be of a different colour, so that a woman might be seen at different times on the same day with a yellow, black, red, or brown wig. Fashion demanded that the colour of the wig should be different from that of the wearer's own hair—fair-haired women wore black wigs and those with dark hair wore blond wigs.

These and other eccentricities of hairdressing came in about 1795 and lasted several years. About 1800 various attempts were made to find some suitable form of hairdressing resembling that of the ancient Greeks. These efforts were not more successful than those which had been made to imitate Grecian styles of dress. The hair above the forehead was curled and coiled, while the back hair was plaited and arranged with the help of combs into a large crown from which numerous small curls—*tire-bouchons*—hung loosely. This fashion also did not last long, and for lack of anything better women began to borrow male fashions, especially the style *à la Titus*. This developed about 1812 into a very simple and becoming *coiffure*. The front hair was parted in the middle of the forehead, combed smoothly toward the sides, and curled, while the back hair was arranged in a coil. With all these *coiffures* some sort of headdress was worn, mostly a turban (Fig. 479). About 1806 a tall ostrich feather came to be stuck perpendicularly in the hair.

Earlier types of hats and bonnets continued to be worn, but fashions were ever changing. Bonnets were smaller, and by 1814 were very tiny, and close-fitting all round. Hat fashions moved in a different direction, and aimed at protection rather than decoration. Except for a few short-lived styles they attained a certain uniformity in keeping with the rest of the attire, but without losing altogether their independent character. The first outbreak of the Revolution left women's hats unchanged. They were already not as large as they had been, although still high in the crown and lavishly trimmed. They formed such a contrast to the simpler attire of those days that they too soon became less ostentatious. The crown was lower, the brim broader, and all the elaborate decoration was reduced to one single upright ostrich feather.

THE PERIOD 1820-70

MEN'S DRESS

THE "*Biedermeier* gentleman"[1] was the embodiment of elegant attire. About the year 1840 knitted breeches disappeared in favour of long trousers wide at the waist. The bell-shaped dress coat alone retained its modish appearance, and offered resistance for a time to the general tendency toward uniformity. The

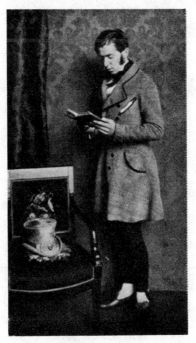

Fig. 499. GREY FROCK COAT, ABOUT 1830

waist of the dress coat gradually came to its natural position, and although for a time the coat continued to be close-fitting middle-class ideas of comfort ultimately triumphed. The elegant curves of the *Biedermeier* style gave place to an outline of manly strength

[1] See p. 50 *n*.—TRANSLATOR.

and practical comfort (see Fig. 499). The turned-down collar decreased in width, and the pocket-flaps were reduced in size. The broad neckcloth of silk or batiste was abandoned in favour of a

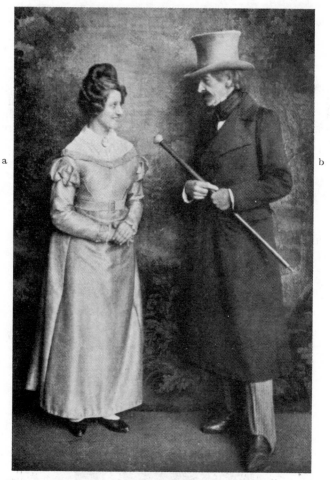

Fig. 500. (*a*) BEIGE-COLOURED DRESS OF BARÈGE WITH TURQUOISE-BLUE TRIMMING. (*b*) COAT OF KING LUDWIG I, ABOUT 1835

tie of narrow ribbon. The fancy waistcoat was the last to yield. A distaste was shown for any style of dress that cramped free movement. The 'choker' gave way about the year 1855 to a stiff, narrow collar.

The old fashions of course continued for a long time to be worn

beside the new. During the Second Empire there was a brief recru-
descence of the striving after elegance, but severity of outline once
more gained the day over the clumsiness that had crept in at the
beginning of the fifties.

The Dress Coat. By the year 1818 the narrow back piece had been
given up, a distinctly wider back piece being substituted. The
shoulders were now broad, and the collar left the back of the neck

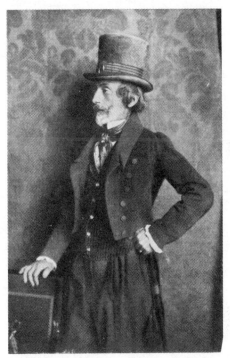

Fig. 501. Brown " Biedermeier " Tail Coat,
about 1835

free. Similarly the coat stood away from the body at the chest,
while it fitted closely above the hips. The tails were narrow and
pointed, and came to below the knees. The sleeves were wide at
the top and very tight at the wrist, but widened again after that,
covering the hand as far as the fingers. This prolongation was open
at the back.

Soon afterward, about 1820, both dress coat and overcoat were
made in a new way (Fig. 475). The tails were cut separately and
sewn separately to the body of the coat. This ensured a better fit,
and the coat now followed the lines of the body even when it was not

405

buttoned. The sleeve had still two seams, and was shaped to the arm. The collar too had a seam down the centre. The front lapels were also cut separately and sewn on, so that they retained their position better. Collar and lapels were suitably stiffened with pad-

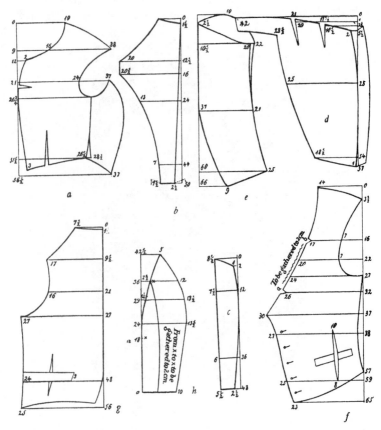

Fig. 502. PATTERN OF DRESS COAT IN 1858

(a) Front; (b) back; (c) collar; (d) tails; (e) sleeve; (f) waistcoat (g) with back; (h) collar of waistcoat.

ding inside. The coat was also padded at breast and hips. The projecting collar of 1818 lay closer to the neck, but it was now nearly high enough to reach the head, and was so broad and stiff that by 1830 it was not unlike the hames of a horse. The ungracefulness of this fashion was soon recognized, and in 1837 both coat and collar were entirely changed, so that the garment had a quite different appearance. The sleeves were as tight and close-fitting as possible, but came only to the wrist. The cut-away of the long, narrow tails began in the middle of the chest, so that the coat could not now be buttoned.

Up to the year 1841 the dress coat was again wide at the waist. The tails, which were the same breadth top and bottom, were sharply cut away in front and squared at the foot. The collar was narrow and low, and the lapels extended nearly to the waist. The sleeves were still tight and short. A favourite style of coat at this time was the riding dress coat, intermediate between a dress coat and a riding coat. The riding dress coat had broader tails than the dress coat ; the tails, however, did not meet all the way as they did in the riding coat, but either only at the top or not at all. These riding dress coats had diagonal pockets in front with broad flaps. Some styles could be buttoned up to the neck.

About 1850 the upper part both of dress coat and coat increased in length. The back was broader, and the tight sleeves were exchanged for wider ones (Fig. 503). At the same time the collar became broader, and came higher up at the neck. The lapels were shortened and the tails more pointed.

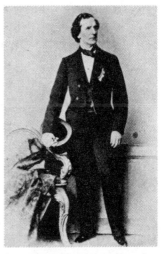

Fig. 503. GENTLEMAN IN TAIL COAT 1860—EMIL DEVRIENT

Some years later the waist of the dress coat was made wider, and the whole garment now bore a closer resemblance to the coat, seeing that it had already adopted many of the changes that had affected the latter. By 1780 the dress coat differed from the coat only in having larger lapels and cut-away tails.

Trousers. The French Revolution had brought about great alterations in men's nether garments. First of all it had abolished knee-breeches and the long stockings worn with them and introduced trousers that reached to the ankles and covered the boot-tops. To distinguish them from breeches they were called *pantalons*, after the merry-andrew of the Italian harlequinade, who always wore garments of this kind.

For several years these *pantalons* changed very little, but about 1800, owing to the shortness of the waistcoats then worn, they had to be much higher at the top. They now came up nearly to the armpits, and as they could not be kept up by means of a draw-string

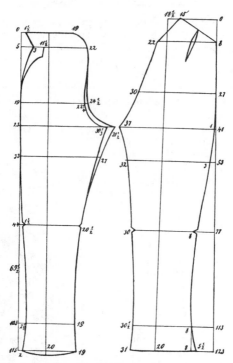

Fig. 504. CUT OF TROUSERS WORN WITH COAT SHOWN IN FIG. 502

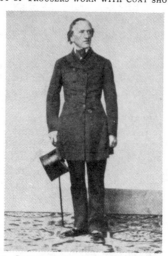

Fig. 505. GENTLEMAN IN FROCK COAT, ABOUT 1860—
PROFESSOR THEODOR KULLACK

—this had been the custom with all earlier styles—recourse was had
to braces—broad tapes passing over the shoulders and buttoned to

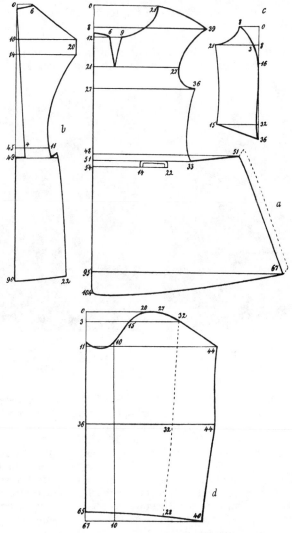

Fig. 506. PATTERN OF A FROCK COAT WITH WIDE SLEEVES
(a) Front; (b) back; (c) side; (d) sleeve.

the trousers at back and front. In 1818 trousers were very short
—hardly ankle-length—and tight at the knees, widening downward.

Seven years later they were tight all the way down, and were kept from riding up by leather straps passing under the soles of the boots. Still later the legs narrowed gradually from top to foot, and were very tight at the ankles. In 1830 they were again tight all the way down. In 1835 they became once more wider, after having been tight as far as the knees and gradually widening below. About this time the narrow front flap, which had come in about 1790, was discarded, and the broader flap reappeared. Horsemen wore white buckskin trousers

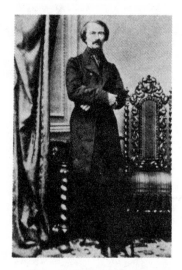

Fig. 507. GENTLEMAN'S COAT, ABOUT 1845

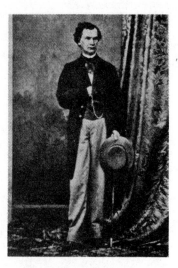

Fig. 508. GENTLEMAN IN COAT AND LIGHT TROUSERS, CARRYING A ROUND HAT, 1865

long enough to cover the boot-tops. About 1840 trousers were tight at the top and the foot, but looser at the knees. During all these minor alterations the straps under the soles were worn continuously. (See Fig. 500.)

From the year 1835 onward black cloth was less and less used for trousers owing to its lack of durability ; its place was taken by coarser, more suitable material, buckskin being a great favourite. Trousers for summer wear were of white English leather, coarse cotton, or real East Indian nankeen. About 1839 ' summer buckskin ' and the various ' greys ' were found more suitable for summer trousers than the usual white or yellow cloths.

About 1850 all the ideas that had long prevailed with regard to what was suitable and stylish were completely discarded. The front flap was abandoned and replaced by the slit opening, which had been completely forgotten since the end of the seventeenth century. The

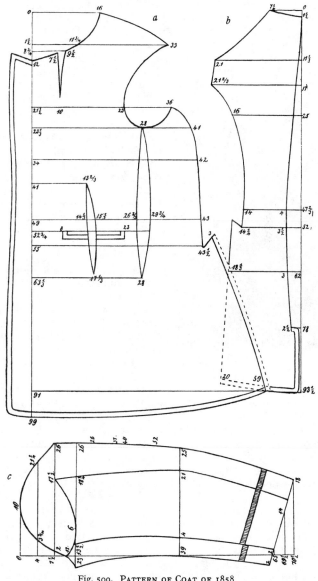

Fig. 509. PATTERN OF COAT OF 1858
(a) Front; (b) back; (c) sleeve.

buttons were hidden by an edging of material. Boot-straps were given up, and the trousers flapped loosely round the legs. In 1865 trouser legs were utterly out of keeping with the outlines of the limbs they were meant to clothe. (See Fig. 508.) They were narrow at the top, wide at the knee, and again tight below the knee—that is to say, the shape from the thigh to the calf of the leg was the exact opposite of the natural contour. In order to retain their columnar shape trousers were made of the coarsest, stiffest material possible.

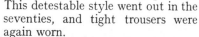

Fig. 510. GENTLEMAN IN COAT AND COLOURED WAISTCOAT, 1858

This detestable style went out in the seventies, and tight trousers were again worn.

The Waistcoat. After 1800 waistcoats had gradually increased in length, and by 1812 they once more came down to the hips. They were made with two rows of buttons—*i.e.*, were double-breasted—and had a broad, stiff, stand up collar. In 1818 they were still as long as in 1812, but they had now a single row of buttons. Up to 1825 the erect collar gradually became narrower, till it was simply the top edge of the waistcoat folded down. From 1818 to 1825 it was the fashion to wear two waistcoats of different colours, but after the latter date the practice was dropped.

For several years there was little change, but in 1836 appeared the roll collar. In this style the whole upper edge of the waistcoat was folded down outward in almost uniform width as far as the breast.

There were numerous minor alterations, but none of any importance. All the continuous changes of fashion produced nothing really novel. From 1836 onward all waistcoats had either the roll collar or a small stand-up collar. (See Fig. 501.) They were either single- or double-breasted, but all came more or less low down the body.

There was greater variety in the materials of which they were made, but even here a certain uniformity had been reached. About the middle of the century fancy waistcoats ceased to be worn (Figs. 508 and 510), and these garments were made of the same material as the trousers or the coat. Velvet waistcoats were still occasionally worn, but they gradually went out also. The light summer waistcoat of washing material continued in favour as at once sensible and suitable.

412

The Cravat and Necktie. About the year 1792 men wore a tie that went twice round the neck and was tied in a bow in front. Before long it became the fashion to tie it behind. A second neckcloth was also worn, and this made the wrap so thick that its circumference was equal to that of the head, and the chin was buried in the neckcloth. The latter was usually black in colour. A narrow edge of the white cravat worn underneath showed over it. About the year 1812, when the under-neckcloth had gone out of fashion and the unbecoming thickness had disappeared, the white edge was supplied by a kind of

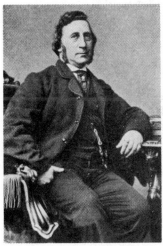

Fig. 511. Gentleman in Coat, and with a Low Style of Collar, 1868 Fig. 512. Gentleman in Coat, Choker Collar, and High Cravat, 1855

collar, whose corners and side-edges were visible beneath the neck-cloth. These under-collars were of linen or even of paper, and were starched so stiffly that they stood up on both sides of the face (see Figs. 499 and 501). From the first decade of the nineteenth century the neckcloth was tied in a bow in front, and in 1818 it had a fairly broad lining, shaped at the sides and stiffened with whalebone or pigs' bristles so that it rose in an arch at the cheeks.

Fashions entirely changed about 1830. Neckcloths were abandoned, and stiffened cravats were worn instead. The stiffening material was covered with satin, camlet, or serge. A bow was sewn on in front, and the whole was fastened behind with a buckle and strap. (See Fig. 512.) At dances and on festive occasions men wore cravats of white satin. Those for everyday wear were made of some dark, cheaper material. These simpler cravats had no bow in front. They consisted of two broad pieces of material filling the open space at the top of the waistcoat and held together by buttons or pins (see Fig. 507). They did away with the need for a white shirt-front. Since the beginning of the eighteenth century men had worn a frill at the breast, but when that fashion went out the shirt-front was not exposed. It was covered by a 'dicky,' which could be more easily changed and more cheaply washed than the whole shirt. This dicky was also made of coarse linen—in the earlier fashion the frill at least had to be of fine linen. About 1835 cravats were still worn, but they were very plain. (See Fig. 501.) The

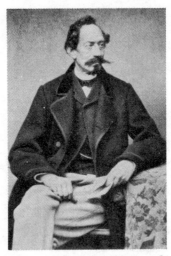

Fig. 513. Gentleman in Overcoat, 1865, with Low Collar and Small Tie—Count William of Würtemberg

shirt-frill was again fashionable, but was not now so wide ; it was fluted as in 1800, not crimped as in the eighteenth century. The 'choker' collar, which had been less popular since 1830, came in again ; it was no longer upright, but was curved outward.

About 1840 neckwear was almost entirely a matter of individual taste. Some men wore cravats, while others preferred the neckcloth tied in a bow in front. About 1848 the neck was almost bare, and in place of cravats (which gradually went out of fashion) men wore narrow ties, the ends of which were fastened in front by a pin or tied in a small bow or knot. (See Figs. 503, 511, and 517.) These ties, over which the shirt-collar was folded, were popular with young men, while older men preferred the neckcloth. The white satin tie continued to be a necessary part of full dress on ceremonious occasions. The separate shirt-front, or dicky, disappeared, and the inset shirt-breast, which was of finer linen than the rest of the shirt, was visible at the waistcoat opening.

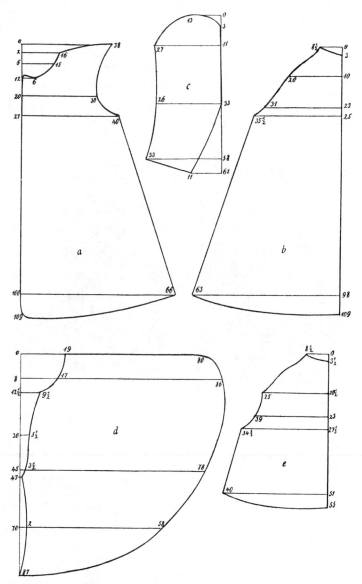

Fig. 514. PATTERN OF PELISSE WITH CAPE, 1858
(a) Front ; (b) back ; (c) collar ; (d) (e) sleeve parts.

The Cloak or Mantle.   Toward the end of the eighteenth century there was a pronounced preference for clothing that was at once convenient and practical.   The cloaks of former days, in spite of their width and large armholes, were felt to be cumbrous and inconvenient. They were now fitted with sleeves, but this was done without robbing them of their characteristic features or transforming them into over-coats.   Both the sleeved cloak and the roomy, sleeveless cloak re-mained in fashion.

The only variations lay in the number and length of the overlapping capes and the width of the garment.   The general cut was unchanged.

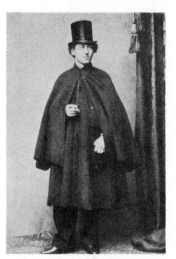

Fig. 515.   Coat and Cape in the Sixties

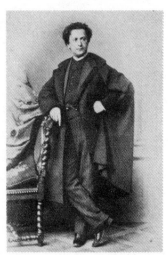

Fig. 516.   Gentleman wearing Cape-shaped Cloak, 1865—A. von Sonnenthal (Actor)

The eighteenth-century style of cape was retained, but a second, larger cape was added, covering shoulders, breast, and back.   About 1780 this cape was much longer behind and in front than at the sides.

About 1800 two or even four capes were added, each being always a little larger than the one over it.   (See Fig. 470.)   The cloak was no longer fastened in front with a single or double row of buttons and buttonholes, but by broad strips of cloth, those on one side holding the buttons and those on the other side containing the buttonholes. This was the fashion till 1830.   When the cloak was merely thrown over the shoulders it was held by a hook and a small chain.

The main body of this cloak gradually lost the circular form it had had since the end of the eighteenth century.   It was now wider at the top and narrower below.   To make the width at the top correspond to that at the neck the material at the neck was arranged in broad

416

pleats. When it was to be worn on horseback the garment had a slit at the back that could be buttoned.

By about 1830 the various capes of the cloak had grown longer, but there were not so many of them. The under one was circular and as long as the sleeves, while the outermost one was far broader than before. The lining was retained, and the cape could if necessary be turned up in cold weather. Cloak capes had long been trimmed with fur. At the back was a cloth strap that could be buttoned, and the cloak, or ulster, could be worn with this either open or fastened.

The cloak was now very convenient and comfortable, but before long it was condemned as inelegant, and ceased to be worn. At the end

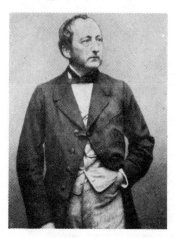

Fig. 517. OVERCOAT WITH LIGHT TROUSERS AND WAISTCOAT, IN THE SIXTIES—A. THALBERG (PIANIST)

of the thirties fashionable men thought it clumsy and heavy, and various attempts were made to adapt it to the changing opinion. It was shortened and made tighter and lighter, but it ultimately disappeared from the wardrobe of men of fashion, and survived only as livery for coachmen and footmen. Even working people ceased to wear it, highly practical as it was in many respects.

About 1840 the cloak had lost most of its peculiar features, and about ten years later it gave place to the top-coat or overcoat. During this decade it appeared in many forms, one part or another being modified as superfluous or inelegant.

About 1836 the mantle, having lost its sleeves and large collar, had become a mere cape. About 1840 it went to the other extreme and assumed the character of a coat. It was closer-fitting and shorter, and had two long openings at the level of the elbows through which the arms could be passed. (See Fig. 516.) To preserve its character as a cloak, however, it had a circular cape as well as a small velvet collar (see Fig. 515). These mantles were fastened with a thick, short bar of wood covered with silk, which was attached to one side of the cape and held in a loop of cord attached to the other side. The long ends of the cord terminated in tassels. Another style of cloak came in at the same time and showed still more clearly the gradual transition to the overcoat. It had no cape. The shoulder and back were

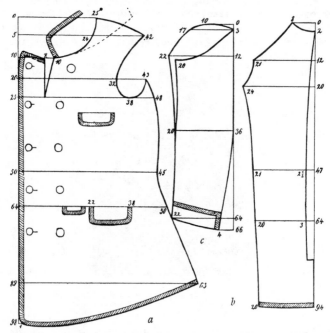

Fig. 518. PATTERN OF OVERCOAT WHICH WAS ALSO WORN AS A COAT, 1858
(a) Front; (b) back; (c) sleeve.

quite plain, and the collar lay quite flat and smooth. The sleeves, open in front down to the elbows, were also plain. This garment was fastened at the neck with bar and loop, and was trimmed with *appliqué* and braid.

Headgear. At the opening of the seventeenth century caps were no longer worn out of doors. Till now they had been far more popular than hats, but the latter now came to be the prevailing fashion. The cap was worn only by the workman at his work and by clergymen, scholars, and officials. It was still frequently worn indoors.

Caps continued to be neglected till the beginning of the nineteenth century, but the inconvenience of the tall silk hat brought them again into fashion. They began to be worn about 1820 as a convenient, light form of headgear, a protection against sun and rain, and as a comfortable head-covering for travelling and hunting. The favourite shape was that of the former *Barett*. The cap consisted of a fairly wide head-piece gathered into a band, and with a leather peak to shield the eyes against the sun.

About 1830 fashion brought in the Russian cap, which was much worn by soldiers, the Orleans cap, and others. (See Fig. 468.) One of the most comfortable was the Austrian cap, but its much smaller peak was a great drawback in strong light. Mention should also be

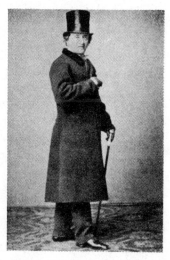

Fig. 519. Gentleman wearing Overcoat, Middle of the Sixties—Grunerth (Actor)

made of a cap worn by coachmen and outriders as part of their livery and by jockeys at races. Indeed, this was for a time an almost essential part of fashionable riding outfit.

About 1848 the cap again went out of fashion, largely because preference was now given to the smarter small, light hat made of felt. By and by this hat was also made of silk or of coarse felt covered with plush. It differed from all previous hats in its height and in its comparatively narrow brim bound with ribbon. At first the height was not excessive ; some styles widened and others narrowed upward. In 1795 both styles were being worn, and in both the brim was slightly curved up at the sides. (See Figs. 471, 478, 500, and 501.)

From the time when it was introduced the round hat underwent many modifications, ranging between the two extremes of cap and tall hat. Ultimately an intermediate form was adopted in which the shape was cylindrical, with a somewhat narrow brim.

419

(See Figs. 515 and 519.) Further changes merely affected its height. For ordinary wear the tall hat had to yield place to the small, comfortable, soft felt hat which came in about the year 1848 (Fig. 508).

WOMEN'S DRESS

The acme of women's fashions and their turning-point can be dated about the year 1820. Short bodices and gusseted skirts were still in

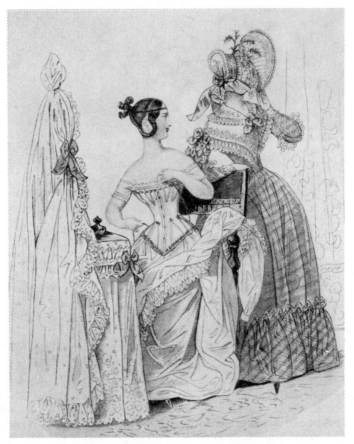

Fig. 520. LADIES DRESSING. CORSETS OF 1834

fashion, but in other particulars the prevailing modes were so numerous and varied that tailors, with a view to the creation of something novel, had to face the question of a radical alteration. Apart from the short bodice and the close-fitting skirt, the main features of the current fashions were a bodice that was half high or high at the neck (ball dresses being very low both in front and at the back), having

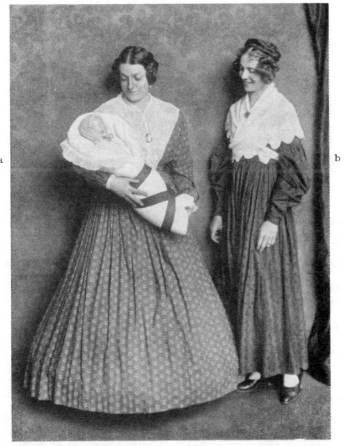

a

b

Fig. 521. (a) HOUSE DRESS OF RUST-BROWN PRINT, ABOUT 1830
(b) BROWN PRINT HOUSE DRESS, ABOUT 1840

sleeves that were very short, close-fitting, and gathered in puffs at the top, and a fairly short skirt hardly reaching the ankles. (See Figs. 482 and 498.) Although white was still much worn, coloured dresses were also fashionable, as were coloured bodices with white skirts. Coloured bodices were mostly high-necked. A waist-belt was worn —coloured if the dress were white.

Shortly after 1820 the styles of dress underwent a radical change, which lasted till about 1830, when fashions again took another

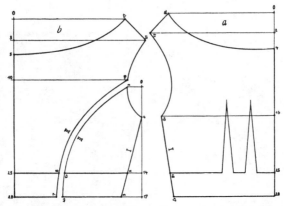

Fig. 522. PATTERN OF THE HOUSE DRESS SHOWN IN FIG. 521, *a*
(*a*) Front ; (*b*) back.

direction. (See Fig. 500.) The innovations affected two items of attire—the short bodice and the excessively tight skirt. Sleeves too were greatly changed.

Bodices had been short, but they were now much longer, and the formerly tight skirts were now somewhat full ; a thinly padded or stiffly starched petticoat was worn (Fig. 521, *a*). The bodice, either fairly low or quite high at the neck, was straight at the foot, and held in place by a waist-belt. The skirt was hardly ankle-length. A characteristic feature at the beginning of the thirties was the so-called 'ham-shaped' sleeves ; these were long and enormously wide at the top, narrower from the elbow down, and tight at the wrists. These sleeves, as well as the very wide, short sleeves of the ball dresses,

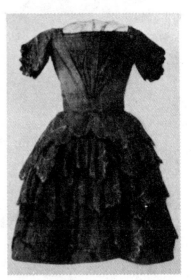

Fig. 523. CHILD'S FROCK OF NATURAL-COLOURED LINEN WITH BEIGE EMBROIDERY, 1845

were kept at their full width by means of wicker frames or feather cushions. Along with the dresses proper, which were fastened at the back, so-called over-dresses were much worn. They differed from the dresses only in being fastened in front. These over-dresses, which

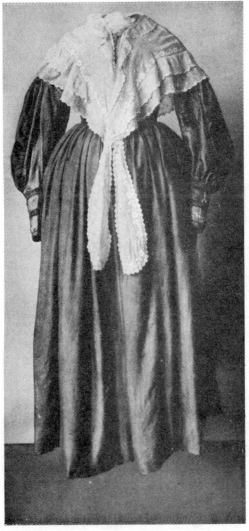

Fig. 524. Dress of Green and Lilac Shot Taffeta, with Fichu
about 1835

reached up to the neck, by and by almost entirely superseded the dresses.

Strong opposition was offered to this style of costume as early as 1835. To do away with the ungraceful 'ham shape,' sleeves were

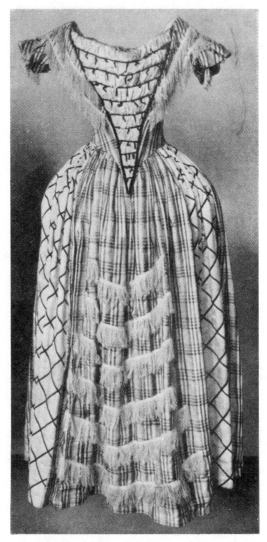

Fig. 525. BALL DRESS, ABOUT 1835

reversed—*i.e.*, they were made tight at the top and wide lower down, but still remained very tight at the wrists. (See Fig. 524.)

424

About 1840 sleeves came in which were tight all the way down
(Fig. 549). The upper part of the bodice was also left free of all the
ornamentation which had exaggerated the breadth of the figure across

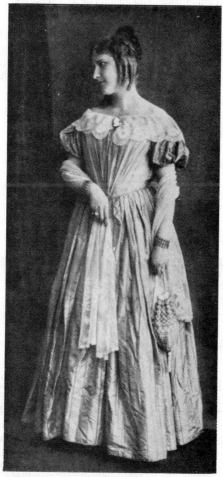

Fig. 526. MAUVE-COLOURED BALL DRESS TRIMMED WITH LACE,
1840

the shoulders, and the bodice was as plain as possible. The waist
was still long, but the neck was much less low. The word 'waist'
came to mean 'bodice.' The skirt grew longer year by year; it was
fastened in front. Women dressed as warmly as possible. Underneath dresses which had the same width at the top and foot and were

425

pleated at the waist women wore five or six petticoats (some of them padded), and in addition they had thick cushions at the hips or at the back.

Owing to all these changes the costume of 1841 had come to be in strong contrast to that of 1830 (Fig. 526). But a firm basis had been laid for further progress. Long, tight sleeves, wide, padded skirts that entirely concealed the feet, and bodices high at the neck and padded in various places—all these constituted a very practical style of dress for women. The tailor's art could not only conceal any personal deformity, but could also make good any natural defect.

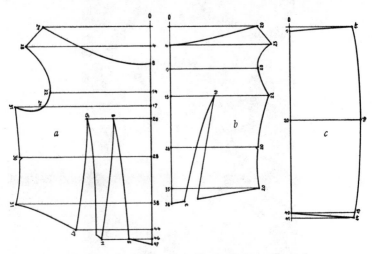

Fig. 527. Pattern of Ball Dress shown in Fig. 526
(a) Front ; (b) back ; (c) sleeve-puff.

It is therefore not surprising that, with advantages like these, high, closed bodices and long, full skirts held the field for a long time. But the girth of the fair sex was destined to be still further increased, without making it necessary for them to burden themselves with numerous petticoats. From about the year 1857 the farthingale was revived under the name of crinoline. (See Figs. 528 and 529.) (The name meant originally an arrangement made of horsehair.) After its reintroduction it passed through many changes, all of them involving an increase in size. Even the crinoline of 1865, which required 8 to 10 metres of material for a dress to go over it, was insufficient for the gusseted skirt of 1866, which required a still more capacious crinoline. (See Figs. 530 and 535.)

The great width of the skirts provided an opportunity for an ever-increasing lavishness of trimming. At one time a third of the length of the dress was adorned with plain strips and puffs ; at another time

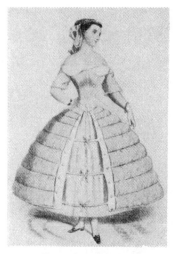

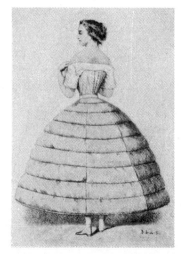

Figs. 528, 529. " The Secrets of the Crinoline," about 1860

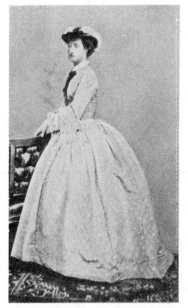

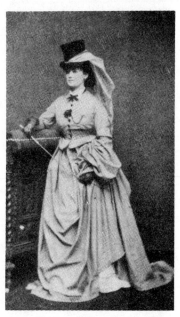

Fig 530. The Empress Eugénie of France, 1865

Fig. 531. Riding Habit, about 1868

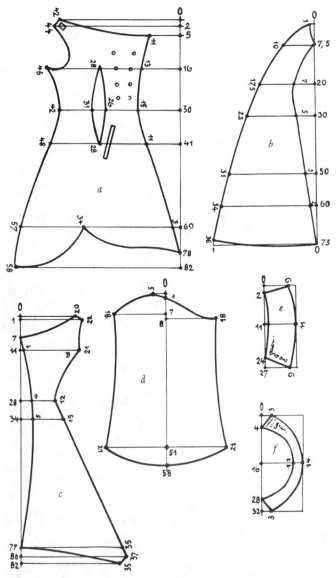

Fig. 532. PATTERN FOR A TUNIC, 1867
(a) Front ; (b) side ; (c) back ; (d) sleeve ; (e) cuff ; (f) collar.

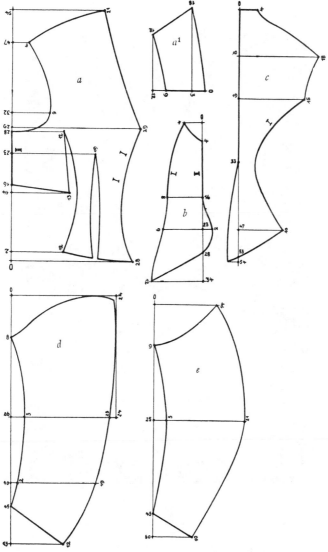

Fig. 533. Pattern of a Long Bodice, 1870
(a) Front ; (a¹) front skirt ; (b) side ; (c) back ; (d) upper sleeve ;
(e) lower sleeve.

429

the dress had several flounces, 25–30 cm. in depth, made of its own
material or of print or embroidered braid, each flounce overlapping
the one below it.   In 1860 the entire dress was trimmed in this way,

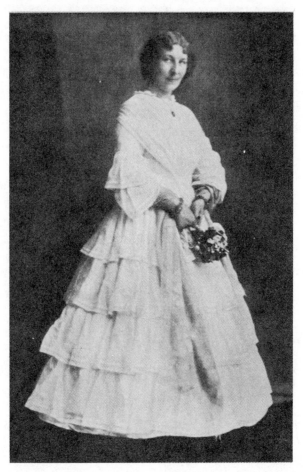

Fig. 534. Ball Dress of White Muslin, 1848

ten or twelve small flounces being not unusual. (See Fig. 534.)
Lace came in again, and was lavishly employed as trimming. As
these flounces were frequently 50–60 cm. in depth very little of the
material of the dress was visible. Some women were not content
with white or black lace, but added tulle embroidered with gold or
silver. To give the skirt the necessary support it was lined with stiff
gauze, and numerous starched white petticoats were worn. Even

Plate XV

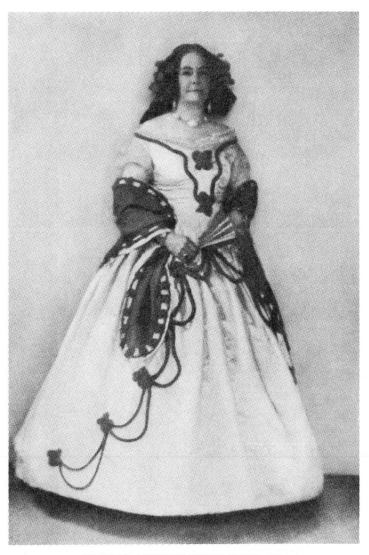

EVENING GOWN OF WHITE SATIN, 1865

ladies' riding habits were fantastically ornamented, and notwithstanding the extremely wide skirts, which may seem ridiculous to our minds, the period produced beautiful and daring horsewomen, like the Empress Elizabeth of Austria. During the Second French Empire this fashion attained such magnificence that the period has been called " the second baroque era." Skirts reached an enormous

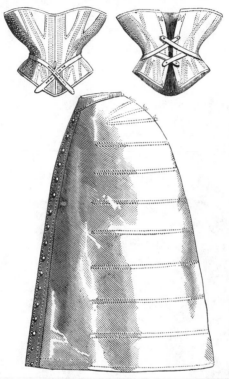

Fig. 535. CRINOLINE UNDER-SKIRT AND CORSET (WITH BACK VIEW),
1868

width (see Fig. 537), but the gathers were pushed mostly to the back ; the width of the skirt at the foot remained the same. Wreaths of tulle were kept in place by broad ribbons, among which were interspersed flowers. The masses of material were distributed by being gathered and held by lace and tassels, while scarves and sashes supplied further ornamentation. (See Plate XV.)

The corset, which in the thirties and forties was still emphasizing the long wasp-waist (see Fig. 520), was now quite small (see Fig. 535), because the upper bust was meant to be visible amid the voluminous folds of the dresses. The bodice had become quite short (Fig. 547).

The ball dress was low-necked, with a broad lace trimming called a
'Berthe,' and was cut to leave the shoulder-line quite clear.   The
sleeves of these evening dresses were also restricted to the smallest

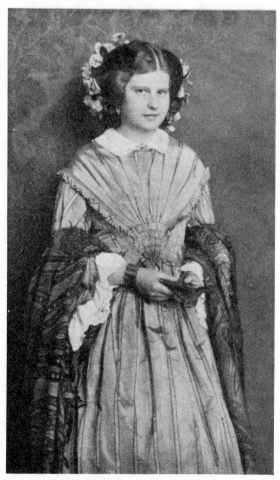

Fig. 536. Brownish-pink Taffeta Dress, 1853

possible proportions.   (See Figs. 556 and 558.)   In the fifties women
were still wearing with high bodices sleeves which were bell-shaped
at the wrist and lavishly embroidered.   From these emerged under-
sleeves (see Fig. 540) about 30 cm. long and 70 cm. broad, made of
finest batiste covered with embroidery   Collars were in keeping
with the sleeves.   Broad at first, they became narrower.   These

432

accessories of embroidered white material lasted till 1870. Blouse-like chemisettes were frequently worn underneath dresses of wool and of silk. These blouses of batiste and lace, kept in place by a waist-belt with buckle, were called *canezous* (Fig. 538). They came in about the forties, and lasted till well on in the seventies. If we are to believe the fashion plates they were even worn as part of summer riding attire.

The lining of the bodice was of white or grey half-linen, with three or four intakes at the back and two in front at right and left. When

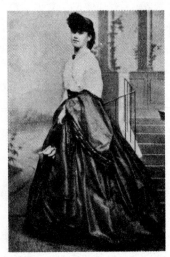

Fig. 537. Taffeta Gown with White Blouse, 1867

the long bodices overlapping the skirt—as in the case of tunics—became fashionable the intakes were cut at the waist-line in order to emphasize the figure at the hips. (See Figs. 532 and 556.) The bodice was stiffened with whalebone, and indeed a tiny bodice like this was a marvel of the dressmaker's art. The neck was still low, and small collars of embroidered batiste or lace were worn, fastened with a brooch. (See Figs. 536 and 545.)

To keep the loose sleeves in position small crinolines were used—frames of ten or twelve wire hoops, open in front at the bend of the arm.

With regard to the underclothing worn by women at this period not much need be said. When the waves of the Revolution had subsided a return was made to the styles usually worn by women of the good middle classes. First of all, the chemise became high-necked, and had sleeves that almost reached the elbows (see Fig. 520). About the beginning of the forties the corset came in again. For

433

nearly a hundred years it had been a decisive element in the dress of women throughout Europe. It was absolutely indispensable for the

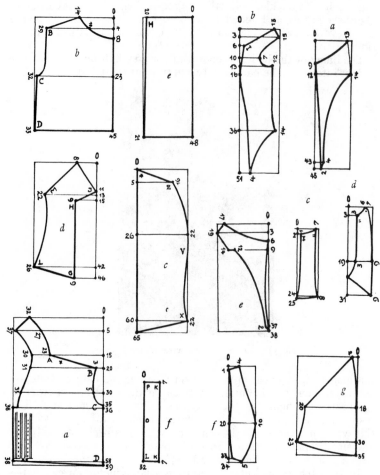

Fig. 538. PATTERN OF A SO-CALLED
" CANEZOU " BLOUSE

(a) Front ; (b) back ; (c) sleeve ; (d) sleeve-flap ;
(e) sleeve-puff ; (f) wristband.

Fig. 539. PATTERN OF A LOW-CUT
BODICE, 1862

(a) Front part I ; (b) front part II ; (c) side-piece I ;
(d) side-piece II ; (e) back ; (f) top of sleeve ;
(g) lower sleeve.

proper outline of the wasp-waist. It was not until the thirties that drawers came to be universally worn by women. A garment of this kind that belonged to Queen Adelaide of England (who was a princess of Saxe-Coburg-Meiningen) still exists in private ownership in

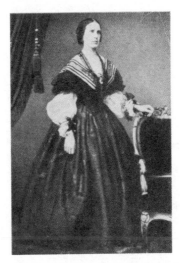

Fig. 540. Dress with Low-cut Bodice and Lower
Sleeve, 1855-60

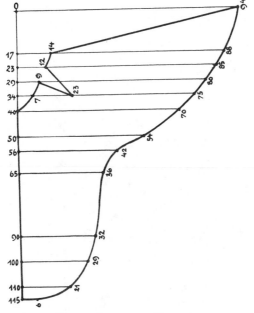

Fig. 541. Pattern of Mantilla

435

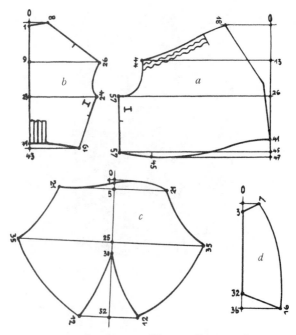

Fig. 542. PATTERN OF A WALKING DRESS OF 1860
(a) Front ; (b) back ; (c) sleeve ; (d) reversed cuff.

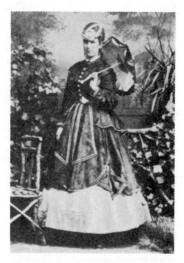

Fig. 543. ANKLE-LENGTH STREET DRESS OF ABOUT 1868

Germany. Had it not been a rarity at the time it would hardly have been so carefully preserved. The legs are extraordinarily long. It

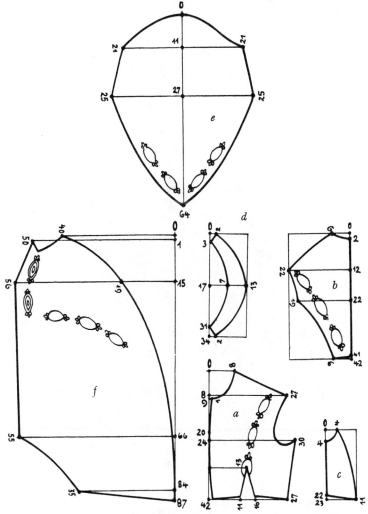

Fig. 544. PATTERN OF LONG BODICE TO ANKLE-LENGTH SKIRT, 1867-68, WITH RICH TRIMMING OF PASSEMENTERIE
To be worn over tight under-sleeves. (a) Front ; (b) back ; (c) side-piece ; (d) collar; (e) cape ; (f) half of tunic.

helps us to imagine the appearance presented by the fair ladies of 1820-29, with this long, tight-fitting, lace-trimmed garment peeping

437

from under their billowy skirts. In previous centuries this had rarely been an integral part of women's dress. It was the Empress Josephine of France who introduced the wearing of white washable clothing of this kind, at the beginning of the nineteenth century

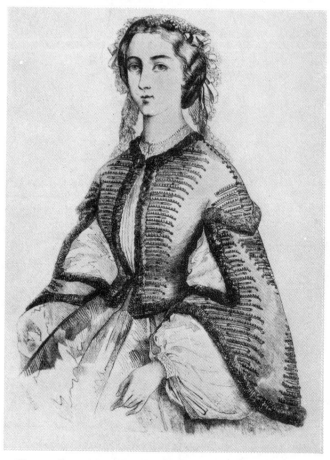

Fig. 545. Zouave Jacket of Black Taffeta with Embroidery and Braid, 1862

Old photographs suggest that this garment was indispensable for well-dressed young girls. Numerous petticoats were worn. First came a thick petticoat of red or white flannel—called in Germany 'Hansel.' In very cold weather it was made of padded silk. Then came several petticoats of strong coloured material trimmed with

Plate XVI

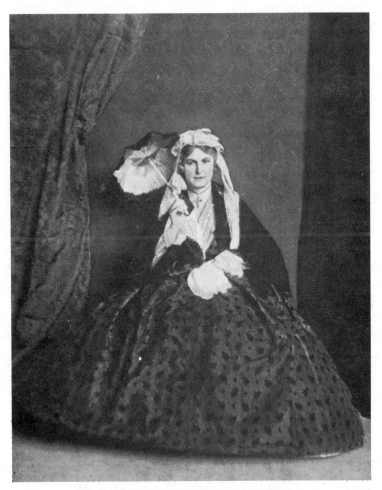

TOWN COSTUME WITH MANTILLA, 1860   438

black braid. Wealthy ladies wore silk and cotton or white embroidered material.

Neckwear and Sleeves. About the year 1818 women were again wearing with high-necked dresses a fairly broad neck-ruff—the *fraise*. With low-necked dresses there was nothing of this kind ; necklets of pearls or other ornaments were worn instead. (See Fig. 496.) A few years later the ruff was replaced by a broad shoulder-cape with a

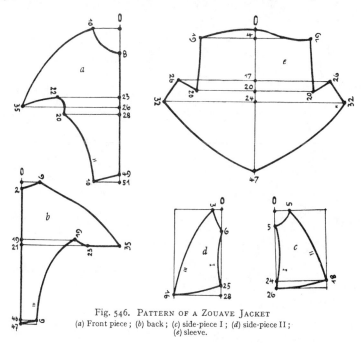

Fig. 546. PATTERN OF A ZOUAVE JACKET
(*a*) Front piece ; (*b*) back ; (*c*) side-piece I ; (*d*) side-piece II ;
(*e*) sleeve.

narrow frill at the top and embroidery at the foot, and this was worn with either high- or low-necked dresses. Various styles of these capes continued to be fashionable for a long time, and it was not till 1830 that any important alteration appeared. The cape was now lengthened in front and behind to a long point which reached to the waist (Fig. 524). It was kept in place by a waist-belt. On the shoulders were broad, often double, strips of material (*epaulettes*) which ran to a sharp point in front and behind and served as trimming for the back and front of the cape. These capes were mostly made of tulle ; they were called fichus. Beneath a small, turned-back fichu, whose place was occasionally taken by a narrow ruff of stiffened strips of tulle, a broad coloured ribbon was worn, tied in a bow in front.

There was greater variety of neck ornament than of neckwear about 1830. Ladies attending balls or other festive functions wore low-

439

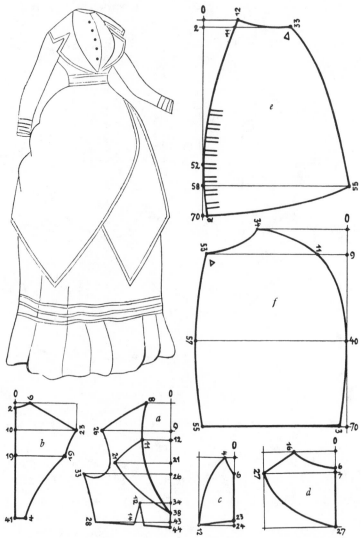

Figs. 547, 548. Sketch and Pattern of a Walking Dress for Winter Wear, 1868

(a) Front piece ; (b) back; (c) side-piece ; (d) collar ; (e) front of tunic ; (f) back of tunic.

necked dresses. As jewellery they wore a plain, broad gold chain or small gold chains connected with diamonds.

In winter, not only out of doors, but also in the ballroom, women wore fur boas several yards in length. These were often of great value, and consisted of countless small pieces of fur (minever, minever tails, marten, fitch, etc.) threaded together on a long cord.

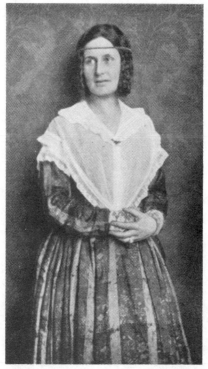

Fig. 549. BROWN SILK DRESS WITH FICHU, ABOUT 1840

In the year 1836 the fichu was out of fashion again. Its place was taken by collars of various kinds. Two of these were far more popular than the rest. One of these came fairly high at the neck and lay over a chemisette worn beneath it ; the other covered only the shoulders, forming little 'epaulettes' like the fichu. This collar was round at the back; but the ends were long and pointed in front (Fig. 521, *b*). They were crossed in front and fastened in the waist-belt. A third variety of this novel neckwear was a much pleated chemisette of tulle or muslin, worn beneath the dress, with a narrow frill down the front and round the neck. Small, light kerchiefs

441

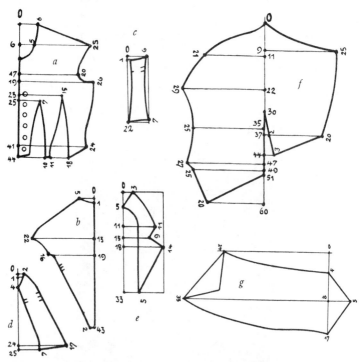

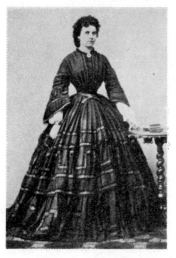

Fig. 550. Cut of a High-necked Bodice with Long, Wide Sleeves, 1862
The bodice could be worn with or without a collar. (a) Front; (b) back; (c) side-piece I;
(d) side-piece II; (e) collar; (f) sleeve; (g) cuff.

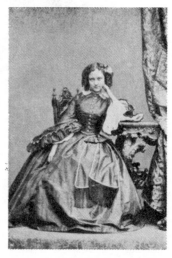

Fig. 551. High-necked Dress, 1864

Fig. 552. High-necked Dress, 1864
Frau Dahn-Haussmann

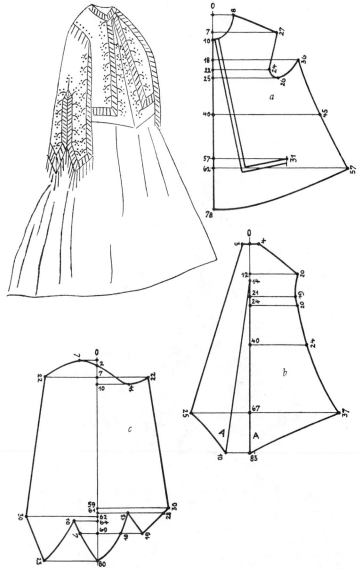

Figs. 553, 554. Sketch and Pattern of a "Don Carlos"
Mantilla, 1868
(a) Front ; (b) side ; (c) sleeve.

443

were also much worn. They were thrown lightly round the neck, the ends being tucked into the waist-belt. The boa had gone quickly out of fashion, but nothing took its place. Neck ornaments were now much simpler. They took the form of a dainty gold chain with a few stones or a string of pearls.

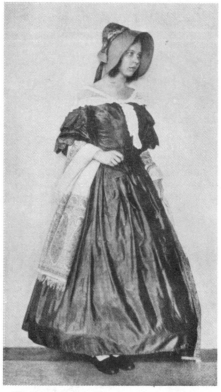

Fig. 555. DRESS OF RED-BLACK TAFFETA, 1840

About 1850 dresses were higher at the neck (Figs. 534, 551, 552), and separate neckwear was unnecessary. Sometimes, however, a narrow collar or a small frill or a small coloured silk kerchief was tied round the neck underneath a narrow collar. And although women always went to dances with neck and shoulders bare, neck ornaments went more and more out of fashion. The sole jewellery worn was a simple brooch pinned in front close to the top of the dress. On the other hand, broad bracelets on both arms were fashionable for many years. (See Plate XV.)

The Cloak. About the year 1830 cloaks returned once more to favour as winter wear, but their shape was a proof that they had been long forgotten. Unlike those of former days, they were not mere

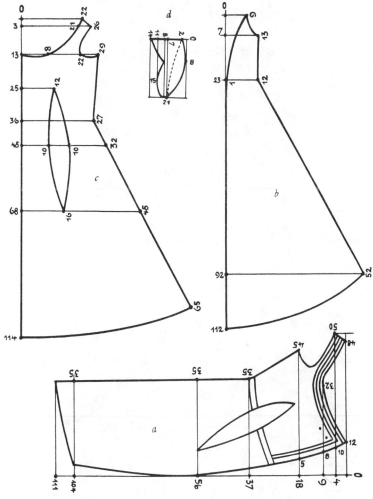

Fig. 556. PATTERN OF AN EVENING GOWN, 1868
(a) Front of tunic; (b) side-piece of tunic; (c) back; (d) sleeve.

wraps, but closely resembled the former overcoat, the only differences being in their greater width and the long cape. Before long, however, the sleeves were omitted, and the garment again became

445

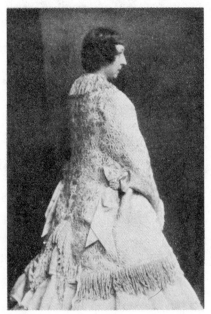

Fig. 557. MANTILLA OF WHITE PATTERNED
SATIN WITH CHENILLE FRINGE, 1850

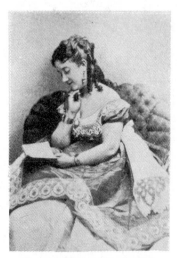

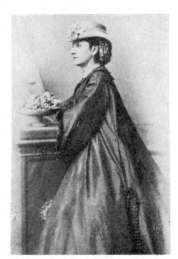

Fig. 558. EVENING GOWN, 1868
ANNA SCHRAMM (ACTRESS)

Fig. 559. LOOSE CLOAK, 1862

a mere ' wrap,' by which name it continued long to be known.   It was in most cases padded and trimmed with fur.   It reached to the ankles.   It was cut in circular shape, and usually had a fairly large cape.   (See Figs. 561 and 562.)

In the year 1856 these wraps were on the whole shorter, and were worn in autumn and spring.   They were no longer so thickly padded,

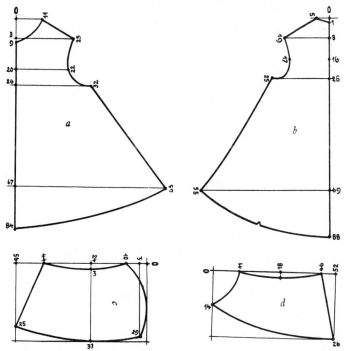

Fig. 560. Pattern of Cloak shown in Fig. 559
(a) Front ; (b) back ; (c) lower sleeve ; (d) upper sleeve.

and lighter materials were used, mostly silk.   Winter wraps were made of fine cloth or velvet.   The lighter capes were trimmed with fringes and other forms of *passementerie*.   About the year 1840 sleeve-holes were made in the wraps or wide sleeves were actually added. This gave them again a cloak-like character, which was soon further emphasized by the omission of the large cape and the addition of a hood.

From this time onward the cloak had a better defined waist.   It was closer-fitting, and as the sleeves also were tighter it was again practically an overcoat.   (See Figs. 563, 566.)

Between the years 1800 and 1835 the shawl and scarf had been

continuously in fashion, one or other being more in favour from time
to time (Figs. 481 and 526). About 1835 mantillas came in again,

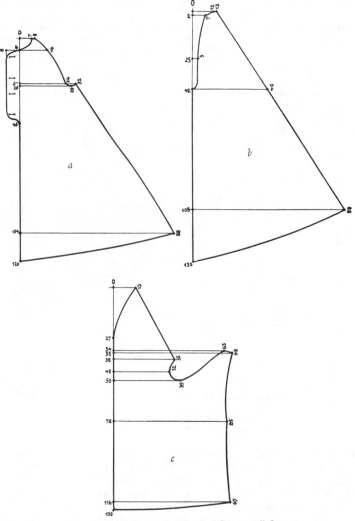

Fig. 561. PATTERN OF SO-CALLED " PARISIAN " CLOAK
(a) Front ; (b) back ; (c) sleeve.

and superseded both shawl and scarf for a considerable time. At
first these were exactly the same as those of the end of the eighteenth
century, and, like them, were made of black silk. Soon, however,

the mantillas were shortened at the back and made wider across the shoulders (see Plate XVI and Fig. 541), so that they now resembled short capes with long ends. Both the foot of the cape and its broad collar were trimmed with a ruff. It was fastened in front.

Although the very high-necked dresses which came in about 1850 made these wraps superfluous, they by no means altogether ceased to be worn. They were made of the same materials as the dresses,

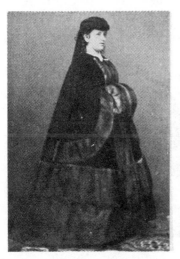 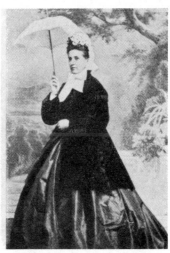

Fig. 562. PARISIAN CLOAK WITH CAPE, 1866

Fig. 563. WALKING DRESS WITH THREE-QUARTER-LENGTH VELVET COAT, END OF THE SIXTIES

and were cut like a mantilla or even like a cape. (See Figs. 553 and 554.)

The elegant shawl of Eastern patterned material was still worn with the walking dress. (See Fig. 536.) Wealthy women selected for evening wear a large triangular piece of black lace, which covered the whole dress. Either it was turned over like an actual shawl covering the shoulders or the upper edge had a trimming of broad coloured silk ribbon.

Hats and Caps. At the turn of the eighteenth century hats had gradually assumed the style of the *capote*, which had appeared first in 1801 and become quite common by 1804. (See Fig. 498.) At first only the back part was of cloth, the peak being made of straw, but by and by the whole hat was made of cloth. These were the first hats with which veils were worn. Veils now became increasingly fashionable for a time, and although they were from time to time less common, they never quite went out. The *capote* was worn in various shapes up till 1815. The style of 1810, with a long, wide

449

peak, was less becoming than some of the others. About this date
the hat itself began to be higher and the peak was much broader
and more perpendicular. An entirely new shape had gradually
evolved by about 1818.

These hats had a stiff frame of wood, covered with velvet or plush,
satin or camlet. The colours were white or grey, blue or green, red
or black, and sometimes the material was striped in two colours.
The trimming consisted of ribbon, flowers, or feathers. There were
also other styles that resembled more or less men's hats. These also
were made of various materials trimmed with flowers or feathers and
occasionally only with ribbon. This men's style developed further,

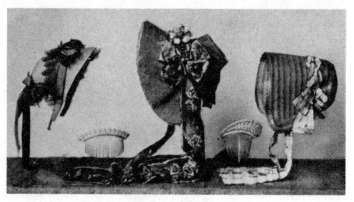

Fig. 564. Hats, about 1830–60

the brim being broadened and the crown heightened. It was, however, unable to compete with its rivals, and ere long it entirely
disappeared.

For a long time the peaked hat had the field to itself. All kinds of
trimming were employed. (See Figs. 564 and 565.) The peak was
widened and was carried down both sides of the face. After 1830
attempts were made to decrease the circumference. The peak was
tied down at the sides, and this raised it in front. This style did not
commend itself, however, although the crown of the hat was lower,
and fitted closer at the neck. The crown was therefore lowered and
the sides lengthened and made pointed, giving rise in 1840 to the
close-fitting hat, a kind of *capote*, which continued without much
change, except in the peak. (See Figs. 555, 564, and 566.)

About 1860 the peak was again raised. The space inside the hat,
so far as it was not occupied by the *coiffure*, was trimmed with lace
and flowers, and lace and flounces of ribbon were added at the nape
of the neck. This part of the hat was called the *bavolet*. This style
was unbecoming, and did not last long.

Up till now women's hats were made only of cloth or straw, but

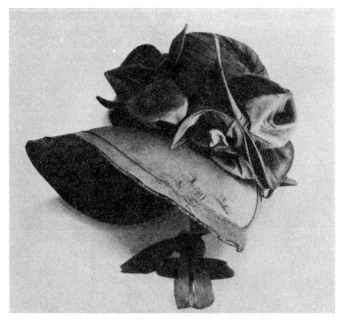

Fig. 565. COAL-SCUTTLE HAT OF GREEN SILK, ABOUT 1830-40

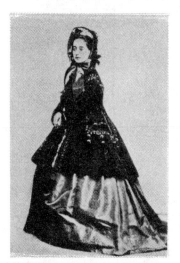

Fig. 566. PHOTOGRAPH OF THE
SINGER PAULINE LUCCA, 1864

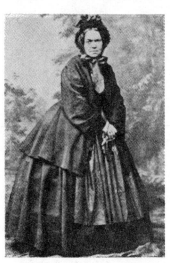

Fig. 567. PHOTOGRAPH OF THE ACTRESS
FRIEDERIKE BLUMENAUER, 1860

during the fifties felt hats with an upright plume came into fashion again. The hat was no longer *capote*-shaped, but round, low in the

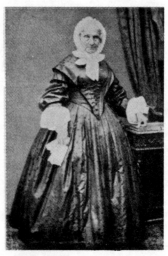

Fig. 568. PHOTOGRAPH OF THE ACTRESS
SOPHIE SCHRÖDER, 1855

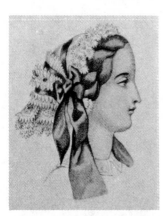

Fig. 569. CAP FROM THE " BAZAR,"
1862

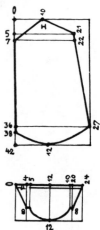

Fig. 570. PATTERN OF THE
CAP SHOWN IN FIG. 569

crown, and with a fairly broad brim. From now onward the two styles prevailed—the close-fitting hat and the round hat. The former was mostly worn by older ladies, and the latter by girls. (Fig. 559.)

Under the Second Empire hats became smaller year by year (Fig. 574). The favourite model was the small shepherdess hat of the early eighteenth century. These small hats, which were shaped like plates or saucers, were placed upright on the hair, rising high at the back. A diameter of 12 to 20 cm. was not unusual. The bent-up brim measured 1½ cm., and the crown was from 2–3 cm. high. Ostrich feathers, flowers, or lace were the usual trimming. From under the brim ribbons or a veil, fixed in position by a few dark red roses, fell to the *chignon.*

During all this time, however, the bonnet had continued to be one

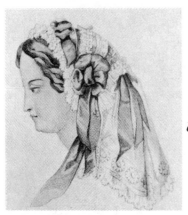

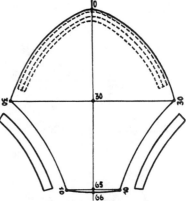

Fig. 571. Cap from the "Bazar," 1862   Fig. 572. Cut of the Cap in Fig. 571

of the most important items of attire. The picturesque element in it constituted an irresistible appeal. True, the bonnet of 1830 with lappets was short-lived. Its grotesque outline and its broad brim of starched lace caused it to lose favour together with the high *coiffure* with which it was worn. In 1840 bonnets were small and close-fitting. To be in keeping with the smooth parting of the hair the lace and ribbons used for trimming were narrower than before. (See Figs. 567 and 568.) When in the sixties the hair was dressed higher at the back of the head the bonnet was altered to suit the change. When it was a question of concealing the lack of their own hair ladies were quick to use arrangements of tulle and lace with long, loose ends. (See Figs. 569 and 571.) Sometimes a silk net was used to enclose the entire hair. A ribbon of black velvet round the head kept this net in position. For the evening *toilette* long garlands of flowers were worn, and these, interspersed with ribbons and lace, surrounded the face and often hung down to the shoulders.

Styles of Hairdressing. When the simple *coiffure* of the Empire ceased to be in keeping with the attire, it had to be made more

453

elaborate. Plaits were still in favour, but the silhouette of the head was entirely altered by the wearing of curls. (See Fig. 521, *b*.) These were now larger and more numerous at the temples, and the plait which began on the top of the head practically disappeared and gave place to puffs and loops kept up by wire frames and held in position at the back of the head by ornamental combs. (See Fig. 500.) On ceremonial occasions, when effective *coiffures* were desirable, artificial puffs were added. These were stiffened with wire and attached as high as possible on the head by means of small, long-toothed

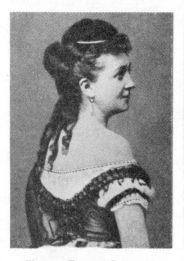 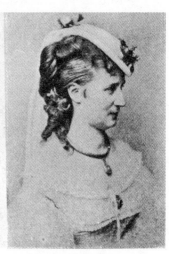

Fig. 573. Evening Coiffure, about 1870   Fig. 574. Lady wearing Hat, 1870

combs. Round these puffs a broad plait was arranged ; flowers and plumes completed the structure. By and by the hair-puffs were replaced by bows of ribbon. The puffs decreased in size, and with them the curls at the front. These curls were replaced by a wide parting, and the hair was dressed in plaits and pendent curls. (See Figs. 526 and 549.) The hair on either side of the parting was smooth or waved or tufted. At balls a single flower was worn—preferably a camelia.

About 1860 women began once more to comb the hair high and to use small foundations. (See Fig. 551.) The hair at the temples was slightly waved and also combed high. (See Figs. 575 and 576.) The back hair was treated less elaborately. It was either arranged in a roll reaching from ear to ear or was enclosed in a net. In 1864 *chignons* came into fashion again, and were very largely worn. For evening wear under the Second Empire round *chignons* were popular, with numerous curls hanging down the back and on the shoulders. This style, embellished still further by garlands of flowers, lace, and long ribbons, suited the lavish style of dress worn at the time.

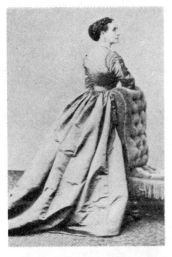

Fig. 575. PHOTOGRAPH OF THE ACTRESS ADELAIDE RISTORI, 1866

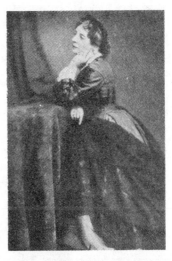

Fig. 576. PHOTOGRAPH OF THE ACTRESS DÉJAZET, ABOUT 1870

Various elaborate styles of hair-dressing, especially those employed for evening wear, had high-sounding names taken from the time of Louis XIV and Louis XV—*e.g.*, *à la Maintenon, à la Pompadour, à la Sévigné*— as well as others taken from mythology, such as *à la Cérès*, and the Apollo knot. Several features were common to them all: the hair was combed away from the forehead, it was not too broad at the temples, and the back hair was arranged in rolls which came down to the nape of the neck. The 'love-locks' were pinned on. All these styles were worn only by mature women. Young girls wore as headdress a circlet of flowers, in keeping with the trimming of their dresses. There was, however, no want of variety. Fashionable adornments included nasturtiums and even thistles.

Footwear. Down to 1860 there was little change in the shape or

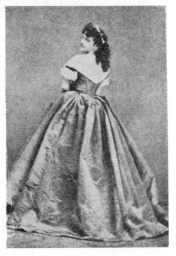

Fig. 577. LADY IN EVENING DRESS, END OF THE SIXTIES

455

material of ladies' footwear. About this time, however, heels came in again, at first for boots and from 1862 onward also for low shoes. Shoes were somewhat plain—the long skirts hindered the display of luxury in this item of attire. The boots came about three fingers' breadth above the ankles. They were rarely of leather, but mostly of silk or cloth, with toes of patent leather. They were buttoned at the side, or had elastic sides, but laced boots were not unknown. A favourite form of shoe-ornamentation was quilted seams of white silk. The tops were trimmed with coloured silk, and the laces were made of ribbon of the same colour. The boots were sometimes of white or grey satin, sometimes of chamois leather or bronze-coloured leather— the last a fashionable novelty. The upper was in one piece. The top was surrounded by a narrow ruche of ribbon. The low shoe was adorned with rosettes or bows kept in place by buckles of lace or leather. With evening dress ladies wore shoes of white satin, and white stockings. The ball dress might be white with a coloured pattern. Stockings with coloured insertions were part of the dinner *toilette*.

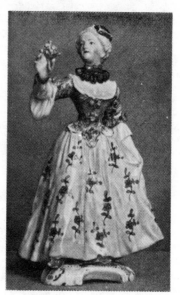

Fig. 578. GIRL WITH FLOWERS

BIBLIOGRAPHY

BISSING, FR. W. FREIHERR VON : *Denkmäler ägyptischer Skulptur* (Munich, 1914).

BOEHN, MAX VON : *Die Mode : Menschen und Moden vom Untergang der alten Welt bis zum Beginn des zwanzigsten Jahrhunderts* (8 vols., Munich, 1907–25).

BOSSERT, HELMUTH TH. : *Alt Kreta, Kunst und Kunstgewerbe im ägäischen Kulturkreise* (Berlin, 1921).

BOYE, VILHELM : *Trouvailles de cercueils en chêne de l'âge de bronze au Danemark* (Copenhagen, 1894).

BRANTING, AGNES : *Das goldene Gewand der Königin Margareta in der Domkirche zu Uppsala* (Stockholm, 1911).

BULLE, OSKAR : *Der schöne Mensch* (Munich, 1912).

BURCKHARDT, RUDOLF F. : *Gewirkte Bildteppiche des fünfzehnten und sechzehnten Jahrhunderts im historischen Museum zu Basel* (Leipzig, 1923).

BUSS, G. : *Das Kostüm in Vergangenheit und Gegenwart* (Bielefeld and Leipzig).

DAYOT, ARMAND : *Le Second Empire* (Paris).

FALKE, J. VON : *Kostümgeschichte der Kulturvölker* (Stuttgart).

FRED, W. : *Psychologie der Mode* (Berlin, 1905).

FURTWÄNGLER, A., and REICHHOLD, K. : *Griechische Vasenmalerei* (Munich, 1909–26).

GIRKE, GEORG : *Die Tracht der Germanen in der vor- und frühgeschicht-lichen Zeit* (Mannus-Bibliothek, 24) (Leipzig, 1922).

HAHNE, HANS. See *Vorzeitfunde aus Niedersachsen.*

HAMDI BEY : *Une Nécropole royale à Sidon* (Paris, 1896).

HEFNER-ALTENECK, J. H. VON : *Trachten, Kunstwerke und Gerätschaften vom frühen Mittelalter bis Ende des achtzehnten Jahrhunderts nach gleichzeitigen Originalen* (Frankfort-on-the-Main).

HEUZY, L. : *Histoire du costume antique* (Paris, 1922).

HEYNE, MORITZ : *Körperpflege und Kleidung bei den Deutschen* (Leipzig, 1903).

HIRSCH : *Das achtzehnte Jahrhundert.*

HOTTENROTH, FRIEDRICH : *Trachten, Haus-, Feld-, und Kriegsgerät-schaften alter und neuer Zeit* (Stuttgart, 1879).

KÖHLER, CARL : *Die Trachten der Völker in Bild und Schnitt* (Dresden, 1871).

—— *Die Entwicklung der Tracht in Deutschland während des Mittelalters und der Neuzeit* (Nürnberg, 1877).

A HISTORY OF COSTUME

LICHTENBERG : *Die ägäische Kultur* (Leipzig, 1918).

LÖWY, E. : *Die griechische Plastik* (Leipzig, 1916).

MOHRBUTTER, A. : *Das Kleid der Frau* (Darmstadt).

MÜTZEL, H. : *Kostümkunde für Sammler* (second edition, Berlin, 1921).

—— *Vom Lendenschurz zur Modetracht* (Berlin, 1926).

RACINET, AUGUSTE : *Le Costume historique* (Paris, 1888).

RIEZLER, WALTER : *Weissgrundige attische Lekythen* (Munich, 1914).

RUMPF, FRITZ : *Der Mensch und seine Tracht* (Berlin, 1905).

SCHMITZ, HERMANN : *Die Kunst des frühen und hohen Mittelalters in Deutschland* (Munich, 1924).

SCHRADER, HANS : *Auswahl archaischer Marmor-Skulpturen im Akropolis-Museum* (Vienna, 1913).

SOMBART, W. : *Wirtschaft und Mode, Grenzfragen des Nerven- und Seelenlebens* (Wiesbaden).

STRATZ, C. H. : *Reform der Frauenkleidung* (Stuttgart).

WINTER, MAX : *Kleidung und Putz der Frau nach den französischen Chansons de Gestes* (Marburg, 1886).

Der Bazar : Illustrierte Damenzeitung (Berlin, 1861–62).

Jahrbuch des deutschen Archäologischen Instituts, vol. xxxiii (Berlin, 1918).

Kongl. Lifrustkammaren (Stockholm, 1897).

Meddelelser om Grønland, vol. lxvii (Copenhagen, 1924).

La Mode (Paris, 1834).

Moden-Telegraph (Nürnberg, 1857–59).

Moniteur de la Mode : Journal du grand Monde (Paris, 1867–68).

Petit Courrier des Dames : Journal des Modes (Paris).

Vorzeitfunde aus Niedersachsen. Part B, *Moorleichenfunde*, by Hans Hahne (Hildesheim, 1923).

INDEX

A HISTORY OF COSTUME

INDEX

Over-dress—*continued*
  in Italy, fourteenth and fifteenth centuries, 203 ; sixteenth century, 280
  in Spain, fourteenth and fifteenth centuries, 213 f. ; sixteenth century, 230 ff. ; seventeenth century, 288

PADDED SHOULDERS, in England, 174
  in France, 167, 168
  in Germany, 273
Pænula, 115 f., 118
Palla, 118
Pallium—see *Pluviale*
Parthians, dress of the, 83 ff.
Pauvre diable, nickname for *redingote*, 383
Peplos, 96, 100 f.
Persians, dress of the, 75 ff.
Petticoats, introduced in France, 360
  in Spain, 288
  much in use in nineteenth century, 438–439
Pieschen, 185
Pluderhose, 266
Pluviale, or *pallium*, part of German royal costume, 148–149
Pourpoint, 151, 161, 166, 167, 168, 293 ff., 335
Priests' costume, Assyrian, 72 f.
  Hebrew, 69
  Median, 77 ff.
Puffjacke, 260

Redingote, 382 ff.
Regalia, Imperial German, 146 ff.
Rennröcklein (racing doublet), 258
Retennu-Tehennu, dress of the, 66 f.
Robe, 162, 168 f., 171
  in England, 178
  in France, 171, 319
Romans, dress of the, 112 ff.

SANDALS, Greek, 106
  Roman, 118
Sarmatians, dress of the, 85 ff.
Sash, 63
Saye, 237
Scarf, 71, 448–449
Scharlach, 181 *n.*
Schaube, 241, 247 ff.
Schlender, 351
Schoszweste, 387
Scythians, dress of the, 81 f.
Seam of sleeve, position of, 139, 153
Shawl, 100 f., 112, 130, 448–449

Shirt, Assyrian, 70
  German, 135
  Hebrew, 68
  Median, 75
  Roman, 112
Shorts,' in Germany, 189
Sinus of Roman toga, 113
Slippers, in France, 353
Sorket, 183
Soutane, 162
Spain, fourteenth century, men's dress, 209 ff. ; women's dress, 212 ff.
  fifteenth century, men's dress, 215 ff.
  sixteenth century, men's dress, 218 ff. ; women's dress, 227 ff.
  seventeenth century, men's dress, 286 ; women's dress, 287 ff.
Stockings, in England, 175
  in France, 305
  part of German royal costume, 249
  in Germany, 269 f. ; for women, 273 f.
  in Spain, 222
Stola, part of German royal costume, 148
  Roman, 117 f.
Stole, Assyrian, 71
Strumpfhosen, 388
Suckenie, or *Sukni*, 141 f.
Sumptuary laws, 289
Surcot, 166, 170 f., 177
Syrians and Phœnicians, dress of the, 64 ff.

Tabard, introduced into England, 174
Tabaré, 234
Tablier, 369
Tappert, 185 f., 196, 200
Tebenna, Etruscan, 111
Teutonic dress, in prehistoric period, 121 f.
  in third and fourth centuries A.D., 123 ff.
Tippet, 352
Toga, Roman, 112 ff.
Toghe, 203
Tonneaux, or *tonnelets*, 235
Trousers, Dacian, 86 f.
  in France, 1790–1820, 388 ; 1820–70, 407 ff.
  Parthian, 83
  Scythian, 81, 82
  in thirteenth century, 153–154
  See also Breeches, Hose, Leg-garments

A CATALOG OF SELECTED DOVER
BOOKS IN ALL FIELDS OF INTEREST

CONCERNING THE SPIRITUAL IN ART, Wassily Kandinsky. Pioneering work by father of abstract art. Thoughts on color theory, nature of art. Analysis of earlier masters. 12 illustrations. 80pp. of text. 5⅜ x 8½.   23411-8 Pa. $4.95

ANIMALS: 1,419 Copyright-Free Illustrations of Mammals, Birds, Fish, Insects, etc., Jim Harter (ed.). Clear wood engravings present, in extremely lifelike poses, over 1,000 species of animals. One of the most extensive pictorial sourcebooks of its kind. Captions. Index. 284pp. 9 x 12.   23766-4 Pa. $14.95

CELTIC ART: The Methods of Construction, George Bain. Simple geometric techniques for making Celtic interlacements, spirals, Kells-type initials, animals, humans, etc. Over 500 illustrations. 160pp. 9 x 12. (USO)   22923-8 Pa. $9.95

AN ATLAS OF ANATOMY FOR ARTISTS, Fritz Schider. Most thorough reference work on art anatomy in the world. Hundreds of illustrations, including selections from works by Vesalius, Leonardo, Goya, Ingres, Michelangelo, others. 593 illustrations. 192pp. 7⅛ x 10¼.   20241-0 Pa. $9.95

CELTIC HAND STROKE-BY-STROKE (Irish Half-Uncial from "The Book of Kells"): An Arthur Baker Calligraphy Manual, Arthur Baker. Complete guide to creating each letter of the alphabet in distinctive Celtic manner. Covers hand position, strokes, pens, inks, paper, more. Illustrated. 48pp. 8¼ x 11.   24336-2 Pa. $3.95

EASY ORIGAMI, John Montroll. Charming collection of 32 projects (hat, cup, pelican, piano, swan, many more) specially designed for the novice origami hobbyist. Clearly illustrated easy-to-follow instructions insure that even beginning papercrafters will achieve successful results. 48pp. 8¼ x 11.   27298-2 Pa. $3.50

THE COMPLETE BOOK OF BIRDHOUSE CONSTRUCTION FOR WOODWORKERS, Scott D. Campbell. Detailed instructions, illustrations, tables. Also data on bird habitat and instinct patterns. Bibliography. 3 tables. 63 illustrations in 15 figures. 48pp. 5¼ x 8½.   24407-5 Pa. $2.50

BLOOMINGDALE'S ILLUSTRATED 1886 CATALOG: Fashions, Dry Goods and Housewares, Bloomingdale Brothers. Famed merchants' extremely rare catalog depicting about 1,700 products: clothing, housewares, firearms, dry goods, jewelry, more. Invaluable for dating, identifying vintage items. Also, copyright-free graphics for artists, designers. Co-published with Henry Ford Museum & Greenfield Village. 160pp. 8¼ x 11.   25780-0 Pa. $10.95

HISTORIC COSTUME IN PICTURES, Braun & Schneider. Over 1,450 costumed figures in clearly detailed engravings—from dawn of civilization to end of 19th century. Captions. Many folk costumes. 256pp. 8⅜ x 11¾.   23150-X Pa. $12.95

STICKLEY CRAFTSMAN FURNITURE CATALOGS, Gustav Stickley and L. & J. G. Stickley. Beautiful, functional furniture in two authentic catalogs from 1910. 594 illustrations, including 277 photos, show settles, rockers, armchairs, reclining chairs, bookcases, desks, tables. 183pp. 6½ x 9¼. 23838-5 Pa. $11.95

AMERICAN LOCOMOTIVES IN HISTORIC PHOTOGRAPHS: 1858 to 1949, Ron Ziel (ed.). A rare collection of 126 meticulously detailed official photographs, called "builder portraits," of American locomotives that majestically chronicle the rise of steam locomotive power in America. Introduction. Detailed captions. xi + 129pp. 9 x 12. 27393-8 Pa. $13.95

AMERICA'S LIGHTHOUSES: An Illustrated History, Francis Ross Holland, Jr. Delightfully written, profusely illustrated fact-filled survey of over 200 American lighthouses since 1716. History, anecdotes, technological advances, more. 240pp. 8 x 10¾.
25576-X Pa. $12.95

TOWARDS A NEW ARCHITECTURE, Le Corbusier. Pioneering manifesto by founder of "International School." Technical and aesthetic theories, views of industry, economics, relation of form to function, "mass-production split" and much more. Profusely illustrated. 320pp. 6⅛ x 9¼. (USO) 25023-7 Pa. $9.95

HOW THE OTHER HALF LIVES, Jacob Riis. Famous journalistic record, exposing poverty and degradation of New York slums around 1900, by major social reformer. 100 striking and influential photographs. 233pp. 10 x 7⅞.
22012-5 Pa. $11.95

FRUIT KEY AND TWIG KEY TO TREES AND SHRUBS, William M. Harlow. One of the handiest and most widely used identification aids. Fruit key covers 120 deciduous and evergreen species; twig key 160 deciduous species. Easily used. Over 300 photographs. 126pp. 5⅜ x 8½. 20511-8 Pa. $3.95

COMMON BIRD SONGS, Dr. Donald J. Borror. Songs of 60 most common U.S. birds: robins, sparrows, cardinals, bluejays, finches, more–arranged in order of increasing complexity. Up to 9 variations of songs of each species.
Cassette and manual 99911-4 $8.95

ORCHIDS AS HOUSE PLANTS, Rebecca Tyson Northen. Grow cattleyas and many other kinds of orchids–in a window, in a case, or under artificial light. 63 illustrations. 148pp. 5⅜ x 8½. 23261-1 Pa. $5.95

MONSTER MAZES, Dave Phillips. Masterful mazes at four levels of difficulty. Avoid deadly perils and evil creatures to find magical treasures. Solutions for all 32 exciting illustrated puzzles. 48pp. 8¼ x 11. 26005-4 Pa. $2.95

MOZART'S DON GIOVANNI (DOVER OPERA LIBRETTO SERIES), Wolfgang Amadeus Mozart. Introduced and translated by Ellen H. Bleiler. Standard Italian libretto, with complete English translation. Convenient and thoroughly portable–an ideal companion for reading along with a recording or the performance itself. Introduction. List of characters. Plot summary. 121pp. 5¼ x 8½.
24944-1 Pa. $3.95

TECHNICAL MANUAL AND DICTIONARY OF CLASSICAL BALLET, Gail Grant. Defines, explains, comments on steps, movements, poses and concepts. 15-page pictorial section. Basic book for student, viewer. 127pp. 5⅜ x 8½.
21843-0 Pa. $4.95

BRASS INSTRUMENTS: Their History and Development, Anthony Baines. Authoritative, updated survey of the evolution of trumpets, trombones, bugles, cornets, French horns, tubas and other brass wind instruments. Over 140 illustrations and 48 music examples. Corrected and updated by author. New preface. Bibliography. 320pp. 5⅜ x 8½. 27574-4 Pa. $9.95

HOLLYWOOD GLAMOR PORTRAITS, John Kobal (ed.). 145 photos from 1926-49. Harlow, Gable, Bogart, Bacall; 94 stars in all. Full background on photographers, technical aspects. 160pp. 8⅜ x 11¼. 23352-9 Pa. $12.95

MAX AND MORITZ, Wilhelm Busch. Great humor classic in both German and English. Also 10 other works: "Cat and Mouse," "Plisch and Plumm," etc. 216pp. 5⅜ x 8½. 20181-3 Pa. $6.95

THE RAVEN AND OTHER FAVORITE POEMS, Edgar Allan Poe. Over 40 of the author's most memorable poems: "The Bells," "Ulalume," "Israfel," "To Helen," "The Conqueror Worm," "Eldorado," "Annabel Lee," many more. Alphabetic lists of titles and first lines. 64pp. 5$\frac{3}{16}$ x 8¼. 26685-0 Pa. $1.00

PERSONAL MEMOIRS OF U. S. GRANT, Ulysses Simpson Grant. Intelligent, deeply moving firsthand account of Civil War campaigns, considered by many the finest military memoirs ever written. Includes letters, historic photographs, maps and more. 528pp. 6⅛ x 9¼. 28587-1 Pa. $12.95

AMULETS AND SUPERSTITIONS, E. A. Wallis Budge. Comprehensive discourse on origin, powers of amulets in many ancient cultures: Arab, Persian Babylonian, Assyrian, Egyptian, Gnostic, Hebrew, Phoenician, Syriac, etc. Covers cross, swastika, crucifix, seals, rings, stones, etc. 584pp. 5⅜ x 8½. 23573-4 Pa. $12.95

RUSSIAN STORIES/PYCCKNE PACCKA3bl: A Dual-Language Book, edited by Gleb Struve. Twelve tales by such masters as Chekhov, Tolstoy, Dostoevsky, Pushkin, others. Excellent word-for-word English translations on facing pages, plus teaching and study aids, Russian/English vocabulary, biographical/critical introductions, more. 416pp. 5⅜ x 8½. 26244-8 Pa. $9.95

PHILADELPHIA THEN AND NOW: 60 Sites Photographed in the Past and Present, Kenneth Finkel and Susan Oyama. Rare photographs of City Hall, Logan Square, Independence Hall, Betsy Ross House, other landmarks juxtaposed with contemporary views. Captures changing face of historic city. Introduction. Captions. 128pp. 8¼ x 11. 25790-8 Pa. $9.95

AIA ARCHITECTURAL GUIDE TO NASSAU AND SUFFOLK COUNTIES, LONG ISLAND, The American Institute of Architects, Long Island Chapter, and the Society for the Preservation of Long Island Antiquities. Comprehensive, well-researched and generously illustrated volume brings to life over three centuries of Long Island's great architectural heritage. More than 240 photographs with authoritative, extensively detailed captions. 176pp. 8¼ x 11. 26946-9 Pa. $14.95

NORTH AMERICAN INDIAN LIFE: Customs and Traditions of 23 Tribes, Elsie Clews Parsons (ed.). 27 fictionalized essays by noted anthropologists examine religion, customs, government, additional facets of life among the Winnebago, Crow, Zuni, Eskimo, other tribes. 480pp. 6⅛ x 9¼. 27377-6 Pa. $10.95

FRANK LLOYD WRIGHT'S HOLLYHOCK HOUSE, Donald Hoffmann. Lavishly illustrated, carefully documented study of one of Wright's most controversial residential designs. Over 120 photographs, floor plans, elevations, etc. Detailed perceptive text by noted Wright scholar. Index. 128pp. 9¼ x 10¾. 27133-1 Pa. $11.95

THE MALE AND FEMALE FIGURE IN MOTION: 60 Classic Photographic Sequences, Eadweard Muybridge. 60 true-action photographs of men and women walking, running, climbing, bending, turning, etc., reproduced from rare 19th-century masterpiece. vi + 121pp. 9 x 12. 24745-7 Pa. $10.95

1001 QUESTIONS ANSWERED ABOUT THE SEASHORE, N. J. Berrill and Jacquelyn Berrill. Queries answered about dolphins, sea snails, sponges, starfish, fishes, shore birds, many others. Covers appearance, breeding, growth, feeding, much more. 305pp. 5¼ x 8¼. 23366-9 Pa. $8.95

GUIDE TO OWL WATCHING IN NORTH AMERICA, Donald S. Heintzelman. Superb guide offers complete data and descriptions of 19 species: barn owl, screech owl, snowy owl, many more. Expert coverage of owl-watching equipment, conservation, migrations and invasions, etc. Guide to observing sites. 84 illustrations. xiii + 193pp. 5⅜ x 8½. 27344-X Pa. $8.95

MEDICINAL AND OTHER USES OF NORTH AMERICAN PLANTS: A Historical Survey with Special Reference to the Eastern Indian Tribes, Charlotte Erichsen-Brown. Chronological historical citations document 500 years of usage of plants, trees, shrubs native to eastern Canada, northeastern U.S. Also complete identifying information. 343 illustrations. 544pp. 6½ x 9¼. 25951-X Pa. $12.95

STORYBOOK MAZES, Dave Phillips. 23 stories and mazes on two-page spreads: Wizard of Oz, Treasure Island, Robin Hood, etc. Solutions. 64pp. 8¼ x 11. 23628-5 Pa. $2.95

NEGRO FOLK MUSIC, U.S.A., Harold Courlander. Noted folklorist's scholarly yet readable analysis of rich and varied musical tradition. Includes authentic versions of over 40 folk songs. Valuable bibliography and discography. xi + 324pp. 5⅜ x 8½. 27350-4 Pa. $9.95

MOVIE-STAR PORTRAITS OF THE FORTIES, John Kobal (ed.). 163 glamor, studio photos of 106 stars of the 1940s: Rita Hayworth, Ava Gardner, Marlon Brando, Clark Gable, many more. 176pp. 8⅝ x 11¼. 23546-7 Pa. $12.95

BENCHLEY LOST AND FOUND, Robert Benchley. Finest humor from early 30s, about pet peeves, child psychologists, post office and others. Mostly unavailable elsewhere. 73 illustrations by Peter Arno and others. 183pp. 5⅜ x 8½. 22410-4 Pa. $6.95

YEKL and THE IMPORTED BRIDEGROOM AND OTHER STORIES OF YIDDISH NEW YORK, Abraham Cahan. Film Hester Street based on Yekl (1896). Novel, other stories among first about Jewish immigrants on N.Y.'s East Side. 240pp. 5⅜ x 8½. 22427-9 Pa. $6.95

SELECTED POEMS, Walt Whitman. Generous sampling from *Leaves of Grass.* Twenty-four poems include "I Hear America Singing," "Song of the Open Road," "I Sing the Body Electric," "When Lilacs Last in the Dooryard Bloom'd," "O Captain! My Captain!"—all reprinted from an authoritative edition. Lists of titles and first lines. 128pp. 5³⁄₁₆ x 8¼. 26878-0 Pa. $1.00

THE BEST TALES OF HOFFMANN, E. T. A. Hoffmann. 10 of Hoffmann's most important stories: "Nutcracker and the King of Mice," "The Golden Flowerpot," etc. 458pp. 5⅜ x 8½. 21793-0 Pa. $9.95

FROM FETISH TO GOD IN ANCIENT EGYPT, E. A. Wallis Budge. Rich detailed survey of Egyptian conception of "God" and gods, magic, cult of animals, Osiris, more. Also, superb English translations of hymns and legends. 240 illustrations. 545pp. 5⅜ x 8½. 25803-3 Pa. $13.95

FRENCH STORIES/CONTES FRANÇAIS: A Dual-Language Book, Wallace Fowlie. Ten stories by French masters, Voltaire to Camus: "Micromegas" by Voltaire; "The Atheist's Mass" by Balzac; "Minuet" by de Maupassant; "The Guest" by Camus, six more. Excellent English translations on facing pages. Also French-English vocabulary list, exercises, more. 352pp. 5⅜ x 8½. 26443-2 Pa. $9.95

CHICAGO AT THE TURN OF THE CENTURY IN PHOTOGRAPHS: 122 Historic Views from the Collections of the Chicago Historical Society, Larry A. Viskochil. Rare large-format prints offer detailed views of City Hall, State Street, the Loop, Hull House, Union Station, many other landmarks, circa 1904-1913. Introduction. Captions. Maps. 144pp. 9⅜ x 12¼. 24656-6 Pa. $12.95

OLD BROOKLYN IN EARLY PHOTOGRAPHS, 1865-1929, William Lee Younger. Luna Park, Gravesend race track, construction of Grand Army Plaza, moving of Hotel Brighton, etc. 157 previously unpublished photographs. 165pp. 8⅞ x 11¾. 23587-4 Pa. $13.95

THE MYTHS OF THE NORTH AMERICAN INDIANS, Lewis Spence. Rich anthology of the myths and legends of the Algonquins, Iroquois, Pawnees and Sioux, prefaced by an extensive historical and ethnological commentary. 36 illustrations. 480pp. 5⅜ x 8½. 25967-6 Pa. $10.95

AN ENCYCLOPEDIA OF BATTLES: Accounts of Over 1,560 Battles from 1479 B.C. to the Present, David Eggenberger. Essential details of every major battle in recorded history from the first battle of Megiddo in 1479 B.C. to Grenada in 1984. List of Battle Maps. New Appendix covering the years 1967-1984. Index. 99 illustrations. 544pp. 6½ x 9¼. 24913-1 Pa. $16.95

SAILING ALONE AROUND THE WORLD, Captain Joshua Slocum. First man to sail around the world, alone, in small boat. One of great feats of seamanship told in delightful manner. 67 illustrations. 294pp. 5⅜ x 8½. 20326-3 Pa. $6.95

ANARCHISM AND OTHER ESSAYS, Emma Goldman. Powerful, penetrating, prophetic essays on direct action, role of minorities, prison reform, puritan hypocrisy, violence, etc. 271pp. 5⅜ x 8½. 22484-8 Pa. $7.95

MYTHS OF THE HINDUS AND BUDDHISTS, Ananda K. Coomaraswamy and Sister Nivedita. Great stories of the epics; deeds of Krishna, Shiva, taken from puranas, Vedas, folk tales; etc. 32 illustrations. 400pp. 5⅜ x 8½. 21759-0 Pa. $12.95

BEYOND PSYCHOLOGY, Otto Rank. Fear of death, desire of immortality, nature of sexuality, social organization, creativity, according to Rankian system. 291pp. 5⅜ x 8½. 20485-5 Pa. $8.95

A THEOLOGICO-POLITICAL TREATISE, Benedict Spinoza. Also contains unfinished Political Treatise. Great classic on religious liberty, theory of government on common consent. R. Elwes translation. Total of 421pp. 5⅜ x 8½. 20249-6 Pa. $9.95

MY BONDAGE AND MY FREEDOM, Frederick Douglass. Born a slave, Douglass became outspoken force in antislavery movement. The best of Douglass' autobiographies. Graphic description of slave life. 464pp. 5⅜ x 8½. 22457-0 Pa. $8.95

FOLLOWING THE EQUATOR: A Journey Around the World, Mark Twain. Fascinating humorous account of 1897 voyage to Hawaii, Australia, India, New Zealand, etc. Ironic, bemused reports on peoples, customs, climate, flora and fauna, politics, much more. 197 illustrations. 720pp. 5⅜ x 8½. 26113-1 Pa. $15.95

THE PEOPLE CALLED SHAKERS, Edward D. Andrews. Definitive study of Shakers: origins, beliefs, practices, dances, social organization, furniture and crafts, etc. 33 illustrations. 351pp. 5⅜ x 8½. 21081-2 Pa. $8.95

THE MYTHS OF GREECE AND ROME, H. A. Guerber. A classic of mythology, generously illustrated, long prized for its simple, graphic, accurate retelling of the principal myths of Greece and Rome, and for its commentary on their origins and significance. With 64 illustrations by Michelangelo, Raphael, Titian, Rubens, Canova, Bernini and others. 480pp. 5⅜ x 8½. 27584-1 Pa. $9.95

PSYCHOLOGY OF MUSIC, Carl E. Seashore. Classic work discusses music as a medium from psychological viewpoint. Clear treatment of physical acoustics, auditory apparatus, sound perception, development of musical skills, nature of musical feeling, host of other topics. 88 figures. 408pp. 5⅜ x 8½. 21851-1 Pa. $11.95

THE PHILOSOPHY OF HISTORY, Georg W. Hegel. Great classic of Western thought develops concept that history is not chance but rational process, the evolution of freedom. 457pp. 5⅜ x 8½. 20112-0 Pa. $9.95

THE BOOK OF TEA, Kakuzo Okakura. Minor classic of the Orient: entertaining, charming explanation, interpretation of traditional Japanese culture in terms of tea ceremony. 94pp. 5⅜ x 8½. 20070-1 Pa. $3.95

LIFE IN ANCIENT EGYPT, Adolf Erman. Fullest, most thorough, detailed older account with much not in more recent books, domestic life, religion, magic, medicine, commerce, much more. Many illustrations reproduce tomb paintings, carvings, hieroglyphs, etc. 597pp. 5⅜ x 8½. 22632-8 Pa. $12.95

SUNDIALS, Their Theory and Construction, Albert Waugh. Far and away the best, most thorough coverage of ideas, mathematics concerned, types, construction, adjusting anywhere. Simple, nontechnical treatment allows even children to build several of these dials. Over 100 illustrations. 230pp. 5⅜ x 8½. 22947-5 Pa. $8.95

DYNAMICS OF FLUIDS IN POROUS MEDIA, Jacob Bear. For advanced students of ground water hydrology, soil mechanics and physics, drainage and irrigation engineering, and more. 335 illustrations. Exercises, with answers. 784pp. 6⅛ x 9¼. 65675-6 Pa. $19.95

SONGS OF EXPERIENCE: Facsimile Reproduction with 26 Plates in Full Color, William Blake. 26 full-color plates from a rare 1826 edition. Includes "TheTyger," "London," "Holy Thursday," and other poems. Printed text of poems. 48pp. 5¼ x 7. 24636-1 Pa. $4.95

OLD-TIME VIGNETTES IN FULL COLOR, Carol Belanger Grafton (ed.). Over 390 charming, often sentimental illustrations, selected from archives of Victorian graphics—pretty women posing, children playing, food, flowers, kittens and puppies, smiling cherubs, birds and butterflies, much more. All copyright-free. 48pp. 9¼ x 12¼. 27269-9 Pa. $7.95

PERSPECTIVE FOR ARTISTS, Rex Vicat Cole. Depth, perspective of sky and sea, shadows, much more, not usually covered. 391 diagrams, 81 reproductions of drawings and paintings. 279pp. 5⅜ x 8½. 22487-2 Pa. $7.95

DRAWING THE LIVING FIGURE, Joseph Sheppard. Innovative approach to artistic anatomy focuses on specifics of surface anatomy, rather than muscles and bones. Over 170 drawings of live models in front, back and side views, and in widely varying poses. Accompanying diagrams. 177 illustrations. Introduction. Index. 144pp. 8⅜ x11¼. 26723-7 Pa. $8.95

GOTHIC AND OLD ENGLISH ALPHABETS: 100 Complete Fonts, Dan X. Solo. Add power, elegance to posters, signs, other graphics with 100 stunning copyright-free alphabets: Blackstone, Dolbey, Germania, 97 more–including many lower-case, numerals, punctuation marks. 104pp. 8⅛ x 11. 24695-7 Pa. $8.95

HOW TO DO BEADWORK, Mary White. Fundamental book on craft from simple projects to five-bead chains and woven works. 106 illustrations. 142pp. 5⅜ x 8. 20697-1 Pa. $4.95

THE BOOK OF WOOD CARVING, Charles Marshall Sayers. Finest book for beginners discusses fundamentals and offers 34 designs. "Absolutely first rate . . . well thought out and well executed."–E. J. Tangerman. 118pp. 7¾ x 10⅝. 23654-4 Pa. $6.95

ILLUSTRATED CATALOG OF CIVIL WAR MILITARY GOODS: Union Army Weapons, Insignia, Uniform Accessories, and Other Equipment, Schuyler, Hartley, and Graham. Rare, profusely illustrated 1846 catalog includes Union Army uniform and dress regulations, arms and ammunition, coats, insignia, flags, swords, rifles, etc. 226 illustrations. 160pp. 9 x 12. 24939-5 Pa. $10.95

WOMEN'S FASHIONS OF THE EARLY 1900s: An Unabridged Republication of "New York Fashions, 1909," National Cloak & Suit Co. Rare catalog of mail-order fashions documents women's and children's clothing styles shortly after the turn of the century. Captions offer full descriptions, prices. Invaluable resource for fashion, costume historians. Approximately 725 illustrations. 128pp. 8⅜ x 11¼. 27276-1 Pa. $11.95

THE 1912 AND 1915 GUSTAV STICKLEY FURNITURE CATALOGS, Gustav Stickley. With over 200 detailed illustrations and descriptions, these two catalogs are essential reading and reference materials and identification guides for Stickley furniture. Captions cite materials, dimensions and prices. 112pp. 6½ x 9¼. 26676-1 Pa. $9.95

EARLY AMERICAN LOCOMOTIVES, John H. White, Jr. Finest locomotive engravings from early 19th century: historical (1804–74), main-line (after 1870), special, foreign, etc. 147 plates. 142pp. 11⅜ x 8¼. 22772-3 Pa. $10.95

THE TALL SHIPS OF TODAY IN PHOTOGRAPHS, Frank O. Braynard. Lavishly illustrated tribute to nearly 100 majestic contemporary sailing vessels: Amerigo Vespucci, Clearwater, Constitution, Eagle, Mayflower, Sea Cloud, Victory, many more. Authoritative captions provide statistics, background on each ship. 190 black-and-white photographs and illustrations. Introduction. 128pp. 8⅞ x 11¾. 27163-3 Pa. $14.95

EARLY NINETEENTH-CENTURY CRAFTS AND TRADES, Peter Stockham (ed.). Extremely rare 1807 volume describes to youngsters the crafts and trades of the day: brickmaker, weaver, dressmaker, bookbinder, ropemaker, saddler, many more. Quaint prose, charming illustrations for each craft. 20 black-and-white line illustrations. 192pp. 4⅝ x 6. 27293-1 Pa. $4.95

VICTORIAN FASHIONS AND COSTUMES FROM HARPER'S BAZAR, 1867–1898, Stella Blum (ed.). Day costumes, evening wear, sports clothes, shoes, hats, other accessories in over 1,000 detailed engravings. 320pp. 9⅜ x 12¼. 22990-4 Pa. $15.95

GUSTAV STICKLEY, THE CRAFTSMAN, Mary Ann Smith. Superb study surveys broad scope of Stickley's achievement, especially in architecture. Design philosophy, rise and fall of the Craftsman empire, descriptions and floor plans for many Craftsman houses, more. 86 black-and-white halftones. 31 line illustrations. Introduction 208pp. 6½ x 9¼. 27210-9 Pa. $9.95

THE LONG ISLAND RAIL ROAD IN EARLY PHOTOGRAPHS, Ron Ziel. Over 220 rare photos, informative text document origin (1844) and development of rail service on Long Island. Vintage views of early trains, locomotives, stations, passengers, crews, much more. Captions. 8⅞ x 11¾. 26301-0 Pa. $13.95

THE BOOK OF OLD SHIPS: From Egyptian Galleys to Clipper Ships, Henry B. Culver. Superb, authoritative history of sailing vessels, with 80 magnificent line illustrations. Galley, bark, caravel, longship, whaler, many more. Detailed, informative text on each vessel by noted naval historian. Introduction. 256pp. 5⅜ x 8½. 27332-6 Pa. $7.95

TEN BOOKS ON ARCHITECTURE, Vitruvius. The most important book ever written on architecture. Early Roman aesthetics, technology, classical orders, site selection, all other aspects. Morgan translation. 331pp. 5⅜ x 8½. 20645-9 Pa. $8.95

THE HUMAN FIGURE IN MOTION, Eadweard Muybridge. More than 4,500 stopped-action photos, in action series, showing undraped men, women, children jumping, lying down, throwing, sitting, wrestling, carrying, etc. 390pp. 7⅞ x 10⅝. 20204-6 Clothbd. $27.95

TREES OF THE EASTERN AND CENTRAL UNITED STATES AND CANADA, William M. Harlow. Best one-volume guide to 140 trees. Full descriptions, woodlore, range, etc. Over 600 illustrations. Handy size. 288pp. 4½ x 6⅜. 20395-6 Pa. $6.95

SONGS OF WESTERN BIRDS, Dr. Donald J. Borror. Complete song and call repertoire of 60 western species, including flycatchers, juncoes, cactus wrens, many more–includes fully illustrated booklet. Cassette and manual 99913-0 $8.95

GROWING AND USING HERBS AND SPICES, Milo Miloradovich. Versatile handbook provides all the information needed for cultivation and use of all the herbs and spices available in North America. 4 illustrations. Index. Glossary. 236pp. 5⅜ x 8½. 25058-X Pa. $7.95

BIG BOOK OF MAZES AND LABYRINTHS, Walter Shepherd. 50 mazes and labyrinths in all–classical, solid, ripple, and more–in one great volume. Perfect inexpensive puzzler for clever youngsters. Full solutions. 112pp. 8⅛ x 11. 22951-3 Pa. $4.95

PIANO TUNING, J. Cree Fischer. Clearest, best book for beginner, amateur. Simple repairs, raising dropped notes, tuning by easy method of flattened fifths. No previous skills needed. 4 illustrations. 201pp. 5⅜ x 8½. 23267-0 Pa. $6.95

A SOURCE BOOK IN THEATRICAL HISTORY, A. M. Nagler. Contemporary observers on acting, directing, make-up, costuming, stage props, machinery, scene design, from Ancient Greece to Chekhov. 611pp. 5⅜ x 8½. 20515-0 Pa. $12.95

THE COMPLETE NONSENSE OF EDWARD LEAR, Edward Lear. All nonsense limericks, zany alphabets, Owl and Pussycat, songs, nonsense botany, etc., illustrated by Lear. Total of 320pp. 5⅜ x 8½. (USO) 20167-8 Pa. $7.95

VICTORIAN PARLOUR POETRY: An Annotated Anthology, Michael R. Turner. 117 gems by Longfellow, Tennyson, Browning, many lesser-known poets. "The Village Blacksmith," "Curfew Must Not Ring Tonight," "Only a Baby Small," dozens more, often difficult to find elsewhere. Index of poets, titles, first lines. xxiii + 325pp. 5⅜ x 8¼. 27044-0 Pa. $8.95

DUBLINERS, James Joyce. Fifteen stories offer vivid, tightly focused observations of the lives of Dublin's poorer classes. At least one, "The Dead," is considered a masterpiece. Reprinted complete and unabridged from standard edition. 160pp. 5³⁄₁₆ x 8¼. 26870-5 Pa. $1.00

THE HAUNTED MONASTERY and THE CHINESE MAZE MURDERS, Robert van Gulik. Two full novels by van Gulik, set in 7th-century China, continue adventures of Judge Dee and his companions. An evil Taoist monastery, seemingly supernatural events; overgrown topiary maze hides strange crimes. 27 illustrations. 328pp. 5⅜ x 8½. 23502-5 Pa. $8.95

THE BOOK OF THE SACRED MAGIC OF ABRAMELIN THE MAGE, translated by S. MacGregor Mathers. Medieval manuscript of ceremonial magic. Basic document in Aleister Crowley, Golden Dawn groups. 268pp. 5⅜ x 8½. 23211-5 Pa. $9.95

NEW RUSSIAN-ENGLISH AND ENGLISH-RUSSIAN DICTIONARY, M. A. O'Brien. This is a remarkably handy Russian dictionary, containing a surprising amount of information, including over 70,000 entries. 366pp. 4½ x 6⅛. 20208-9 Pa. $9.95

HISTORIC HOMES OF THE AMERICAN PRESIDENTS, Second, Revised Edition, Irvin Haas. A traveler's guide to American Presidential homes, most open to the public, depicting and describing homes occupied by every American President from George Washington to George Bush. With visiting hours, admission charges, travel routes. 175 photographs. Index. 160pp. 8¼ x 11. 26751-2 Pa. $11.95

NEW YORK IN THE FORTIES, Andreas Feininger. 162 brilliant photographs by the well-known photographer, formerly with *Life* magazine. Commuters, shoppers, Times Square at night, much else from city at its peak. Captions by John von Hartz. 181pp. 9¼ x 10¾. 23585-8 Pa. $12.95

INDIAN SIGN LANGUAGE, William Tomkins. Over 525 signs developed by Sioux and other tribes. Written instructions and diagrams. Also 290 pictographs. 111pp. 6⅛ x 9¼. 22029-X Pa. $3.95

ANATOMY: A Complete Guide for Artists, Joseph Sheppard. A master of figure drawing shows artists how to render human anatomy convincingly. Over 460 illustrations. 224pp. 8⅜ x 11¼. 27279-6 Pa. $11.95

MEDIEVAL CALLIGRAPHY: Its History and Technique, Marc Drogin. Spirited history, comprehensive instruction manual covers 13 styles (ca. 4th century thru 15th). Excellent photographs; directions for duplicating medieval techniques with modern tools. 224pp. 8⅜ x 11¼. 26142-5 Pa. $12.95

DRIED FLOWERS: How to Prepare Them, Sarah Whitlock and Martha Rankin. Complete instructions on how to use silica gel, meal and borax, perlite aggregate, sand and borax, glycerine and water to create attractive permanent flower arrangements. 12 illustrations. 32pp. 5⅜ x 8½. 21802-3 Pa. $1.00

EASY-TO-MAKE BIRD FEEDERS FOR WOODWORKERS, Scott D. Campbell. Detailed, simple-to-use guide for designing, constructing, caring for and using feeders. Text, illustrations for 12 classic and contemporary designs. 96pp. 5⅜ x 8½. 25847-5 Pa. $3.95

SCOTTISH WONDER TALES FROM MYTH AND LEGEND, Donald A. Mackenzie. 16 lively tales tell of giants rumbling down mountainsides, of a magic wand that turns stone pillars into warriors, of gods and goddesses, evil hags, powerful forces and more. 240pp. 5⅜ x 8½. 29677-6 Pa. $6.95

THE HISTORY OF UNDERCLOTHES, C. Willett Cunnington and Phyllis Cunnington. Fascinating, well-documented survey covering six centuries of English undergarments, enhanced with over 100 illustrations: 12th-century laced-up bodice, footed long drawers (1795), 19th-century bustles, 19th-century corsets for men, Victorian "bust improvers," much more. 272pp. 5⅜ x 8¼. 27124-2 Pa. $9.95

ARTS AND CRAFTS FURNITURE: The Complete Brooks Catalog of 1912, Brooks Manufacturing Co. Photos and detailed descriptions of more than 150 now very collectible furniture designs from the Arts and Crafts movement depict davenports, settees, buffets, desks, tables, chairs, bedsteads, dressers and more, all built of solid, quarter-sawed oak. Invaluable for students and enthusiasts of antiques, Americana and the decorative arts. 80pp. 6½ x 9¼. 27471-3 Pa. $8.95

HOW WE INVENTED THE AIRPLANE: An Illustrated History, Orville Wright. Fascinating firsthand account covers early experiments, construction of planes and motors, first flights, much more. Introduction and commentary by Fred C. Kelly. 76 photographs. 96pp. 8¼ x 11. 25662-6 Pa. $8.95

THE ARTS OF THE SAILOR: Knotting, Splicing and Ropework, Hervey Garrett Smith. Indispensable shipboard reference covers tools, basic knots and useful hitches; handsewing and canvas work, more. Over 100 illustrations. Delightful reading for sea lovers. 256pp. 5⅜ x 8½. 26440-8 Pa. $7.95

FRANK LLOYD WRIGHT'S FALLINGWATER: The House and Its History, Second, Revised Edition, Donald Hoffmann. A total revision—both in text and illustrations—of the standard document on Fallingwater, the boldest, most personal architectural statement of Wright's mature years, updated with valuable new material from the recently opened Frank Lloyd Wright Archives. "Fascinating"—*The New York Times.* 116 illustrations. 128pp. 9¼ x 10¾. 27430-6 Pa. $12.95

PHOTOGRAPHIC SKETCHBOOK OF THE CIVIL WAR, Alexander Gardner. 100 photos taken on field during the Civil War. Famous shots of Manassas Harper's Ferry, Lincoln, Richmond, slave pens, etc. 244pp. 10⅝ x 8¼. 22731-6 Pa. $9.95

FIVE ACRES AND INDEPENDENCE, Maurice G. Kains. Great back-to-the-land classic explains basics of self-sufficient farming. The one book to get. 95 illustrations. 397pp. 5⅜ x 8½. 20974-1 Pa. $7.95

SONGS OF EASTERN BIRDS, Dr. Donald J. Borror. Songs and calls of 60 species most common to eastern U.S.: warblers, woodpeckers, flycatchers, thrushes, larks, many more in high-quality recording. Cassette and manual 99912-2 $9.95

A MODERN HERBAL, Margaret Grieve. Much the fullest, most exact, most useful compilation of herbal material. Gigantic alphabetical encyclopedia, from aconite to zedoary, gives botanical information, medical properties, folklore, economic uses, much else. Indispensable to serious reader. 161 illustrations. 888pp. 6½ x 9¼. 2-vol. set. (USO) Vol. I: 22798-7 Pa. $9.95
Vol. II: 22799-5 Pa. $9.95

HIDDEN TREASURE MAZE BOOK, Dave Phillips. Solve 34 challenging mazes accompanied by heroic tales of adventure. Evil dragons, people-eating plants, blood-thirsty giants, many more dangerous adversaries lurk at every twist and turn. 34 mazes, stories, solutions. 48pp. 8¼ x 11. 24566-7 Pa. $2.95

LETTERS OF W. A. MOZART, Wolfgang A. Mozart. Remarkable letters show bawdy wit, humor, imagination, musical insights, contemporary musical world; includes some letters from Leopold Mozart. 276pp. 5⅜ x 8½. 22859-2 Pa. $7.95

BASIC PRINCIPLES OF CLASSICAL BALLET, Agrippina Vaganova. Great Russian theoretician, teacher explains methods for teaching classical ballet. 118 illustrations. 175pp. 5⅜ x 8½. 22036-2 Pa. $5.95

THE JUMPING FROG, Mark Twain. Revenge edition. The original story of The Celebrated Jumping Frog of Calaveras County, a hapless French translation, and Twain's hilarious "retranslation" from the French. 12 illustrations. 66pp. 5⅜ x 8½. 22686-7 Pa. $3.95

BEST REMEMBERED POEMS, Martin Gardner (ed.). The 126 poems in this superb collection of 19th- and 20th-century British and American verse range from Shelley's "To a Skylark" to the impassioned "Renascence" of Edna St. Vincent Millay and to Edward Lear's whimsical "The Owl and the Pussycat." 224pp. 5⅜ x 8½. 27165-X Pa. $5.95

COMPLETE SONNETS, William Shakespeare. Over 150 exquisite poems deal with love, friendship, the tyranny of time, beauty's evanescence, death and other themes in language of remarkable power, precision and beauty. Glossary of archaic terms. 80pp. 5 3/16 x 8¼. 26686-9 Pa. $1.00

BODIES IN A BOOKSHOP, R. T. Campbell. Challenging mystery of blackmail and murder with ingenious plot and superbly drawn characters. In the best tradition of British suspense fiction. 192pp. 5⅜ x 8½. 24720-1 Pa. $6.95

THE WIT AND HUMOR OF OSCAR WILDE, Alvin Redman (ed.). More than 1,000 ripostes, paradoxes, wisecracks: Work is the curse of the drinking classes; I can resist everything except temptation; etc. 258pp. 5⅜ x 8½.   20602-5 Pa. $5.95

SHAKESPEARE LEXICON AND QUOTATION DICTIONARY, Alexander Schmidt. Full definitions, locations, shades of meaning in every word in plays and poems. More than 50,000 exact quotations. 1,485pp. 6½ x 9¼. 2-vol. set.
Vol. 1: 22726-X Pa. $17.95
Vol. 2: 22727-8 Pa. $17.95

SELECTED POEMS, Emily Dickinson. Over 100 best-known, best-loved poems by one of America's foremost poets, reprinted from authoritative early editions. No comparable edition at this price. Index of first lines. 64pp. 5³⁄₁₆ x 8¼.
26466-1 Pa. $1.00

CELEBRATED CASES OF JUDGE DEE (DEE GOONG AN), translated by Robert van Gulik. Authentic 18th-century Chinese detective novel; Dee and associates solve three interlocked cases. Led to van Gulik's own stories with same characters. Extensive introduction. 9 illustrations. 237pp. 5⅜ x 8½.   23337-5 Pa. $7.95

THE MALLEUS MALEFICARUM OF KRAMER AND SPRENGER, translated by Montague Summers. Full text of most important witchhunter's "bible," used by both Catholics and Protestants. 278pp. 6⅝ x 10.   22802-9 Pa. $12.95

SPANISH STORIES/CUENTOS ESPAÑOLES: A Dual-Language Book, Angel Flores (ed.). Unique format offers 13 great stories in Spanish by Cervantes, Borges, others. Faithful English translations on facing pages. 352pp. 5⅜ x 8½.
25399-6 Pa. $8.95

THE CHICAGO WORLD'S FAIR OF 1893: A Photographic Record, Stanley Appelbaum (ed.). 128 rare photos show 200 buildings, Beaux-Arts architecture, Midway, original Ferris Wheel, Edison's kinetoscope, more. Architectural emphasis; full text. 116pp. 8¼ x 11.   23990-X Pa. $9.95

OLD QUEENS, N.Y., IN EARLY PHOTOGRAPHS, Vincent F. Seyfried and William Asadorian. Over 160 rare photographs of Maspeth, Jamaica, Jackson Heights, and other areas. Vintage views of DeWitt Clinton mansion, 1939 World's Fair and more. Captions. 192pp. 8⅞ x 11.   26358-4 Pa. $12.95

CAPTURED BY THE INDIANS: 15 Firsthand Accounts, 1750-1870, Frederick Drimmer. Astounding true historical accounts of grisly torture, bloody conflicts, relentless pursuits, miraculous escapes and more, by people who lived to tell the tale. 384pp. 5⅜ x 8½.   24901-8 Pa. $8.95

THE WORLD'S GREAT SPEECHES, Lewis Copeland and Lawrence W. Lamm (eds.). Vast collection of 278 speeches of Greeks to 1970. Powerful and effective models; unique look at history. 842pp. 5⅜ x 8½.   20468-5 Pa. $14.95

THE BOOK OF THE SWORD, Sir Richard F. Burton. Great Victorian scholar/adventurer's eloquent, erudite history of the "queen of weapons"—from prehistory to early Roman Empire. Evolution and development of early swords, variations (sabre, broadsword, cutlass, scimitar, etc.), much more. 336pp. 6⅛ x 9¼.
25434-8 Pa. $9.95

AUTOBIOGRAPHY: The Story of My Experiments with Truth, Mohandas K. Gandhi. Boyhood, legal studies, purification, the growth of the Satyagraha (nonviolent protest) movement. Critical, inspiring work of the man responsible for the freedom of India. 480pp. 5⅜ x 8½. (USO)   24593-4 Pa. $8.95

CELTIC MYTHS AND LEGENDS, T. W. Rolleston. Masterful retelling of Irish and Welsh stories and tales. Cuchulain, King Arthur, Deirdre, the Grail, many more. First paperback edition. 58 full-page illustrations. 512pp. 5⅜ x 8½.   26507-2 Pa. $9.95

THE PRINCIPLES OF PSYCHOLOGY, William James. Famous long course complete, unabridged. Stream of thought, time perception, memory, experimental methods; great work decades ahead of its time. 94 figures. 1,391pp. 5⅜ x 8½. 2-vol. set.
Vol. I: 20381-6 Pa. $13.95
Vol. II: 20382-4 Pa. $14.95

THE WORLD AS WILL AND REPRESENTATION, Arthur Schopenhauer. Definitive English translation of Schopenhauer's life work, correcting more than 1,000 errors, omissions in earlier translations. Translated by E. F. J. Payne. Total of 1,269pp. 5⅜ x 8½. 2-vol. set.
Vol. 1: 21761-2 Pa. $12.95
Vol. 2: 21762-0 Pa. $12.95

MAGIC AND MYSTERY IN TIBET, Madame Alexandra David-Neel. Experiences among lamas, magicians, sages, sorcerers, Bonpa wizards. A true psychic discovery. 32 illustrations. 321pp. 5⅜ x 8½. (USO)   22682-4 Pa. $9.95

THE EGYPTIAN BOOK OF THE DEAD, E. A. Wallis Budge. Complete reproduction of Ani's papyrus, finest ever found. Full hieroglyphic text, interlinear transliteration, word-for-word translation, smooth translation. 533pp. 6½ x 9¼.
21866-X Pa. $11.95

MATHEMATICS FOR THE NONMATHEMATICIAN, Morris Kline. Detailed, college-level treatment of mathematics in cultural and historical context, with numerous exercises. Recommended Reading Lists. Tables. Numerous figures. 641pp. 5⅜ x 8½.
24823-2 Pa. $11.95

THEORY OF WING SECTIONS: Including a Summary of Airfoil Data, Ira H. Abbott and A. E. von Doenhoff. Concise compilation of subsonic aerodynamic characteristics of NACA wing sections, plus description of theory. 350pp. of tables. 693pp. 5⅜ x 8½.   60586-8 Pa. $14.95

THE RIME OF THE ANCIENT MARINER, Gustave Doré, S. T. Coleridge. Doré's finest work; 34 plates capture moods, subtleties of poem. Flawless full-size reproductions printed on facing pages with authoritative text of poem. "Beautiful. Simply beautiful."–*Publisher's Weekly.* 77pp. 9¼ x 12.   22305-1 Pa. $7.95

NORTH AMERICAN INDIAN DESIGNS FOR ARTISTS AND CRAFTSPEOPLE, Eva Wilson. Over 360 authentic copyright-free designs adapted from Navajo blankets, Hopi pottery, Sioux buffalo hides, more. Geometrics, symbolic figures, plant and animal motifs, etc. 128pp. 8⅜ x 11. (EUK)   25341-4 Pa. $8.95

SCULPTURE: Principles and Practice, Louis Slobodkin. Step-by-step approach to clay, plaster, metals, stone; classical and modern. 253 drawings, photos. 255pp. 8⅛ x 11.
22960-2 Pa. $11.95

THE INFLUENCE OF SEA POWER UPON HISTORY, 1660–1783, A. T. Mahan. Influential classic of naval history and tactics still used as text in war colleges. First paperback edition. 4 maps. 24 battle plans. 640pp. 5⅜ x 8½. 25509-3 Pa. $14.95

THE STORY OF THE TITANIC AS TOLD BY ITS SURVIVORS, Jack Winocour (ed.). What it was really like. Panic, despair, shocking inefficiency, and a little heroism. More thrilling than any fictional account. 26 illustrations. 320pp. 5⅜ x 8½. 20610-6 Pa. $8.95

FAIRY AND FOLK TALES OF THE IRISH PEASANTRY, William Butler Yeats (ed.). Treasury of 64 tales from the twilight world of Celtic myth and legend: "The Soul Cages," "The Kildare Pooka," "King O'Toole and his Goose," many more. Introduction and Notes by W. B. Yeats. 352pp. 5⅜ x 8½. 26941-8 Pa. $8.95

BUDDHIST MAHAYANA TEXTS, E. B. Cowell and Others (eds.). Superb, accurate translations of basic documents in Mahayana Buddhism, highly important in history of religions. The Buddha-karita of Asvaghosha, Larger Sukhavativyuha, more. 448pp. 5⅜ x 8½. 25552-2 Pa. $12.95

ONE TWO THREE . . . INFINITY: Facts and Speculations of Science, George Gamow. Great physicist's fascinating, readable overview of contemporary science: number theory, relativity, fourth dimension, entropy, genes, atomic structure, much more. 128 illustrations. Index. 352pp. 5⅜ x 8½. 25664-2 Pa. $8.95

ENGINEERING IN HISTORY, Richard Shelton Kirby, et al. Broad, nontechnical survey of history's major technological advances: birth of Greek science, industrial revolution, electricity and applied science, 20th-century automation, much more. 181 illustrations. ". . . excellent . . ."–*Isis.* Bibliography. vii + 530pp. 5⅜ x 8¼. 26412-2 Pa. $14.95

DALÍ ON MODERN ART: The Cuckolds of Antiquated Modern Art, Salvador Dalí. Influential painter skewers modern art and its practitioners. Outrageous evaluations of Picasso, Cézanne, Turner, more. 15 renderings of paintings discussed. 44 calligraphic decorations by Dalí. 96pp. 5⅜ x 8½. (USO) 29220-7 Pa. $4.95

ANTIQUE PLAYING CARDS: A Pictorial History, Henry René D'Allemagne. Over 900 elaborate, decorative images from rare playing cards (14th–20th centuries): Bacchus, death, dancing dogs, hunting scenes, royal coats of arms, players cheating, much more. 96pp. 9¼ x 12¼. 29265-7 Pa. $12.95

MAKING FURNITURE MASTERPIECES: 30 Projects with Measured Drawings, Franklin H. Gottshall. Step-by-step instructions, illustrations for constructing handsome, useful pieces, among them a Sheraton desk, Chippendale chair, Spanish desk, Queen Anne table and a William and Mary dressing mirror. 224pp. 8⅛ x 11¼. 29338-6 Pa. $13.95

THE FOSSIL BOOK: A Record of Prehistoric Life, Patricia V. Rich et al. Profusely illustrated definitive guide covers everything from single-celled organisms and dinosaurs to birds and mammals and the interplay between climate and man. Over 1,500 illustrations. 760pp. 7½ x 10⅛. 29371-8 Pa. $29.95

Prices subject to change without notice.

Available at your book dealer or write for free catalog to Dept. GI, Dover Publications, Inc., 31 East 2nd St., Mineola, N.Y. 11501. Dover publishes more than 500 books each year on science, elementary and advanced mathematics, biology, music, art, literary history, social sciences and other areas.

8/04 (5) 3/04

5/10 (8) 2/9

5/12 (11)
11/17 (13) 12/15.